Manual of Lifestyle Medicine

Lifestyle Medicine

Series Editor: *James M. Rippe*

Professor of Medicine, University of Massachusetts Medical School

Led by James M. Rippe, MD, founder of the Rippe Lifestyle Institute, this series is directed to a broad range of researchers and professionals consisting of topical books with clinical applications in nutrition and health, physical activity, obesity management, and applicable subjects in lifestyle medicine.

Increasing Physical Activity: *A Practical Guide*
James M. Rippe

Manual of Lifestyle Medicine
James M. Rippe

For more information, please visit: www.routledge.com/Lifestyle-Medicine/book-series/CRCLM

Manual of Lifestyle Medicine

James M. Rippe

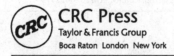

CRC Press
Taylor & Francis Group
Boca Raton London New York

CRC Press is an imprint of the
Taylor & Francis Group, an **informa** business

First edition published 2021
by CRC Press
6000 Broken Sound Parkway NW, Suite 300, Boca Raton, FL 33487-2742

and by CRC Press
2 Park Square, Milton Park, Abingdon, Oxon, OX14 4RN

Library of Congress Cataloging-in-Publication Data

Names: Rippe, James M., author.
Title: Manual of lifestyle medicine / James M. Rippe.
Description: First edition. | Boca Raton : CRC Press, 2021. | Includes
bibliographical references and index.
Identifiers: LCCN 2020052978 (print) | LCCN 2020052979 (ebook) | ISBN
9780367481315 (pbk) | ISBN 9780367489649 (hbk) | ISBN 9781003043706
(ebk)
Subjects: MESH: Primary Prevention | Health Promotion | Health Behavior |
Life Style
Classification: LCC RA776 (print) | LCC RA776 (ebook) | NLM WA 108 | DDC
613--dc23
LC record available at https://lccn.loc.gov/2020052978
LC ebook record available at https://lccn.loc.gov/2020052979

ISBN: 9780367489649 (hbk)
ISBN: 9780367481315 (pbk)
ISBN: 9781003043706 (ebk)

Typeset in Times
by Deanta Global Publishing Services, Chennai, India

To my wonderful wife, Stephanie Hart Rippe, and our amazing children Hart, Jaelin, Devon, and Jamie, who give meaning and purpose to my life.

Contents

Preface

What each of us does in our daily lives profoundly impacts our short- and long-term health and quality of life. This is the fundamental premise of lifestyle medicine. The evidence supporting these assertions comes from literally thousands of studies in the areas of physical activity, nutrition, weight management, and avoiding cigarette-smoking and tobacco products, in general.

More and more clinicians are engaging in lifestyle medicine. Some have devoted their entire careers to this discipline, while others are seeking to incorporate components of lifestyle medicine into their daily practices. It is encouraging to see that numerous medical schools around the country have established at least a few courses in the area of lifestyle practices and health and many more are contemplating this. It is my hope and belief that this will encourage more medical students to embrace these principles as key components of their medical practices. The *Manual of Intensive Care Medicine* is intended to be a clinically oriented summary of many of the disciplines that comprise the study of lifestyle medicine. It is intended to provide a point of entry to individuals who are either starting their career in lifestyle medicine or contemplating using lifestyle medicine concepts as components of their practice.

This manual provides key summaries with an emphasis on clinical factors in lifestyle medicine. For the individual seeking more detailed evidence behind each of these areas, I would refer them to the 3rd edition of my *Lifestyle Medicine* textbook. This comprehensive textbook, which was published in 2019, provides detailed evidence from over 150 experts from around the world in various aspects of lifestyle medicine and health.

There is no longer any serious doubt that lifestyle practices and habits profoundly impact on health. These concepts are central to the evidence-based guidelines from multiple prestigious organizations in the areas of prevention and treatment of disease, including the following:

- JNC VIII Guidelines for Hypertension, Prevention, and Treatment
- ACC/AHA Guidelines for the Prevention, Detection, Evaluation, and Treatment of High Blood Pressure
- NCEP (ATP IV) Guidelines for Blood Cholesterol
- Institute of Medicine Guidelines for Obesity Treatment
- ACC/AHA Scientific Consensus Statement on the Treatment for Blood Cholesterol, 2018
- Guidelines from the American Diabetes Association for the Management of Diabetes
- Dietary Guidelines for Americans 2015–2020 and 2020-2025.
- American Heart Association Nutrition Implementation Guidelines
- Guidelines from the American Academy of Pediatrics for the Prevention and Treatment of Childhood Obesity

- Guidelines from the American Academy of Pediatrics for the Treatment of Pediatric Blood Pressure
- Guidelines from the American Academy of Pediatrics for the Treatment of Lipids
- Guidelines from the American Heart Association and the American Academy of Pediatrics for the Prevention and Treatment of the Metabolic Syndrome
- American Heart Association Strategic Plan for 2020
- Joint Statement from the American Heart Association and American Cancer Society for the Prevention of Heart Disease and Cancer
- Presidential Advisory from the AHA and American Stroke Association on Optimizing Brain Health
- AHA/ACC/TOS Guidelines for the Management of Overweight and Obesity in Adults
- ACS/ADA/AHA Scientific Statement on Preventing Cancer, Cardiovascular Disease, and Diabetes
- Physical Activity Guidelines for Americans Scientific Advisory Committee Report of 2018
- The American Heart Association Impact Goal 2030

Despite the enormous body of information linking lifestyle habits and practices to good health, we are still falling dramatically short in terms of convincing the public at large to adopt these principles and practices. In fact, when the American Heart Association listed their components for "ideal" cardiovascular health, which includes many lifestyle practices such as increased physical activity, healthy nutrition, avoiding tobacco products, and maintaining a healthy body weight, they noted that only 5% of individuals in the United States follow all of the components to generate "ideal" cardiovascular health.

Moreover, it is sad to note that most physicians are not incorporating counseling about these habits and practices in their daily clinical work or incorporating them in their own lives. A number of studies have indicated that only 30–40% of physicians counsel patients on lifestyle practices, whether it be physical activity, weight management, or healthy nutrition. This is unfortunate given that over 70% of adults in the United States visit a physician at least once a year. We simply have to do better!

We live in an era where non-communicable diseases (NCDs) far exceed communicable diseases in terms of their impact on morbidity and mortality, as well as health care costs. It has been estimated that over 80% of all chronic diseases have a significant lifestyle component. The WHO has sounded the alarm in this area and listed nine areas of NCDs where it is hoped that clinicians and public health officials will devote significant resources. These include heart disease, diabetes, lack of physical activity, obesity, and excessive alcohol consumption.

The current manual focuses on two interrelated aspects of lifestyle medicine. The first enumerates the practices and habits which we should be encouraging all of our patients to observe such as healthy nutrition, physical activity and health, and other aspects of behavior change. The second major emphasis is on how lifestyle medicine practices can impact on specific diseases. These include cardiovascular disease, diabetes, cancer, obesity, and pulmonary disease. In addition, there are chapters focused on specific areas of medical practice such as obstetrics and gynecology.

While much of the structure of the *Manual of Lifestyle Medicine* mirrors that of the 3rd edition of *Lifestyle Medicine*, there are a number of new areas of information which have arisen over the last several years which are given particular emphasis in the manual. One of these is the Physical Activity Guidelines for Americans 2018 Scientific Report. This magnificent compilation of information provides overwhelming evidence of the role of physical activity throughout the lifespan and also touches upon most areas of medicine. In addition, the American Heart Association (AHA) and the American Stroke Association (ASA) joined forces to issue a Presidential Advisory in the area of "Optimal Brain Health." This document provides an important framework for how lifestyle practices and habits can impact on helping individuals maintain strong cognition throughout their lifespan and lower the risk of decreased brain function, including many forms of dementia and Alzheimer's disease.

There are important data available now about how lifestyle practice and habits impact on individuals throughout every stage of their lives. With this in mind, I have devoted a whole chapter to lifestyle medicine in the pediatric age group, as well as a chapter on lifestyle medicine for people over the age of 65. Also included are other areas of lifestyle medicine where clinicians have not been involved as we should have been. An example of this is in the area of injury prevention, which is the leading cause of morbidity and mortality for individuals under the age of 44. I have devoted an entire chapter to this.

Lifestyle medicine does not exist in a vacuum. It is important to recognize that multiple factors impact the area of lifestyle medicine. Because of this, I have devoted a whole chapter on public policy and environmental supports for lifestyle medicine. As more clinicians consider making lifestyle medicine practices a key component of their medical careers, it is important to understand resources that are available to help in the area of lifestyle medicine. With this in mind, I have devoted a whole chapter providing a framework for the practice of lifestyle medicine, including guidelines and educational resources.

It is important to note that most adults spend at least half of their waking hours in the work environment. To address this issue, I have devoted an entire chapter to health promotion with a specific emphasis on the workplace, which has been an area of active interest and progress for many decades in our country.

The manual concludes with two chapters looking toward growth and the future. As lifestyle medicine has spread around the world, there is an increasing number of individuals and organizations devoted around the globe to supporting the area of lifestyle medicine. I have devoted an entire chapter to how lifestyle medicine continues to grow around the world.

The *Manual of Lifestyle Medicine* concludes with a chapter on the future of lifestyle medicine. While enormous progress has been made, there are still significant challenges in front of us. We need to work hard to help individuals understand the power of their daily habits and practices so that we can close the gap between current knowledge and what people are actually doing in their lives. Furthermore, it will be important for lifestyle medicine practitioners to understand that subspecialties such as cardiology and endocrinology are now increasingly embracing lifestyle practices. It will be incumbent upon lifestyle medicine practitioners to seek collaborations with those individuals.

Research areas which will increasingly interact with lifestyle medicine include the emerging data in the area of epigenetics where initial studies have suggested that many of our daily lifestyle habits and practices profoundly impact on the way that DNA is ultimately modified through the process of epigenetics. Another area that is important for lifestyle medicine practitioners to assess are emerging technologies such as smartphones and wearable devices, both of which can provide greater avenues for dissemination of information and also motivation for individuals through direct feedback as well as social interactions through the internet.

The future of lifestyle medicine is indeed bright. It will be essential for all individuals engaged in the area of lifestyle medicine to continue to educate themselves and advocate for the importance of daily lifestyle habits and actions for reducing the great burden of NCDs around the world. I hope that the *Manual of Lifestyle Medicine* will assist individuals in continuing to gain knowledge and clinical expertise in the vitally important area of lifestyle medicine.

James M. Rippe, M.D.
Boston, Massachusetts

Acknowledgments

Textbook writing and editing are collaborative efforts that involve the hard work, passion, and commitment from a number of individuals. Many people have stimulated my thinking about the interaction between lifestyle and health over many years. These individuals are too numerous to acknowledge all by name. I would, however, like to particularly thank a few individuals who played specific and important roles in the creation of the *Manual of Lifestyle Medicine*.

First, my long-time Editorial Director, Beth Grady, who plays a vital role in all my book writing and editorial efforts. The *Manual of Lifestyle Medicine* is one of over 56 books that Beth has either managed or helped generate through our organization. She also helps provide editorial support for two major academic textbooks that I am involved in, *Irwin & Rippe's Intensive Care Medicine* (now in its 8th edition) and *Lifestyle Medicine*, 3rd edition, published in 2019. Beth also helps provide editorial direction to the two academic journals which I edit, the *Journal of Intensive Care Medicine*, which is now in its 35th year of publication, and the *American Journal of Lifestyle Medicine*, which is now in its 15th year of publication. Beth also helps coordinate numerous other academic endeavors. She possesses superb editorial skills and combines her enormous efforts with unfailing good humor to coordinate these complex and difficult projects.

I would also like to express my appreciation to my office support staff, including my Executive Assistant, Carol Moreau, who seamlessly coordinates my schedule and travel plans to free up the time for large writing and publishing projects. In addition, she has word processed a number of chapters in the *Manual of Lifestyle Medicine* and helped track down hundreds of references. Our Office Assistant, Deb Adamonis, assists all of us in the daily tasks required to expedite diverse projects in our office and has also played a specific and important role in tracking down references and word processing chapters for the current book. Our Chief Financial Officer, Connie Martell, makes sure that the financial processes are in place to support all of our projects in order for them to move forward smoothly. Our research team at Rippe Lifestyle Institute has always contributed enormous insights to help clarify my thinking about numerous aspects of lifestyle medicine, particularly our Director of Marketing and Client Services, Amy Continelli, who coordinates the day-to-day interactions with multiple research sponsors.

I would also like to thank the outstanding editorial team at Taylor & Francis Group/CRC Press, including Randy Brehm, Senior Editor, who has been an early and key supporter of our textbooks. Julia Tanner, Editorial Assistant, provided assistance with the logistical details of this book every step of the way and Rachael Panthier, Production Editor, at CRC Press for helping bring this book to fruition.

The project manager, Keith Emmanual Arnold, at Deanta Global managed the copyediting and typesetting of this book with great skill. Marsha Hecht at Taylor & Francis oversaw the proofing process.

Finally, I am deeply grateful to my family, including my loving wife, Stephanie Hart Rippe, and our four beautiful daughters Hart, Jaelin, Devon, and Jamie, who love and support me through the arduous process of writing and editing many major textbooks and journals, and my other diverse, professional responsibilities which I juggle along with my family life.

I take full responsibility for any errors or omissions in the *Manual of Lifestyle Medicine*. If there is credit due for this project, it belongs to the numerous people who have made substantial contributions along the way.

James M. Rippe, M.D.
Boston, Massachusetts

Author Bio

JAMES M. RIPPE, M.D.

Dr. Rippe is a graduate of Harvard College and Harvard Medical School with post-graduate training at Massachusetts General Hospital. He is currently Founder and Director of the Rippe Lifestyle Institute and Professor of Medicine at the University of Massachusetts Medical School.

Over the past 25 years, Dr. Rippe has established and run the largest research organization in the world exploring how daily habits and actions impact short- and long-term health and quality of life. This organization, Rippe Lifestyle Institute (RLI), has published hundreds of papers that form the scientific basis for the fields of lifestyle medicine and high-performance health. Rippe Lifestyle Institute also conducts numerous studies every year on physical activity, nutrition, and healthy weight management. Dr. Rippe has written over 500 academic papers and research abstracts and also written or edited 56 books, including 33 for health care professionals and 23 for the general public.

A lifelong and avid athlete, Dr. Rippe maintains his personal fitness with a regular walk, jog, swimming, and weight training program. He holds a black belt in karate and is an avid wind surfer, skier, and tennis player. He lives outside of Boston with his wife, television news anchor Stephanie Hart, and their four children, Hart, Jaelin, Devon, and Jamie.

1 Lifestyle Challenges and Opportunities

KEY POINTS

- The study of how daily habits and actions impact on long- and short-term health and quality of life is the core concept in lifestyle medicine.
- There is no longer any serious doubt that positive habits and actions significantly impact on reduction of risk of disease as well as its treatment.
- Such modalities as increased physical activity, proper nutrition, weight management, avoidance of tobacco products, and sleep and stress reduction, all significantly impact both quality of life and likelihood of developing disease.

1.1 INTRODUCTION

An overwhelming body of scientific and medical literature supports the concept that daily habits and actions exert an enormous impact on short- and long-term health and quality of life (1). Thousands of studies supply evidence that engaging in regular physical activity, following sound nutritional practices, maintaining a healthy body weight, not smoking cigarettes or using other tobacco products, and other health promoting practices, all powerfully influence health and quality of life. These habits and practices have formed the basis of the emerging medical subspecialty of lifestyle medicine.

The strength of the scientific literature supporting the positive health impact of these daily habits and actions is underscored by their incorporation into virtually every evidence-based clinical guideline from organizations involved in the prevention and treatment of metabolically related diseases (2). Some of these guidelines and consensus statements from these prestigious medical organizations are found in Table 1.1.

All of these statements emphasize positive lifestyle habits and practices as key components of prevention and treatment of disease, sometimes in conjunction with surgical and medical therapies.

Despite the widespread recognition in the scientific and medical communities of the important role of lifestyle measures and practices as key components of the treatment of various metabolic diseases, it has been frustratingly difficult to achieve improvements in the habits and actions of the American public. Numerous studies have shown that a distinct minority of adults in the United States follow some or all of the recommended positive lifestyle habits and practices.

TABLE 1.1

Consensus Statements from Various Organizations which feature Lifestyle Modalities

- JNC VIII Guidelines for Hypertension, Prevention and Treatment
- ACC/AHA Guidelines for the Prevention, Detection, Evaluation and Treatment of High Blood Pressure
- NCEP (ATP IV) Guidelines for Blood Cholesterol
- Institute of Medicine Guidelines for Obesity Treatment
- ACC/AHA Scientific Consensus Statement on the Treatment for Blood Cholesterol
- Guidelines from the American Diabetes Association for the Management of Diabetes
- Dietary Guidelines for Americans 2015–2020 and 2020-2015
- American Heart Association Nutrition Implementation Guidelines
- Guidelines from the American Academy of Pediatrics for the Prevention and Treatment of Childhood Obesity
- Guidelines from the American Academy of Pediatrics for the Treatment of Pediatric Blood Pressure
- Guidelines from the American Academy of Pediatrics for the Treatment of Lipids
- Guidelines from the American Heart Association and the American Academy of Pediatrics for the Prevention and Treatment of the Metabolic Syndrome
- American Heart Association Strategic Plan for 2020
- Joint Statement from the American Heart Association and American Cancer Society for the Prevention of Heart Disease and Cancer
- Presidential Advisory from the AHA and American Stroke Association
- AHA/ACC/TOS Guideline for the Management of Overweight and Obesity in Adults
- ACS/ADA/AHA Scientific Statement on Preventing Cancer, Cardiovascular Disease and Diabetes
- Physical Activity Guidelines Advisory Committee Report of 2018.

Rippe JM. Lifestyle Medicine (3rd edition). CRC Press (Boca Raton), 2019.

For example, the Strategic Plan for 2020, which was released by American Heart Association (AHA), stated that only 5% of the adult population in the United States practice the positive lifestyle measures or have the health parameters which are clearly shown to significantly reduce the risk of developing cardiovascular disease (CVD) (3).

Numerous studies, including randomized control trials and a variety of cohort studies, have uniformly demonstrated the enormous power of positive lifestyle habits and practices. For example, the Nurses' Health Study, which is a study of over 100,000 female nurses followed for more than 20 years, showed that over 80% of all heart disease and over 91% of all diabetes in women could be eliminated if these individuals would adopt a cluster of positive lifestyle practices, including regular physical activity (30 minutes or more of moderate intensity physical activity on most or all days), maintenance of healthy body mass index (BMI of 19–25 kg/m^2), not smoking cigarettes, and following a few simple nutritional practices such as consuming more fruits and vegetables and increasing whole grains (4). The U.S. Professional Health Study, which is a long-term study of male health professionals, showed similar dramatic reductions in risk of chronic diseases in men who followed the same behaviors (5). In fact, in both studies, individuals who adopted only one of these positive behaviors were able to reduce their risk of developing coronary heart disease (CHD) in half.

While the medical community is generally aware of the wealth of information in this area, a distinct minority of physicians has incorporated it in their medical practices. Physicians agree that we should practice "evidence-based medicine," and yet in the area of lifestyle practices and habits we in the medical community have been relatively slow to apply this standard to preserving good health (6). Virtually every physician would agree with the premise that weight management, sound nutrition, regular physical activity, and not smoking cigarettes all result in health benefits. Less than 40% of physicians regularly counsel patients in these areas.

The purpose of the *Manual of Lifestyle Medicine* is to bring key summaries of lifestyle medicine habits and practices into a user-friendly format to the medical community. This book is an outgrowth of the major academic textbook, *Lifestyle Medicine* 3rd Edition, CRC Press, which I have the honor of editing. This larger text was published in 2019.

The *Manual of Lifestyle Medicine* distills some of the similar information, adds studies which have been published since the 3rd edition of *Lifestyle Medicine*, and puts it in a shorter, perhaps more user-friendly, format for practicing physicians and other health care professionals.

Optimally, individuals will utilize the *Manual of Lifestyle Medicine* in conjunction with my major academic textbook to not only refer to the practical guidelines but also have in-depth summaries of the evidence supporting the power of daily lifestyle habits and actions.

1.2 WHAT IS LIFESTYLE MEDICINE?

I had the privilege of editing the first multiauthored academic textbook in lifestyle medicine. In fact, this textbook, which was published in 1999, introduced the term "Lifestyle Medicine" into the academic literature (7). We defined lifestyle medicine as "the discipline of studying how daily habits and practices impact both on the prevention and treatment of disease often in conjunction with pharmaceutical or surgical therapy to provide an important adjunct to overall health." This initial textbook has continued to expand as the field of lifestyle medicine has continued to grow and mature. The 3rd edition of *Lifestyle Medicine* was published in 2019 and represents the combined wisdom of over 200 scientists and physicians in a 1,500-page double-column textbook (1).

Of course, many investigators have been involved in the diverse areas which are included under the umbrella of lifestyle medicine such as nutrition, physical activity, weight management, and smoking cessation. It is clear, however, that the study of these individual modalities when combined will coalesce around the term of lifestyle medicine.

For example, the AHA changed the name of one of its councils from the "Council on Nutrition, Physical Activity and Metabolism" to "Council on Lifestyle and

Cardiometabolic Health" in 2013 (8). In addition, both the *American College of Preventive Medicine* and the *American Academy of Family Practice* have established working groups and educational tracks in the area of lifestyle medicine.

Representatives from a variety of organizations, including the *American Academy of Pediatrics*, *American College of Sports Medicine*, the *Academy of Nutrition and Dietetics*, the *American Academy of Family Practice*, and the *American College of Preventive Medicine* all sent representatives to a working group which established the first academic summary of competencies for physicians who wish to practice lifestyle medicine which was published in the *Journal of American Medical Association* (9). Recently, the "Competencies for Advanced Knowledge and Intensive Lifestyle Medicine" was published in the *American Journal of Lifestyle Medicine* (10) and expands the prior summary to define the parameters of advanced lifestyle medicine.

Importantly, a new health care organization called The American College of Lifestyle Medicine (ACLM), which was established in 2004, has over the last 16 years rapidly expanded (11). This organization has doubled its membership each year over the last five years. ACLM has also spawned important initiatives to develop curricula and encourage education and certification in the area of lifestyle medicine. Lifestyle medicine has also become an international movement with the inauguration of the Lifestyle Medicine Global Alliance (12).

As already indicated, an academic peer-reviewed journal has been established in lifestyle medicine called the *American Journal of Lifestyle,* where I serve as Editor-in-Chief (13). This journal provides a forum for individuals interested in exchanging academic information in the growing field of lifestyle medicine. AJLM, which is in its 16th year of publication, has over 13,000 subscribers and in 2019 had over 100,000 downloads full text articles. AJLM is listed on PubMed, which assures wide dissemination of important literature in the field of lifestyle medicine.

The name "lifestyle medicine" is appropriate for a variety of reasons. Perhaps, on the most fundamental level, it is the combination of lifestyle and its relationship to health. Clearly, this is an important component of medicine, hence the term "lifestyle medicine" is particularly apt and supported by an enormous body of scientific literature.

1.3   THE POWER OF LIFESTYLE AND ITS PRACTICES TO PROMOTE GOOD HEALTH

The first section of this manual will deal with a number of key issues related to daily lifestyle habits and practices and their impact on short- and long-term health and quality of life. Specifically, I will focus on the following six daily lifestyles issues: physical activity, nutrition, weight management, use of tobacco products, stress, anxiety and depression, and sleep.

- *Physical Activity*
  Physical activity is an extremely important component for overall health and the prevention and treatment of various diseases. Physical activity has specifically demonstrated to reduce the risk of multiple diseases such as

CVD, type 2 diabetes (T2DM), metabolic syndrome, obesity, and certain types of cancer (14,15). In addition, regular physical activity is important for brain function and cognition, as well as mental health, and lowers the risks of anxiety and depression as well as assisting in the reduction of symptoms of stress.

Regular physical activity is important to lower the risk of age-related conditions and is vitally important at every stage of the life span from youth to old age. Regular physical activity is also very important for women's health at all stages of their life span, including pregnancy, postpartum, and menopause. Regular physical activity plays an essential role in optimizing brain health and improving cognition and lowering the risk of various dementias, including Alzheimer's disease. The important role of physical activity in these conditions has been underscored by its prominent role in multiple evidence-based guidelines and consensus statements from virtually every organization that deals with chronic disease.

The recently released 2018 Physical Activity Guidelines Advisory Committee Scientific Report emphasizes that increased physical activity carries multiple benefits both for individuals and public health (14). In addition to lowering the risk of chronic diseases, the report also catalogs that regular physical activity powerfully contributes to improved quality of life by improving sleep, as well as feelings of well-being and daily functioning. As the report emphasizes, some of these benefits occur immediately, while others require ongoing regular performance of physical activity.

Physical activity has also been shown to prevent or minimize excessive weight gain both in children and in adults. Other conditions where regular physical activity results in benefits include osteoarthritis (the leading cause of chronic disability in individuals over the age of 65) and hypertension, the most chronic medical condition in the United States.

For all these reasons, regular physical activity should be recommended to every patient that physicians see. An entire chapter of this book will be devoted to the most recent evidence concerning physical activity and its benefits for multiple conditions (see Chapter 3).

- *Nutrition*

Sound nutrition plays a key role in lifestyle habits and practices that affect virtually every chronic disease. This is spelled out in great detail in the Dietary Guidelines for Americans 2015–2020 (DGA) and 2020-2025 (16). There is strong evidence that proper nutrition lowers the risk of CVD, T2DM, obesity, and cancer and many other conditions.

Virtually every major organization recommends proper nutrition, which includes increase in consumption of fruits and vegetables, whole grains (particularly, high fiber), nonfat dairy, seafood, legumes, and nuts. The guidelines further uniformly recommend that those who consume alcohol (among adults) use it in moderation. Also recommended are diets that are lower in red and processed meats, refined grains, sugar sweetened foods, and saturated and trans fats. The guidelines all emphasize the importance of balancing calories and regular physical activity as a strategy of maintaining healthy weight and lowering the risk of various chronic diseases. These issues will all be discussed in Chapter 2.

• *Weight Management*

Overweight and obesity are extremely common in the United States, with approximately 70% of people falling into these categories (17). In many ways, overweight and obesity represent quintessential lifestyle diseases. Even small amounts of excess weight or weight gain have been associated with many chronic diseases, including CVD, T2DM, some forms of cancer, musculo-skeletal disorders, arthritis, and many other diseases and conditions. The cornerstones of obesity treatment rely on lifestyle measures that contribute to balancing energy to prevent weight gain or creating energy deficits to achieve weight loss. These factors will be discussed in detail in Chapter 8.

• *Tobacco Products*

There is overwhelming evidence from multiple sources that cigarette smoking and second-hand exposure to cigarette smoke both significantly increase the risk of multiple chronic diseases, including CVD, stroke, T2DM, and cancer (18). In the 1950s, over half of both men and women smoked cigarettes. The prevalence of cigarette smoking has declined dramatically over the last 50 years. However, unfortunately, it seems to have leveled off with approximately 15% of individuals currently smoking cigarettes.

• *Stress, Anxiety, and Depression*

Stress is endemic in our modern fast paced world. It has been estimated that over 30% of individuals experience enough stress in daily lives to negatively impact their life at home or at work (19). Multiple lifestyle practices and strategies are available to help in the reduction of stress and its impact. Anxiety is the most common affective disorder in the United States, with almost 20% of individuals experiencing high enough levels of anxiety to impact their daily life. Depression is the second most common effective disorder, with 10% of the population experiencing major depressive episodes on an annual basis.

• *Sleep*

Healthy sleep is extremely important both for risk factor reduction and for improved quality of life. It has been estimated that 15–30% of individuals experience significant sleep disorders (20). In addition, difficulty in sleeping may contribute to fatigue, which in turn may contribute to motor vehicle accidents. The National Highway Transportation Council has estimated that 2–3% of all fatal accidents occur because of drowsiness. Some investigators have suggested that the prevalence of sleep-related fatal accidents may be significantly higher, perhaps as high as 15–20%.

1.4 BEHAVIORAL CHANGE

In many instances, adopting more positive lifestyle practices and habits will require changes in behavior (21). Behavior is often very ingrained, and behavior change is difficult. It is, however, possible. A robust science concerning behavior change has arisen with multiple frameworks and strategies that have been demonstrated to help people effectively change their behaviors. Since this is so important in lifestyle medicine, a whole chapter will be devoted to this (see Chapter 4).

1.5 LIFESTYLE MEDICINE AND CHRONIC DISEASE REDUCTION

As already indicated, lifestyle modalities play a critically important role in risk reduction and treatment of various chronic diseases: cardiovascular disease (CVD), T2DM and prediabetes, cancer, obesity and weight management, and dementia. Separate chapters will be devoted to each of these chronic diseases.

1.6 LIFESTYLE PRACTICES AND IMPROVED HEALTH

In addition to the central role that lifestyle practices play in the disease reduction, lifestyle habits also impact on multiple other medical areas. These include immunology and infectious disease, pulmonary medicine, obstetrics and gynecology, and brain health. Separate chapters will be devoted to each of these. In addition, lifestyle practices and habits significantly impact on the health of both women and men, and separate chapters will be devoted to each of these important areas.

1.7 LIFESTYLE MEDICINE ACROSS THE LIFE SPAN

Healthy lifestyle habits and practices are important throughout one's life span. For this reason, separate chapters will be devoted to lifestyle medicine in youth (22) and lifestyle medicine in older adults (23). In addition, lifestyle practices and habits are essential in preventing injuries, which is an extremely important area that is often neglected when habits and actions are considered, and a separate chapter is devoted to this area. Lifestyle habits and practices can also play a very significant role in reducing the likelihood of substance abuse and addiction and a whole chapter is devoted to this.

1.8 THE PRACTICE OF LIFESTYLE MEDICINE

As lifestyle medicine has grown and matured, an increasing number of physicians have chosen to include lifestyle medicine modalities within the context of their overall practice or even devoted their entire practice to lifestyle medicine (24). A robust body of information is now available about key factors related to the practice of lifestyle medicine. An entire chapter will be devoted to this emerging area, including educational resources for those who wish to pursue more advanced knowledge in lifestyle medicine.

1.9 PUBLIC POLICY AND ENVIRONMENTAL SUPPORT

The practice of lifestyle medicine does not occur in a vacuum. There are multiple interactions with not only individuals but also families, communities, national policies, and the built environment. For this reason, an entire chapter is devoted to this important area.

1.10   LIFESTYLE MEDICINE AROUND THE WORLD

The practice of lifestyle medicine has important implications throughout every country in the world. The lifestyle movement has expanded to include many countries and a whole chapter is devoted to how lifestyle medicine has advanced around the world, including both specific challenges and opportunities.

1.11   THE FUTURE OF LIFESTYLE MEDICINE

As the field of lifestyle medicine continues to advance, it will be important to examine where additional research is important and how various emerging technologies can play central roles in the advancement of lifestyle medicine. An entire chapter is devoted to this.

1.12   HOW TO USE THIS BOOK

The intent of the *Manual of Lifestyle Medicine* is to provide a user-friendly, practical basis for those who wish to improve their knowledge of lifestyle medicine and put its concepts into practice. With this in mind, the emphasis throughout this book will be on application of lifestyle medicine to various population groups and conditions and specific pathways to increase lifestyle medicine in the clinical practice of medicine. While evidence will be presented for the benefits of lifestyle medicine, those who wish to have a much more in-depth exploration of this knowledge are encouraged to combine the use of this manual with the much more extensive 3rd edition of my textbook *Lifestyle Medicine*.

1.13   PRACTICAL APPLICATIONS

- The *Manual of Lifestyle Medicine* is intended to provide a practical and user-friendly approach to incorporation of lifestyle medicine and its principles into the practice of medicine.
- Modalities of lifestyle medicine are discussed as well as the impact of lifestyle medicine habits and practices on chronic disease reduction.
- Individuals who wish to have a more in-depth knowledge of the evidence base behind lifestyle medicine are encouraged to utilize the *Manual of Lifestyle Medicine* in conjunction with the 3rd edition of my major textbook, *Lifestyle Medicine* (CRC Press, 2019).

REFERENCES

1. Rippe JM. *Lifestyle Medicine* (3rd edition). CRC Press (Boca Raton), 2019.
2. Rippe J. Lifestyle Medicine: The Health Promoting Power of Daily Habits and Practices [published online July 20, 2018].
3. Lloyd-Jones D, Hong Y, Labarthe D, Mozaffarian D, Appel L, Van Horn L, et al. Defining and Setting National Goals for Cardiovascular Health Promotion and Disease Reduction: The American Heart Association's Strategic Impact Goal through 2020 and Beyond. *Circulation*. 2010;121:586–613.

4. Colditz G, Hankinson S. The Nurses' Health Study: Lifestyle and Health among Women. *Nature Reviews Cancer.* 2005;5(5):388–96.
5. U.S. National Library of Medicine. Clinical Trials.gov. Health Professionals Follow Up Study. https://clinicaltrials.gov/ct2/show/NCT00005182. Accessed June 29, 2020.
6. Frank E, Holmes D. *Physician Health Practices and Lifestyle. In Rippe JM: Lifestyle Medicine* (3rd edition). CRC Press (Boca Raton), 2019.
7. Rippe JM. *Lifestyle Medicine.* Blackwell Science, Inc. (London), 1999.
8. American Heart Association. Council on Lifestyle and Cardiometabolic Health. https://professional.heart.org/professional/MembershipCouncils/ScientificCouncils/UCM_322856_Council-on-Lifestyle-and-Cardiometabolic-Health.jsp. Accessed June 29, 2018.
9. Lianov L, Fredrickson B, Barron C, et al. Positive Psychology in Lifestyle Medicine and Health Care: Strategies for Implementation. *American Journal of Lifestyle Medicine.* 2019;(13)5:480–486.
10. Kelly J, Shull J. A Comprehensive Clinical Lifestyle Medicine Specialty Fellowship Program: What Intensive Lifestyle Treatment Can Do. *American Journal of Lifestyle Medicine.* 2017;(11)5:414–418.
11. American College of Lifestyle Medicine. https://www.lifestylemedicine.org/. Accessed June 29, 2020.
12. Lifestyle Medicine Global Alliance. https://lifestylemedicineglobal.org/Accessed June 29, 2020.
13. American Journal of Lifestyle Medicine. https://journals.sagepub.com/home/ajl. Accessed June 29, 2020.
14. *2018 Physical Activity Guidelines Advisory Committee. 2018 Physical Activity Guidelines Advisory Committee Scientific Report.* U.S. Department of Health and Human Services (Washington, DC), 2018.
15. Rippe J. *Increasing Physical Activity: A Practical Guide.* CRC Press (Boca Raton), 2020 (in press).
16. U.S. Department of Health and Human Services and U.S. Department of Agriculture. *2015–2020 Dietary Guidelines for Americans* (8th edition). December 2015. Available at http://health.Gov/dietaryguidelines/2015/guidelines/ and . U.S. Department of Health and Human Services and U.S. Department of Agriculture. 2020–2025 Dietary Guidelines for Americans (8th edition). December 2020.
17. Day S. *Epidemiology of Adult Obesity. Lifestyle Medicine* (3rd edition). CRC Press (Boca Raton), 2019.
18. Ciccolo J, SantaBarbara N, Busch A. *Behavioral Approaches to Enhancing Smoking Cessation. Lifestyle Medicine* (3rd edition). CRC Press (Boca Raton), 2019.
19. Loiselle E, Mehta D, Proszynski J. *Chapter 23: Behavioral Approaches to Manage Stress. Lifestyle Medicine* (3rd edition). CRC Press (Boca Raton), 2019.
20. Brain Health. *2018 Physical Activity Guidelines Advisory Committee. 2018 Physical Activity Guidelines Advisory Committee Scientific Report.* U.S. Department of Health and Human Services (Washington, DC), 2018;F3-1–F3-49.
21. Frates E, Eubanks J. *Behavior Change. Lifestyle Medicine* (3rd edition). CRC Press (Boca Raton), 2019.
22. Miller J, Boles R, Daniels S. *Pediatric Lifestyle Medicine. Lifestyle Medicine* (3rd edition). CRC Press (Boca Raton), 2019.
23. Leon A, Tate C. *Lifestyle Medicine and the Older Population: Introductory Framework. Lifestyle Medicine* (3rd edition). CRC Press (Boca Raton), 2019.
24. Guthrie G. *Definition of Lifestyle Medicine. Lifestyle Medicine* (3rd edition). CRC Press (Boca Raton), 2019.

2 Nutrition in Lifestyle Medicine

KEY POINTS

- Nutrition plays a significant role in seven out of the ten leading causes of death worldwide.
- Sound nutritional practices are central to the prevention and treatment of many chronic diseases as is emphasized in multiple evidence-based guidelines from various scientific organizations.
- There is widespread consensus among healthy nutrition guidelines, all of which emphasize increasing consumption of fruits and vegetables, whole grains, and low-fat dairy as well as recommending decreased consumption of red meat, processed meats, and sugar-sweetened beverages.
- The influences on eating behavior are complex, including individual, family, community, and public policy factors.
- Key challenges include making existing knowledge on sound nutrition more accessible to help individuals implement this knowledge into their daily lives.
- Additional education of physicians to improve knowledge in the area of nutrition will be vital to meeting this challenge.

2.1 INTRODUCTION

An overwhelming body of scientific literature supports the power of daily habits and actions to lower the risk of chronic disease and improve short- and long-term health and quality of life: (1) Thousands of studies support the evidence that maintaining healthy weight, following sound nutrition practices, engaging in regular physical activity, not smoking cigarettes, and other health-promoting practices profoundly impact on health and quality of life. Nutrition, in particular, plays a very prominent role in multiple aspects of positive lifestyle and good health. In fact, there is a nutritional component in seven out of the ten leading causes of death worldwide (2).

Nutritional practices are a central component along with other lifestyle habits and practices in the field that is called "Lifestyle Medicine." Eating behavior and other aspects of nutrition are complex, including individual, family, community, and public health factors. However, a considerable amount of science-based evidence exists in this area. A key challenge remains to apply this existing knowledge concerning sound nutrition to help people implement this knowledge in their daily lives (3).

Despite an abundance of knowledge, it has been frustratingly difficult to improve nutritional practices in the American population. Consider the following:

- Almost 70% of the adult population in the United States is either overweight or obese. (There has been a staggering 40% increase in obesity over the past 20 years.)
- Less than one-third of the adult population in the United States consumes adequate servings of fruits and vegetables and follows other simple evidence-based nutritional practices for good health (4).
- The prevalence of diabetes in the United States has doubled in the past 20 years.
- Over 40% of the adult population in the United States has high blood pressure, yet less than 20% of individuals with high blood pressure follow the Dietary Approach to Stop Hypertension (DASH) diet which has been demonstrated to clearly help in the control and reduction of blood pressure (5).
- Despite improvements in the last 20 years, cardiovascular disease (CVD) remains the leading killer of men and women in the United States, resulting in 37% of mortality each year. Multiple nutritional practices impact on the likelihood of developing CVD (6).

Finding practical strategies to help individuals make proper nutritional choices in their lives is an urgent mandate in the United States and in many other countries. Unfortunately, many individuals in the health care community do not have adequate skills or background knowledge to provide nutritional counseling and/or do not incorporate this information into the regular practice of medicine.

All of these issues will be discussed in more detail in this chapter and also in chapters on specific disease entities found throughout this book.

2.2 WIDESPREAD CONSENSUS

Numerous scientific organizations have published guidelines concerning the important role of positive nutritional habits in the prevention or treatment of disease. Among these organizations, there is widespread agreement (2). Major authoritative guidelines which incorporate an important role for nutritional practices include the following:

- Dietary Guidelines for Americans 2015–2020
- National Cholesterol Education Program
- JNC VII and JNC VIII evidence-based guidelines for blood pressure control
- 2017 Guidelines for Prevention and Management of Hypertension
- Institute of Medicine Guidelines for the Management of Obesity
- Lifestyle Management Guidelines from the American Diabetes Association
- Numerous guidelines from the American Heart Association

In addition, virtually every scientific body that deals with metabolic diseases has recommended sound nutrition as a cornerstone for the prevention and treatment of various diseases. A list of some of these guidelines is found in Table 2.1.

TABLE 2.1

Nutrition Guidelines from Various Scientific Organizations

AHA Guidelines for the Prevention and Management of Coronary Artery Disease

AHA Nutrition Implementation Guidelines

AHA 2020 Strategic Impact Goals

Guidelines from the American Diabetes Association for the Management of Diabetes

American Academy of Pediatrics Guidelines for Prevention and Treatment of Childhood Obesity

American Academy of Pediatrics for Heart Disease Risk Factor Reduction in Children

AHA and AAP Guidelines for Prevention and Treatment of Metabolic Syndrome

AHA and American Cancer Society Joint Statement on Prevention of Heart Disease and Cancer

Source: Rippe JM. Nutrition in Lifestyle Medicine: Overview. *Nutrition in Lifestyle Medicine.* Springer International Publishing, Cham, 2017:3-12.

Thus, the role of nutrition and positive lifestyle is built on a broad consensus of scientific statements and authoritative guidelines.

2.3 BACKGROUND

Consensus statements and recommendations from a variety of organizations over the past ten years on the relationship between nutrition and metabolic health are very similar. These recommendations have been drawn from similar data bases and large epidemiological studies. These published consensus statements form the basis of the recommendations made in this chapter:

- Diet and lifestyle recommendations revision 2006: The Scientific Statement from the American Heart Association Nutrition Committee (7)
- Dietary Guidelines for Americans 2015–2020 (8)
- Defining and Setting National Goals for Cardiovascular Health Promotion and Disease Reduction: The American Heart Association Strategic Impact Goals through 2020 and Beyond (9)
- 2013 AHA/ACC Guidelines for Lifestyle Management to Reduce Cardiovascular Risk: The Report of the American College of Cardiology/AHA Task Force on Practice Guidelines (10)
- The American Dietetic Association Practice Guidelines, Evidence-Based Nutrition Practice Guidelines for Diabetes and Scope and Standards of Practice. *Journal of the American Dietetic Association.* 2008;108:S52-58 (11)
- 2017 ACC/AHA Guidelines for Prevention, Detection, Evaluation, and Management of High Blood Pressure in Adults (12)
- 2018 AHA/ACC Guidelines for the Management of Blood Cholesterol (13)

These consensus statements consistently recommend a dietary pattern that is high in fruits and vegetables, whole grains (particularly high fiber), nonfat dairy, seafood, legumes, and nuts. The guidelines also consistently recommend diets that are lower in red and processed meats, refined grains, sugar-sweetened foods, and saturated or trans fat (TFA). The guidelines further recommend that those who consume alcohol (among adults) do so in moderation. The guidelines also emphasize the importance of balancing calories and physical activity as a strategy to maintain healthy weight, thereby reducing the risk of obesity and various other metabolic conditions.

In the area of nutrition, the AHA Strategic Plan for 2020 gives specific guidance. The document recognizes that the optimal nutritional pattern for CVD reduction is complicated but states that with regard to dietary goals, the recommendation is "in the context of a diet that is appropriate in energy balance pursuing an overall dietary pattern consistent with DASH (Dietary Approach to Stop Hypertension)."(5) This diet makes the following recommendations for consumption:

- Consume fruits and vegetables ≥4.5 cups a day
- Consume fish ≥2 or 2½ ounce servings per week (preferably oil fish)
- Whole grain ≥1.1 g of fiber/10 g carbohydrates, 3 one ounce equivalent servings per day
- Sodium ≤1500 mg/day
- Sugar-sweetened beverages ≤460 calories or 36 ounces per week

While recognizing that comprehensive nutrition guidelines are more detailed than this, these recommendations represent a reasonable starting point.

Dietary guidelines over the past 20 years have moved from recommendations related to specific nutrients or specific foods to a greater emphasis on dietary patterns. This will be the approach taken in this chapter as well.

An additional emphasis in nutritional guidelines has shifted to include the critical aspect of implementation. This will also be discussed toward the end of this chapter. An example of the implementation problem is that with regard to nutrition and hypertension, less than 20% of individuals with high blood pressure currently follow the recommended DASH diet. An example is that it has been estimated that less than 30% of adults in the United States consume the recommended number of fruits and vegetables. Thus, the emphasis on nutrition now includes how to help people meet the current and existing guidelines.

2.4   DIETARY PATTERNS

The 2015–2020 Dietary Guidelines for Americans provided a variety of sources of information to integrate scientific research, food pattern modeling, and the analysis of the current intake of population to develop "healthy US style eating pattern." This approach allowed a blending of a variety of components of a diet with health outcomes. In addition, this approach allowed more flexibility in terms of the amounts of food from all food groups to establish healthy eating patterns and also meet nutrient needs and accommodated limitations in saturated fats, sugar, and sodium. With this approach the Dietary Guidelines for 2015–2020 indicated the following (8):

Within the body of evidence, higher intakes of vegetables and fruits consistently have been identified as characteristics of healthy eating patterns: whole grains have been identified as well, although with slightly less consistency. Other characteristics of healthy eating patterns have been identified with less consistency including fat free or low-fat dairy, seafood, legumes, and nuts. Lower intakes of meat including processed meats, poultry, sugar-sweetened foods, particularly beverages and refined grains have also been identified as characteristics of healthy eating patterns.

Some examples of healthy eating patterns include the following:

* Healthy U.S. Style Eating Pattern

    Utilizing the guidelines outlined in the preceding paragraph, the DGA 2015–2020 developed the Healthy U.S. Style Eating Pattern for the 2000-calorie diet, including daily or weekly amounts of various food groups and components. These are found in Table 2.2.

    The DGA 2015–2020 also emphasizes that it is important to balance the intake of calories and that added sugars, saturated fats, and alcohol should be limited and not exceed acceptable macronutrient distribution ranging from protein, carbohydrates, and total fats. The Healthy U.S. Style Eating

TABLE 2.2
Healthy U.S.-Style Eating Pattern at the 2,000-Calorie Level, with Daily or Weekly Amounts from Food Groups, Subgroups, and Components

Food Group[1]	Amount* in the 2.000-Calorie-Level Pattern
Vegetables	**2$^{1/2}$c-eq/day**
Dark Green	1$^{1/2}$c-eq/wk
Red and Orange	5$^{1/2}$c-eq/wk
Legumes (Beans and Peas)	1$^{1/2}$c-eq/wk
Starchy	5 c-eq/wk
Other	4 c-eq/wk
Fruits	**2 c-eq/day**
Grains	**6 oz-eq/day**
Whole Grains	≥3 oz-eq/day
Refined Grains	≤3 oz-eq/day
Dairy	**3 c-eq/day**
Protein Foods	**5$^{1/2}$ oz-eq/day**
Seafood	8 oz-eq/wk
Meats, Poultry and Eggs	26 oz-eq/wk
Nuts, Seeds and Soy Products	5 oz-eq
Oils	**27 g/day**

Source: U.S. Department of Health and Human Services and U.S. Department of Agriculture. *2015–2020 Dietary Guidelines for Americans*, 8th edition. 2015:144

Pattern was also designed to meet recommended daily allowances (RDA) and adequate intakes of potential nutrients set by the Food Nutrition Board of the Institute of Medicine. This dietary pattern was also flexible to allow minor modifications to accommodate the Mediterranean (14) or DASH diets to be followed within these overall guidelines.

- Low-Fat Diet

  Lower fat consumption in the diet has been generally accepted in clinical guidelines for lowering the risk of a variety of chronic diseases, including CVD prevention, diabetes, and obesity. Numerous other diets discussed in this chapter basically follow the concept of low-fat diets (15). These diets are based on consumption of total fat of not more than 25–35% of total calories and saturated fat (SFA) not more than 7–10% and TFA less than 1%. Monounsaturated fats (MUFA), omega-3, or polyunsaturated fat (N-3 PUFA) consist of the rest of the calories from fat. This diet also calls for dietary cholesterol less than 300 mg per day. These recommendations can be met by following the Healthy U.S. Style Eating Pattern and emphasizing fruits, vegetables, low-fat dairy products, and low-fat cuts of meat. Some controversy exists about the type and amount of carbohydrates consumed. It also should be noted that the food matrix for SFAs has been an area of recent research with some suggestion that SFAs which comes from dairy products are less likely to increase risk factors to heart disease compared to other sources of SFAs.

- Low-Carbohydrate Diet

  Low-carbohydrate diets have been advocated as one possible approach to achieving weight loss. These diets are defined as containing less than 45% of total calories from carbohydrates (less than 130 g of carbohydrates/day). These diets have been shown to assist with weight loss and also in the reduction of triglycerides (TGs) and an increase in HDL cholesterol (HDL-C). One study showed that low-carbohydrate diets (DIRECT study) yielded equivalent short-term weight loss compared to the Mediterranean diet and decreased triglycerides and increased HDL-C. In a four-year follow-up, however, there were no differences in comparing low-fat to low-carbohydrate or the Mediterranean diet. In a four-year follow-up, however, there were no significant differences. There are insufficient data from the long-term trials to demonstrate the benefits of low-carbohydrate diet compared to low-fat or Mediterranean diets for reduction of risk factors for CVD.

- Mediterranean Diet

  The Mediterranean diet was originally described as the one typically consumed in countries bordering the Mediterranean Sea (14). This diet is characterized by relatively high fat intake (40–50% of total daily calories with SFA comprising ≤8% and MUFA 15–25% of calories). The Mediterranean diet also has high omega-3 fatty acids from fish and low omega-6–omega 3 fat ratios. It features seasonal local fresh vegetables, fruits, whole-grain bread, legumes, nuts, and olive oil. Red meat is avoided. Moderate amounts of low-fat dairy products as well as eggs, chicken, and fish are allowed. Moderate amounts of wine are allowed to be consumed in meals except in Islamic countries. A recent multicenter randomized trial in Spain of the Mediterranean diet was conducted in individuals with high cardiovascular risk but no evidence of active CVD (14). The Mediterranean diet supplemental with extra virgin olive oil or mixed nuts resulted in decreases of approximately 30% of major cardiovascular events compared to control diet.

- DASH Diet

  DASH diet was originally formulated in the 1990s and has undergone several modifications since then. This diet was designed to lower blood pressure and CVD incidence by nutritional means. The DASH diet features low-fat dairy products, vegetables and fruits, whole grains, chicken, fish, and nuts and is low in fat, red meats, sweets, and soft drinks. Typical DASH diet composition is found in Table 2.3.

  Subsequent additions to DASH diet included substituting some of the carbohydrates with MUFAs and further decreases in sodium in the diet. These modified DASH diets have significantly reduced both systolic and diastolic blood pressures by 7–9 mmHg compared to the typical western diet. A study that used the DASH diet in conjunction with the lifestyle program designed to lower weight and increase physical activity (the PREMIER Trial) showed additional decreases in both systolic and diastolic blood pressures, which were reduced by 14.2 and 17.4 mmHg, respectively. Unfortunately, even with individuals who have high blood pressure, less than 20% are currently following the DASH diet.

- Vegetarian Diets

  A variety of vegetarian diets are available, including vegan (consuming no animal products), lacto-ovo vegetarian (consuming milk and eggs), and pesco (individuals who consume fish along with a vegetarian diet). The data exist to suggest that no one form of the vegetarian diet is superior to others with regard to CVD risk. A few studies are available which compare vegetarian diets to western diets. Some data suggest that vegetarians have improved health outcomes compared to non-vegetarians; however, these studies are typically confounded by the fact that vegetarians are often more health conscious in general than other individuals.

- Plant-Based Diets

  There has been a recent interest and evidence in publications concerning plant-based diets. These diets emphasize on plants, including fruits and vegetables and whole grains. Basically low-fat diets and low-carbohydrate diets can be considered plant-based diets. Mediterranean diet, DASH diet, and vegetarian and Japanese diets are all, in essence, plant-based diets since they all emphasize fruits and vegetables, legumes, and nuts and limit the amount of red meat, processed meats, sweets, and oils.

- Japanese Diet

  There has been recent interest in Japanese diets, particularly in those in Okinawa, which has the lowest CVD rates in the world. Traditional Japanese

TABLE 2.3

Following the DASH Eating Plan (http://bloodpressureplan.com/download-free-dash-diet-cookbook-with-weekly-meal-plan-to-lower-blood-pressure-naturally/?utm_source=adwords&utm_medium=search&utm_term=exact&utm_content=1&utm_campaign=dash&gclid=CN-os8ng0dMCFZVXDQodC8sPQQ)

Food Group	Servings Per Day			Serving Sizes	Examples and Notes	Significance of Each Food Group to the DASH Eating Plan
	1,600 Calories	2,000 Calories	2,600 Calories			
Grains*	6	6–8	10–11	1 slice bread 1 oz dry cereal† ½ cup cooked rice, pasta, or cereal	Whole wheat bread and rolls, whole wheat pasta, English muffin, pita bread, bagel, cereals, grits, oatmeal, brown rice, unsalted pretzels, and popcorn	Major sources of energy and fiber
Vegetables	3–4	4–5	5–6	1 cup raw leafy vegetable ½ cup cut-up raw or cooked vegetable ½ cup vegetable juice	Broccoli, carrots, collards, green beans, green peas, kale, lima beans, potatoes, spinach, squash, sweet potatoes, tomatoes	Rich sources of potassium, magnesium, and fiber
Fruits	4	4–5	5–6	1 medium fruit ¾ cup dried fruit ½ cup fresh, frozen, or canned fruit ½ cup fruit juice	Apples, apricots, bananas, dates, grapes, oranges, grapefruit, grapefruit juice, mangoes, melons, peaches, pineapples, raisins, strawberries, tangerines	Important sources of potassium, magnesium, and fiber
Fat-free or low-fat milk and milk products	2–3	2–3	3	1 cup milk or yogurt 1 ½ oz cheese	Fat-free (skim) or low-fat (1%) milk or buttermilk; fat-free, low-fat, or reduced-fat cheese; fat-free or low-fat regular or frozen yogurt	Major sources of calcium and protein
Lean meats, poultry, and fish	3–6	6 or less	6	1 oz cooked meats, poultry, or fish 1 egg»	Select only lean meats; trim away visible fat: broil, roast, or poach; remove skin from poultry	Rich sources of protein and magnesium

(Continued)

TABLE 2.3 (CONTINUED)
Following the DASH Eating Plan (http://bloodpressureplan.com/download-free-dash-diet-cookbook-with-weekly-meal-plan-to-lower-blood-pressure-naturally/?utm_source=adwords&utm_medium=search&utm_term=exact&utm_content=1&utm_campaign=dash&gclid=CN-os8ng0dMCFZVXDQodC8sPQQ)

Food Group	Servings Per Day			Serving Sizes	Examples and Notes	Significance of Each Food Group to the DASH Eating Plan
	1,600 Calories	2,000 Calories	2,600 Calories			
Nuts, seeds, and legumes	3 per week	4–5 per week	1	½ cup or 1½ oz nuts 2 Tbsp peanut butter 2 Tbsp or ½ oz seeds ½ cup cooked legumes (dry beans and peas)	Almonds, hazelnuts, mixed nuts, peanuts, walnuts, sunflower seeds, peanut butter, kidney beans, lentils, split peas	Rich sources of energy, magnesium, protein, and fiber
Fats and oils*	2	2–3	3	1 tsp soft margarine 1 tsp vegetable oil Tbsp mayonnaise 2 Tbsp salad dressing	Soft margarine, vegetable oil (such as canola, corn, Olive, or safflower), low-fat mayonnaise, light salad dressing	The DASH study had 27 percent of calories as fat, including fat in or added to foods
Sweets and added sugars	0	5 or less per week	≤2	1 Tbsp sugar 1 Tbsp jelly or jam ½ cup sorbet, gelatin 1 cup lemonade	Fruit-flavored gelatin, fruit punch, hard candy, jelly, maple syrup, sorbet and ices, sugar	Sweets should be low in fat

Source: Your Guide to Lowering Your Blood Pressure with DASH https://www.nhlbi.nih.gov/files/docs/public/heart/dash_brief.pdf
https://bloodpressureplan.com/download-free-dash-diet-cookbook-with-weekly-meal-plan-to-lower-blood-pressure-naturally/?utm_source=adwords&utm_medium=search&utm_ter=exact

* Whole grains are recommended for most grain servings as a good source of fiber and nutrients.

† Serving sizes vary between ½ cup and 1¼ cups, depending on cereal type. Check the product's Nutrition Facts label.

‡ Because eggs are high in cholesterol, limit egg yolk intake to no more than four per week; two egg whites have the same protein content as 1 oz of meat.

§ Fat content charges serving amount for fats and oils. For example, 1 Tbsp of regular salad dressing equals one serving; 1 Tbsp of a low-fat dressing equals one-half serving; 1 Tbsp of a fat-free dressing equals zero servings.

Abbreviations: oz = ounce; Tbsp = tablespoon; tsp = teaspoon diets emphasize fish, soy products, seaweed, vegetables, fruits, and green tea, and low consumption of meat. It should be noted that Japanese diets often have high sodium from soy sauce and have been linked to a higher risk of strokes. There have been few studies of Japanese diets, so a number of these issues remain to be determined.

- Prudent Diet

    In essence, the low-fat diet, Mediterranean diet, DASH diet, and vegetarian diet all fit in what the American Health Association has simply called the "Prudent Diet" category. All of these diets contain high levels of fruits, vegetables, legumes, fish, poultry, and other grains compared to a western dietary pattern, which contains higher intakes of red meats, processed meat, refined grains, French fries, and sweets/desserts. Prudent diets have been shown to decrease mortality from CVD, cancer, and all-cause mortality.

2.5   INDIVIDUAL FOOD ITEMS (15)

A number of randomized controlled trials (RCTs) and cohort studies provide evidence for the effects on CVD and other metabolic diseases of certain foods in contrast to individual nutrients. Foods which fit into dietary patterns that have been demonstrated to lower the risk of various metabolic diseases will be emphasized in this section.

- Fruits and Vegetables

    RCTs with diets that emphasize the consumption of fruits and vegetables have repeatedly been shown to produce substantial improvements in risk factors for CVD, T2DM, and obesity. Reduction of such risk factors as lipid levels, blood pressure, insulin resistance, inflammatory biomarker levels, and weight control have been demonstrated from fruits and vegetables. These benefits, however, have not been duplicated with supplements. These benefits appear to be a result of the combination of phytochemicals and fiber found in fruits and vegetables, the combination of which may increase the bioavailability of these nutrients. Ongoing research is exploring which types of fruits and vegetables are most beneficial to lower the risk of CVD and other metabolic diseases.

- Whole Grains and Fiber

    Whole grains contain the endosperm, bran (the outer layer of whole grain), and germ in relative proportions as they exist in the intact grain. Refined grains in contrast retain only the endosperm. Dietary fiber consists of the portion of plant-derived food, including lignin, polysaccharides, and associated substances that are resistant to digestion in the gastrointestinal tract by enzymes. Fiber includes insoluble fiber (including cellulose and lignin), which is found in some vegetables and fruits and whole grains. Soluble fiber includes pectin, guar gum, and mucilage. Soluble fiber is also found in bran and legumes. The National Cholesterol Education Program (ATPIII), American Heart Association, and the Academy of Nutrition and

Dietetics (AND) have all recommended increased fiber intake. The Dietary Reference Intakes (DRI) recommends 25 g of fiber for adult women and 38 g of fiber for men. Unfortunately, at present, adults in the United States consume less than 50% of the recommended fiber.

- Fish

  Fish and other seafoods contain a variety of health-promoting substances, including unsaturated fat, vitamin D, selenium, and long-chain omega-3 polyunsaturated fatty acids (PUFAs). Some studies have suggested that fish oil has anti-arrhythmic effects. Fish oil has also been shown to lower triglyceride levels, systolic and diastolic blood pressure, and resting heart rate. For all these reasons, the AHA dietary recommendations include the consumption of two fish meals (preferably oily fish) per week.

- Nuts

  Nuts, including tree nuts and peanuts, are nutrient-dense foods, which are high in unsaturated fats and other bioactive compounds as well as high-quality vegetable protein, fiber, minerals, tocopherols and phytosterols, and phenolic compounds. Epidemiological studies have consistently shown a negative association between nut consumption and CVD risk.

- Meat

  Dietary patterns that include lower consumption of red meat have consistently been demonstrated to lower the risk of CVD and cancer. Consumption of red meat and processed meat has also been associated with weight gain, which may also increase the risk of CVD. A recent meta-analysis has suggested current evidence does not strongly support limiting the consumption of red meat; however, these data have been challenged on multiple fronts and do not represent the consensus of scientific studies.

- Dairy Products

  Dairy products are rich in minerals such as calcium, potassium, and magnesium; protein (casein and whey); and vitamins (riboflavin and vitamin B-12), and may yield a reduction in risk of both CVD and T2DM. The current guidance from the DGA 2015–2020 recommends low-fat dairy products rather than full-fat dairy products. It should be noted that recent research has suggested that the matrix in dairy products may make the SFAs in them less hazardous than other SFAs. The DGA 2015–2020 recommends that adults consume three cups of low-fat milk or the equivalent on a daily basis. This is far greater than the average serving of one cup per day currently consumed by adults in the United States. Children and adolescents also consume far below recommended levels. The health effects of other dairy products such as yogurt, cheese, and butter are subjects of considerable research and require further study.

- Sugar-Sweetened Beverages

  The effect of sugar-sweetened beverages on the risk of various chronic disease has been subject to a great deal of research and controversy. Some studies have reported that consumption of SSBs may increase the risk of heart disease and other metabolic abnormalities. There are other studies that held that most of the findings relate to increased caloric consumption rather than SSBs per se. The AHA currently recommends no more than 360 kcal/week from sugar-sweetened beverages. The DGA 2015–2020 recommends no more than 10% of calories from added sugars. This recommendation is exceeded by over 80% of the population in the United States.

- Alcohol

  Alcohol consumption in some studies has been shown to yield beneficial effects on cardiovascular outcome. However, heavy alcohol consumption (three alcoholic drinks/day or more for men and two or more alcoholic drinks/day for women) has been associated with increased risk of various cardiac arrhythmias and a variety of other adverse health consequences such as motor vehicle accidents, liver failure, and weight gain. Moderate alcohol consumption (up to two drinks/per day for men and one drink/day for women) has been shown to lower the incidence of CVD and T2DM. These effects may be the result of increasing HDL-C, reducing systematic inflammation, or improving insulin resistance.

- Coffee and Caffeine

  Coffee throughout the world is the leading source of caffeine. Other sources of caffeine include tea, cocoa products, cola beverages, and energy drinks. Recent evidence has suggested that coffee consumption may actually generate a protective effect on CVD mortality. Studies have also shown that T2DM is lower in individuals who consume four or more cups of coffee a day compared to those who drink less than two cups per day.

- Tea

  Tea is also widely consumed throughout the world. Several studies have suggested that tea consumption may protect against the incidence and progression of CVD. These findings may be the result of improved endothelial function produced by the interaction between various tea components (such as polyphenols) and nitric oxide (NO). NO plays a significant role in endothelial function and arterial dilation.

- Eggs

  For many years, the public was cautioned to limit egg consumption due to high-cholesterol content of egg yolks and the potential association with CVD. Some recent studies, however, have suggested that the cholesterol in eggs may actually have minimal effects on blood cholesterol. Eggs are also a good source of high-value protein and a variety of vitamins and minerals. A recent study, however, suggested that consumption of even two eggs a day increases the risk of heart disease. The DGA 2015–2020 has continued to recommend restriction of dietary cholesterol to less than 300 mg/day.

- Garlic

  Garlic preparations have been investigated for both prevention and treatment of cardiovascular disease. Long-term observational studies of garlic consumption, however, are not available. Some short-term studies have suggested that garlic may reduce platelet aggregation, but any potential benefit of garlic on CVD risk factors is controversial.

- Chocolate

  Cocoa is similar to green tea with regard to the content of polyphenols. It should be noted that cocoa powder and chocolate are not identical. The polyphenols from cocoa may have some benefit for reducing risk factors for heart disease and also improving cognitive function. It is more appropriate to recommend cocoa consumption rather than chocolate due to the increased calories from sugar and fat in chocolate.

2.6 NUTRITIONAL SUPPLEMENTS

- Salt and Sodium

  Virtually every heart-healthy dietary plan recommends a reduction in sodium. Sodium in the diet can come from a variety of sources. A major source is processed food but, of course, salt can also come from table salt and snacks. Increase in dietary sodium increases blood pressure. A number of studies have shown that reduction in salt intake lowers the risk of CVD. The AHA has established the interim goal of 2300 mg/day of sodium and ultimately restricted it to less than 1500 mg/day in individuals with hypertension, African Americans, and middle or older age Americans. The average intake of sodium in the United States is currently 3400 mg/day. Several studies have suggested that the current level is optimum in terms of decreasing the risk of CVD and is better than lower or higher intakes of salts. Thus, the appropriate level of sodium consumption remains a somewhat controversial topic.

- Vitamin D

  Vitamin D consumption plays a role in decreasing the risk of bone disease based on a number of well-designed studies. There is some evidence that vitamin D also plays a role in decreasing the risk of other chronic diseases such as CVD. However, at present, there are insufficient data to recommend increased consumption of vitamin D as a strategy for lowering the risk of heart disease.

- Antioxidant Vitamins E and C

  Some initial observational studies suggested that antioxidant vitamins E and C lowered the risk of inflammation and, therefore, lowered the risk of CVD. However, RCTs in this area have not confirmed these findings. In fact, in several instances, consumption of vitamin E and C as supplements increased mortality from CVD and cancer.

2.7 (AHA) DIET AND LIFESTYLE RECOMMENDATIONS

The guidance and lifestyle recommendations from the AHA are based on Scientific Statement from the AHA Nutrition Committee (7) and were extended and updated in 2013 AHA/ACC Guidelines for Lifestyle Management to Reduce Cardiovascular Risk (9). These lifestyle recommendations are also very consistent with all of the other lifestyle recommendations from major organizations when dealing with chronic metabolic diseases, such as T2DM, metabolic diseases, and obesity. The recommendations are as follows:

- Consume an overall healthy diet
- Aim for a healthy body weight
- Aim for a desirable lipid profile
- Aim for a normal blood pressure
- Be physically active
- Avoid use and exposure to tobacco products

2.8   TRANSLATING GUIDELINES INTO INDIVIDUAL BEHAVIOR (3)

Recommendations for nutritional practices for Americans have remained relatively constant for over 20 years. Despite the long-standing and consistent recommendations, it has been difficult to help Americans change their habits and practices. For example, in 2018, 70% of adult Americans were overweight or obese. In 2017, only 25% of U.S. adults aged 18 or older engaged in enough regular physical activity to meet the recommendations from the CDC and the PAGA 2018 Scientific Report. Numerous studies have documented that only 25–30% of U.S. adults consume the recommended serving amounts of fruits and vegetables.

With the demonstrated gap between recommendations and implementation, a number of professional organizations have now focused on translating guidelines, particularly in the area of nutrition to help people implement healthier habits in their daily lives. A recent summary from the American Heart Association divides the impact of various factors which influence individual's likelihood of changing nutrition (3). A similar framework was listed in the PAGA 2018 guidelines for factors that influence an individual's likelihood of increasing their physical activity. These are divided into the following four domains.

- Individual
- Social/family and close peer environment
- Community environments/school/workplace/restaurants/neighborhood (e.g., access to healthful foods) and built environment
- Macro public environment/public policy, corporate policy, and marketing, transportation, popular media/communications, and economic factors

These domains from a Scientific Statement from the AHA entitled "Implementing the American Heart Association Pediatric and Adult Nutrition Guidelines" have been outlined in considerable detail. As already indicated, they are divided into four basic factors:

- Individual Influences
    These include convenience, eating patterns and social factors, psychological factors, need, taste, knowledge/ignorance of helpful recommendations, costs, and access.

- Family Food Influences

  This area is divided into economic factors, parental modeling, family eating patterns, family (nutritional gatekeeper), physical activity modeling, and parental children feeding practices.

- Community Food Influence

  This area is divided into economic factors, work food environment, school environment, food availability, peer modeling, and built environment.

- Macro Public Environment

  This influencing factor is divided into public policy, economic factors, food marketing, corporate policy and practice, cultural norms and values, transportation, and communication/media.

2.9 HYDRATION (16)

While discussion on nutrition simply focus on solid foods, it is important to also include hydration. Water is essential for life, and the body water content is normally tightly regulated, thus remaining relatively constant throughout the day. Water losses of less than 2% of total body water can result in significant declines in both mental and physical performance. Water losses are increased as ambient temperature rises as well as humidity and also by increased levels of physical activity. A variety of foods and beverages normally contribute to the total body water intake. Thus, when individuals are engaged in weight loss strategies, it is important that they consume extra water to make up for the water that they are no longer taking by decreasing the amount of solid foods in their diet.

2.10 DIABETES AND PREDIABETES (17)

Dramatic increases in diabetes (T2DM) have occurred around the world in the past two decades. Lifestyle medicine modalities prevent or treat diabetes focusing on nutrition therapy, physical activity, and education counseling and support. Nutrition therapy has been a mainstay of diabetes therapy for many years. Medical Nutrition Therapy (MNT) is the centerpiece for nutritional therapy for diabetes. MNT promotes healthful eating patterns, emphasizing a variety of nutrient-dense foods at appropriate levels with a goal of achieving and maintaining a healthy weight, maintaining glycemic control, blood pressure, and lipid goals, and delaying or preventing complications of diabetes. There is not one ideal percentage of calories from carbohydrate, protein, or fat for all people with diabetes. A variety of eating patterns are acceptable for the management of diabetes, including the Mediterranean, DASH, and other plant-based diets. All of these have been shown to achieve benefits for people with diabetes.

Weight management and, if necessary, reduction of weight are also important, particularly for overweight and obese people with diabetes. Weight loss can be achieved with 500–700 kcal daily reduction in both men and women adjusted for individuals based on body weight for many individuals with T2DM. Weight loss of greater than 5% is necessary to achieve beneficial outcomes for glycemic control, lipids, and blood pressure, while sustained weight loss of greater than 7% is optimal.

Proper nutrition is also vital for individuals with prediabetes. In the Diabetes Prevention Program (DPP), individuals with prediabetes who engaged in regular physical activity and lost on average 5–7 pounds, the incidence of type 2 diabetes was reduced by 58% over three years. The nutrition plan for DPP focused on reducing calorie intake in order to achieve weight loss, if needed. The recommended diet was consistent with both Mediterranean/DASH eating patterns. Conversely, sugar-sweetened beverages and red meats were minimized, since they were associated with increased risk of diabetes. More information about nutritional effects of T2DM based on lifestyle measures is found in Chapter 6.

2.11   WEIGHT GAIN/OBESITY (18)

It is currently estimated that more than 70% of individuals in the United States are overweight, obese, or severely obese. Both the DPP program and the Look AHEAD Trial showed that weight loss of 7% in obese individuals resulted in significant improvement in risk factors for both heart disease and diabetes.

Nutrition represents a cornerstone in the treatment of overweight and obesity. Dietary treatments for obesity are typically based on MNT, which is also used for a variety of other medical conditions. There is strong evidence that MNT improves waist circumference, waist-to-hip ratio, fasting blood sugar, low-density lipoprotein cholesterol, and blood pressure. Typical nutritional interventions for weight loss in obese individuals involve sustaining an average daily choleric acid of 500 kcal. Recommendations also emphasize that intake should not be less than 1200 calories per day for either male or female adults in order to achieve adequate nutrient intake.

A variety of evidence-based diets had been demonstrated to assist in healthy weight loss. These include the Mediterranean diet, DASH diet, and the Healthy U.S. Style Eating Pattern. It has also been demonstrated that differences in macronutrient composition of weight loss plan (e.g., low fat versus low carb) do not yield different results in studies lasting longer than one year. In both the DPP and the Look AHEAD Trial, individuals were able to keep off greater than 90% of the weight that they lost over three to four years. In the National Weight Control Registry which has over 10,000 individuals who have lost greater than 50 pounds and have kept it off for over one year, regular attention to monitoring nutrition as well as regular physical activity is the key component of how these individuals have been able to maintain weight loss.

2.12   CANCER (19)

The World Cancer Research Fund and the American Institute for Cancer Research (WCRF/AICR) evaluated over 7000 studies and concluded that diet and physical activity were major determinants of cancer risk. In addition, the AICR and IARC (International Agency for Research in Cancer) concluded that there is sufficient evidence to link 13 human malignancies to excess body fat. The Nutrition Guidelines for Cancer Prevention and Treatment are very similar to those for healthy eating in general, although some modifications may be necessary to protect against certain cancers, and/or treat various side effects of cancer therapy such as excessive weight loss.

General lifestyle nutrition measures for cancer prevention involve increasing consumption of foods that have been shown to decrease cancer risk, which include whole grains, vegetables and fruits, and legumes. In addition, individuals should decrease consumption of food associated with increased cancer risk such as processed meat (including ham and bacon), red meat (such as beef, pork, and lamb) and also decrease alcoholic beverages and salt-preserved foods. Furthermore, individuals should eat a healthy diet rather than relying on supplements to protect against cancer. More information about lifestyle issues in the Prevention and Treatment of Cancer can be found in Chapter 7.

2.13 CHILDREN (20)

There is now abundant evidence that many metabolic conditions that are manifested in adults have their roots in childhood. Specifically, there has been a dramatic increase in the prevalence of overweight and obesity as well as T2DM and hypertension in the pediatric population. In general, nutritional recommendations for adults are also applicable to children and are found in detail in DGA 2015–2020. More information on the lifestyle measures in children may be found in Chapter 16.

2.14 OLDER ADULTS (21)

In 2015, there were approximately 65 million adults in the United States over the age of 65. This number is anticipated to double by the year 2050, which will be about 24% of the general population.

General guidance for nutrition in older individuals are quite similar to those under the age of 65. It should be emphasized that diet quality is directly related to optimal physical and cognitive function in older adults. Thus, recommendations to increase fruit and vegetable as well as whole grain consumption apply equally to adults over the age of 65. Nutrient requirements for individuals over the age of 65 either stay the same or increase with advancing years, while energy requirements decline, thereby increasing the importance of making nutrient-dense food choices.

Nutrition in older individuals must overcome changes in sensory perception and the onset of chronic diseases and changes in dentition. In addition, alterations in social environments, including isolation, may create challenges in the ability and desire to obtain, prepare, and consume high-quality diets, so these conditions must also be taken into account when prescribing nutrition to older adults. More detail on issues related to lifestyle measures in adults is found in Chapter 20.

2.15 PHYSICIAN EDUCATION

Despite the multiple known benefits of proper nutrition, most physicians feel they do not have adequate education in this area. Of all physicians, 22% reported receiving no nutrition education in medical school and 35% reported that nutrition education came in a single lecture or in a single section (22). In addition, 70% of residents surveyed felt they received minimum or no education in nutrition during medical residency.

While in the United States, 67% of physicians indicate they have nutrition counseling sessions for patients. These are usually focused on high consumption of sodium, sugar, and fried foods. It should be noted that only 21% of patients feel they received effective communication in the area of nutrition from their physicians. Clearly, there is a need to make significant improvements in physician education in the area of nutrition.

2.16 SUMMARY

There is no longer any serious doubt that proper nutrition can significantly improve the health of individuals who have multiple conditions as well as lower the risk factors for such conditions as CVD, T2DM, obesity, cancer, and perhaps even dementia. Conversely, poor eating habits can significantly increase the risk of all these conditions. We are now entering an era where the importance of nutrition and good health is increasingly being understood by all segments of the health care community. Not only will we need to emphasize the core understanding of healthy nutrition, but also develop effective strategies to help individuals implement nutritional guidelines in their daily lives. The role of physicians is extremely important in this area. Improved education among physicians will be a key moving forward.

2.17 CLINICAL APPLICATIONS

- Physicians should become knowledgeable about counseling on healthy nutrition for all patients.
- Plant-based diets from American Heart Association, American College of Cardiology, and Dietary Guidelines for Americans are largely consistent with each other and will lower the risk of various metabolic diseases.
- The DASH diet and the Mediterranean diet both have been shown to effectively lower blood pressure in individuals with hypertension and also improve a variety of parameters in individuals with T2DM.
- Nutrition plays a key role in lowering the risk of multiple metabolic conditions and should be combined with other aspects of positive lifestyle, including regular physical activity, weight management, and avoidance of tobacco products.
- Clinicians should routinely recommend that individuals follow diets that are high in fruits and vegetables, whole grains, seafood (preferably oily fish), legumes, and nuts and nonfat dairy products while lowering consumption of red meats, processed meats, sugar-sweetened beverages, and refined grains to reduce the risk of various metabolic diseases, including CVD, T2DM, cancer, and obesity.

REFERENCES

1. Rippe JM. *Lifestyle Medicine* (3rd edition). CRC Press (Boca Raton), 2019.
2. Rippe JM. Nutrition in Lifestyle Medicine: Overview. In: Rippe JM, ed., *Nutrition in Lifestyle Medicine*. Springer International Publishing (New York, NY); 2017.

3. Gidding SS, Lichtenstein AH, Faith MS, et al. Implementing American Heart Association Pediatric and Adult Nutrition Guidelines: A Scientific Statement from the American Heart Association Nutrition Committee of the Council on Nutrition, Physical Activity and Metabolism, Council on Cardiovascular Disease in the Young, Council on Arteriosclerosis, Thrombosis and Vascular Biology, Council on Cardiovascular Nursing, Council on Epidemiology and Prevention, and Council for High Blood Pressure Research. *Circulation*. 2009;119:1161–75.

4. Schiller JS, Lucas JW, Ward BW, et al. Summary Health Statistics for U.S. Adults: National Health Interview Survey, 2010. *Vital Health Stat 10*. 2012;252:1–207. Epub 2012/07/28.

5. Appel LJ, Brands MW, Daniels SR, et al. Dietary Approaches to Prevent and Treat Hypertension: A Scientific Statement from the American Heart Association. *Hypertension*. 2006;47(2):296–308.

6. Lloyd-Jones D, Adams RJ, Brown TM, et al. Executive Summary: Heart Disease and Stroke Statistics--2010 Update: A Report from the American Heart Association. *Circulation*. 2010;121(7):948–54. Epub 2010/02/24.

7. Gidding SS, Lichtenstein AH, Faith MS, et al. Implementing American Heart Association Pediatric and Adult Nutrition Guidelines: A Scientific Statement from the American Heart Association Nutrition Committee of the Council on Nutrition, Physical Activity and Metabolism, Council on Cardiovascular Disease in the Young, Council on Arteriosclerosis, Thrombosis and Vascular Biology, Council on Cardiovascular Nursing, Council on Epidemiology and Prevention, and Council for High Blood Pressure Research. *Circulation*. 2009;119:1161–175.

8. U.S. Department of Health and Human Services and U.S. Department of Agriculture. *2015–2020 Dietary Guidelines for Americans* (8th edition), 2015:144.

9. Lloyd-Jones DM, Hong Y, Labarthe D, et al. Defining and Setting National Goals for Cardiovascular Health Promotion and Disease Reduction: The American Heart Association's Strategic Impact Goal through 2020 and Beyond. *Circulation*. 2010;121:586–613.

10. Eckel RH, Jakicic JM, Ard JD, et al. 2013 AHA/ACC Guideline on Lifestyle Management to Reduce Cardiovascular Risk. *Circulation*. 2014;129 Supplement 2:S76–S99.

11. Evidence-Based Nutrition Practice Guidelines for Diabetes and Scope and Standards of Practice. *Journal of the American Dietetic Association*. 2008;108 Supplement 1:S52–58.

12. Whelton PK, Carey RM, Aronow WS, et al. 2017 ACC/AHA/AAPA/ABC/ACPM/AGS /APHA/ASH/ASPC/NMA/PCNA Guideline for the Prevention, Detection, Evaluation, and Management of High Blood Pressure in Adults: A Report of the American College of Cardiology/American Heart Association Task Force on Clinical Practice Guidelines. *Journal of the American College of Cardiology*. 2018;71:e127–e248.

13. Grundy SM, Stone NJ, Bailey AL, Beam C, Birtcher KK, Blumenthal RS. 2018 AHA/ ACC/AACVPR/AAPA/ABC/ACPM/ADA/AGS/APHA/ASPC/NLA/PCNA Guideline on the Management of Blood Cholesterol: A Report of the American College of Cardiology/American Heart Association Task Torce on Clinical Practice Guidelines. *Journal of the American College of Cardiology* 2019;73:e285–e350.

14. Estruch R, Ros E, Salas-Salvadó J, Covas M-I, Corella D, Arós F. Primary Prevention of Cardiovascular Disease with a Mediterranean Diet. *New England Journal of Medicine*. 2013;368:1279–1290.

15. Mozaffarian D. Nutrition and Cardiovascular Disease. In: Bonow R, Mann D, Zipes D, Libby P. eds., *Braunwald's Heart Disease: A Textbook of Cardiovascular Medicine*. Elsevier (Philadelphia, PA), 2012.

16. Evans GH, Maughan RJ, Shirreffs SM. Effects of an Active Lifestyle on Water Balance and Water Requirements. In: Rippe JM, ed., *Lifestyle Medicine* (3rd edition). CRC Press (Boca Raton), 2019.

17. Franz MJ. Lifestyle Therapies for the Management of Diabetes. In: Rippe JM, ed., *Lifestyle Medicine* (3rd edition). CRC Press (Boca Raton), 2019.

18. Crowley N, Arlinghaus KR, Stellefson Myers E. Dietary Management of Overweight and Obesity. In: Rippe JM, ed., *Lifestyle Medicine* (3rd edition). CRC Press (Boca Raton), 2019.

19. Kaur S, Trujillo E. Nutrition Therapy for the Cancer Patient. In Rippe JM, ed., *Lifestyle Medicine* (3rd edition). CRC Press (Boca Raton), 2019.

20. Hildebrandt JL, Couch SC. Cardiovascular Risk and Diet in Children. In Rippe JM, ed., *Lifestyle Medicine* (3rd edition). CRC Press (Boca Raton), 2019.

21. Lichtenstein AH. Optimal Nutrition Guidance for Older Adults. In Rippe JM, ed., *Lifestyle Medicine* (3rd edition). CRC Press (Boca Raton), 2019.

22. Rippe JM. Lifestyle Medicine: The Health Promoting Power of Daily Habits and Practices. *American Journal of Lifestyle Medicine*. 2018;12:499–512.

3 Physical Activity and Health

KEY POINTS

- Increased physical activity lowers the risk of various chronic diseases and can also serve as an adjunct to treatment.
- Increased physical activity plays crucial roles for individuals at all stages of their lives.
- The recently released Physical Activity Guidelines 2018 Scientific Report (PAGA 2018) provides an important summary of the benefits of physical activity for multiple individuals at all stages of their lives and various physical conditions.
- Physicians play a critically important role in urging their patients to make positive decisions in their lives concerning physical activity.
- Recommendations from the PAGA 2018 include that individuals should be encouraged to participate in 150 minutes or more of moderate to vigorous physical activity each week and strength training sessions twice a week with at least one day separated between the two sessions.
- Only 25% of individuals engage in regular levels of physical activity necessary to meet the guidelines from the Centers for Disease Control and the American College of Sports Medicine (ACSM) and PAGA 2018.

3.1 INTRODUCTION

What individuals do in their daily lives profoundly impacts on short- and long-term health and quality of life. This is the essence of lifestyle medicine. These habits include proper nutrition, regular physical activity, weight management, avoiding tobacco products, and many other practices—all of which we have lumped together under the umbrella term "lifestyle medicine" (1).

Among the many important practices that individuals can perform in their daily lives, there is no single lifestyle habit or practice more powerfully associated with improved short- and long-term health and quality of life than regular physical activity.

An enormous and compelling literature generated over the past two decades documents that moderate or vigorous physical activity profoundly lowers the likelihood of developing chronic disease and exerts a powerful impact on quality of life. In addition, regular physical activity has been found in multiple studies to not only play a role in reducing the risk of chronic diseases but also act as a component of their treatment.

For all of these reasons, regular physical activity is a cornerstone in the prevention and treatment of chronic diseases. This is acknowledged in the guidelines of numerous professional organizations ranging from the American Heart Association (AHA) (2) to the American Academy of Pediatrics (AAP) (3) to the American Diabetes Association (ADA) (4) and many others. Regular physical activity is also a cornerstone to the recommendations for Healthy People 2020 (5) and a key factor in the framework that has been established for the Healthy People 2030 guidelines (6).

Recently, the Physical Activity Guidelines Advisory Committee for Americans 2018 Scientific Report was released, and it provided an enormous and compelling body of evidence about the multiple benefits of regular physical activity (7). These benefits extend throughout the life span and for multiple chronic diseases as well as issues related to quality of life. The American College of Sports Medicine (ACSM) has been a leader for many decades in this area (8). The American College of Lifestyle Medicine (ACLM) (9) and the AHA have also played very significant roles in advocating more physical activity and have recommended regular physical activity as a key component for preserving health and improving quality of life.

Despite the enormous evidence now available concerning the positive relationship between physical activity and health, the medical community has been slow to embrace this concept as an important component of routine health care. It has been estimated that less than 40% of physicians regularly counsel their patients on the importance of regular physical activity. This is a wasted opportunity since over 70% of individuals see their primary care physician at least once per year!

The American public has also been slow to embrace the habit of regular physical activity. It has been estimated that less than 25% of adults in the United States meet the recommended levels of physical activity, including 30 minutes of moderate intensity physical activity on most if not all days and two sessions of musculoskeletal strength training on a weekly basis separated by one day. These are the guidelines that are recommended by the PAGA 2018.

This chapter will summarize key elements of how physical activity plays an important role in health and quality of life.

3.2 THE RELATIONSHIP BETWEEN MODERATE TO VIGOROUS PHYSICAL ACTIVITY AND THE RISK OF DEVELOPING CHRONIC DISEASES

Enormous data are available across a wide spectrum of chronic diseases, showing that individuals who are physically active decrease their risk of these conditions compared to inactive individuals. Recently, the PAGA 2018 provided a wealth of evidence across numerous chronic conditions, showing the benefits of regular physical activity in both lowering the risk of chronic diseases and assisting in their treatment (7). Some of the benefits of physical activity occur after an acute bout, while others require a consistent increase in physical activity throughout the life span.

Among the conditions where physical activity can benefit are cardiovascular disease (CVD), cancer, diabetes (T2DM), dementia, brain health, risk of falling, and other injuries, particularly in older individuals. Importantly, benefits of physical activity occur in children as young as 3 years old all the way up through adolescents and are also prominent in adults and even individuals over the age of 65.

TABLE 3.1

Physical Activity-Related Health Benefits for the General Population and Selected Populations Documented by the 2018 Physical Activity Guidelines Advisory Committee

Children

3–6 Years of Age	**Improved bone health and weight status**
6–17 years of age	**Improved cognitive function (ages 6–13 years)**
	Improved cardiorespiratory and muscular fitness Improved bone health
	Improved cardiovascular risk factor status Improved weight status or adiposity
	Fewer symptoms of depression

Adults, all ages

All-cause mortality	Lower risk
Cardiometabolic conditions	Lower cardiovascular incidence and mortality (including heart disease and stroke)
	Lower incidence of hypertension
	Lower incidence of type 2 diabetes
Cancer	Lower incidence of **bladder,** breast, colon, **endometrium, esophagus, kidney, stomach, and lung cancers**
Brain health	**Reduced risk of dementia**
	Improved cognitive function
	Improved cognitive function following bouts of aerobic activity
	Improved quality of life
	Improved sleep
	Reduced feelings of anxiety and depression in healthy people and in people with existing clinical syndromes
	Reduced incidence of depression
Weight status	**Reduced risk of excessive weight gain**
	Weight loss and the prevention of weight regain following initial weight loss when a sufficient dose of moderate-to-vigorous physical activity is attained
	An additive effect on weight loss when combined with moderate dietary restriction

From the 2018 Physical Activity Guidelines Advisory Committee Submits Scientific Report. Office of Disease Prevention and Health Promotion, Washington, DC. 2018.

A summary of the physical activity-related health benefits that are documented in the 2018 PAGA Scientific Report is given in Table 3.1.

There is also a strong relationship between increased physical activity and multiple components of improved quality of life. Individuals who are physically active have less anxiety, depression, and stress in general, and feel better and sleep better. All of these improvements result in higher quality of life in individuals who participate in regular physical activity.

Some people have written that physical activity is like a "polypill" that can contribute to multiple health benefits. These individuals argue that if exercise were actually a pharmaceutical treatment, it would be hard for the pharmaceutical industry to keep it in supply!

3.3 PHYSICAL ACTIVITY AND CHRONIC DISEASES

CARDIOVASCULAR DISEASE

Regular physical activity significantly reduces the risk of cardiovascular disease and all-cause mortality. As recommended by PAGA 2018 and various documents from ACSM and the AHA, the recommendation of 150 minutes of moderate intensity physical activity per week as well as two strength training sessions per week will substantially lower the risk of cardiovascular disease and all-cause mortality as indicated in Figure 3.1.

Further reductions are also available for individuals who engage in physical activity above 150 minutes per week, as indicated in Figure 3.1.

It is important to point out, however, that even small amounts of physical activity can result in significant lowering of both CVD and all-cause mortality. As indicated in Figure 3.1, there is no lower threshold of benefit for increased physical activity in regard to reduction of risk of all-cause mortality. Even individuals who engage in moderate to vigorous physical activity for as low as 30 minutes per week achieve about a 20% reduction in the risk of cardiovascular disease. Unfortunately, only approximately 25% of adults meet the minimum recommendations from the PAGA 2018 and CDC of 150 minutes of moderate intensity physical activity per week.

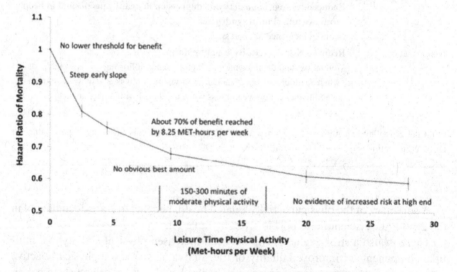

FIGURE 3.1 Relationships of moderate-to-vigorous physical activity to all-cause mortality, with highlighted characteristics common to studies of this type. *Source:* From the 2018 Physical Activity Guidelines Advisory Committee Scientific Report. Adapted from date found in Moore SC, et al. Leisure time physical activity of moderate to vigorous intensity and mortality: A large pooled cohort analysis. *PLoS Med.* 2012;9(11):e1001335.

Young people are even less likely to follow the recommended standards. Fewer than 20% of adolescents perform the recommended 60 minutes or more of daily physical activity from the PAGA 2018.

If individuals who are very physically active are compared for risk of CHD with sedentary individuals, the sedentary individuals show 150–240% higher risk. It should be noted that regular physical activity also lowers the risk of adult weight gain and helps to control high blood pressure, thus reducing the risk of developing hypertension. Increasing amounts of physical activity also lower the risk of stroke and heart failure in a dose-dependent relationship.

Despite these known benefits, physicians have typically not emphasized the role of regular physical activity in reducing the risk of heart disease. In one survey of 175 primary care physicians, only 12% were aware of the recommendations from ACSM or those from PAGA 2018, which are quite similar to ACSM recommendations.

Physical Activity and Diabetes, Prediabetes, and the Metabolic Syndrome (10)

Lifestyle modalities, including physical activity, are the cornerstone of diabetes care. The recommendations for people with diabetes from the PAGA 2018 are similar to those for reducing the risk of CHD. The guidelines from the American Diabetes Association recommend physical activity sessions should be at least 10 minutes, with the goal of 30 minutes per day or more on most days of the week. These are a little bit more rigorous recommendations than PAGA 2018.

In addition, individuals with diabetes should be encouraged to reduce the time spent on sedentary activities such as working at a computer, watching TV, or other activities while sitting or lying down (except sleep). This is based on good data that associate sedentary activities with increased risk of diabetes.

According to the ADA Consensus Report on Physical Activity and Diabetes, prior to starting an exercise program medical providers should perform a history of cardiovascular risk factors in order to customize physical activity regimens to individual needs (10). The American Diabetes Association as well as the PAGA 2018 provides detailed recommendations for physical activity in individuals with diabetes.

In addition, physical activity plays an important role in preventing prediabetes from turning into diabetes. The Diabetes Prevention Program (DPP) (11), the Da Qing Study (12), and the Finnish Diabetes Prevention Study (13) all showed significant reductions of prediabetes turning into diabetes for individuals who were engaged in regular physical activity. In the DPP, individuals who engaged in 150 minutes per week of physical activity and, in addition, lost an average of 7% weight, lowered their risk of their prediabetes progressing into diabetes by 58%.

The metabolic syndrome also benefits from increased physical activity. The metabolic syndrome is a cluster of metabolic abnormalities that significantly increase the risk of CVD. Core interventions for individuals with the metabolic syndrome include the following: regular physical activity at the same levels of recommendation for CHD and diabetes, and following proper nutrition such as DASH or Mediterranean or comparable diets. A detailed summary of physical activity and other lifestyle modalities for diabetes, prediabetes, and the metabolic syndrome is found in Chapter 6.

Physical Activity, Weight Gain, and Obesity (14)

It is currently estimated that approximately 70% of adults in the United States are either overweight (BMI ≥ 25–<30 kg/m^2) or obese (BMI ≥30 kg/m^2), or severely obese (BMI ≥ 35 kg/m^2). Regular physical activity reduces the likelihood of weight gain, and it is also vitally important for maintaining weight loss. The most effective regimens involve the combination of physical activity and moderate dietary restrictions. More details on physical activity, weight gain, and obesity are found in Chapter 8.

3.4 PHYSICAL ACTIVITY AND WOMEN'S HEALTH, INCLUDING PREGNANCY

Regular physical activity is a vitally important lifestyle behavior for women throughout their life span. Guidelines from the AHA, ASCM, PAGA 2018, and American College of Obstetrics and Gynecology (ACOG) (15), all recommend 30 minutes of moderate intensity physical activity on most days of the week with the goal of accumulating 150 minutes of moderate intensity physical activity per week. Numerous studies have shown that women who engage in regular physical activity lower their risk of heart disease. For example, women who engage in exercise 1.5 hours or more per week reduced their risk of heart disease by 30%. Multiple other studies have shown similar reductions in the risk of heart disease and other chronic illnesses. More details about the relationship between regular physical activity and women's health can be found in Chapter 12.

3.5 PHYSICAL ACTIVITY AND ITS RELATIONSHIP TO BRAIN HEALTH AND COGNITION

As the population in the United States and other industrialized countries continues to grow older, finding cost-effective ways of improving brain health and cognition assumes ever-increasing importance. A significant relationship exists between physical activity and various aspects of cognition and brain health (7). This relationship is often underestimated by both physicians and patients.

Regular physical activity has been demonstrated to improve cognition and lower the risks of various forms of dementia in Alzheimer's disease. The PAGA 2018 as well as the Presidential Advisory from the American Heart Association and the American Stroke Association (ASA) both recommend physical activity as a key morality in improving brain health.

Regular physical activity improves sleep and has been demonstrated to reduce feelings of anxiety and depression in healthy people and those with significant clinical affective symptoms. Both the PAGA 2018 and the Presidential Advisory from the AHA and the ASA recommend regular physical activity as a modality in improving brain health. In fact, the AHA/ASA Presidential Advisory entitled "Optimizing Brain Health" includes physical activity as a key recommendation (16). The relationship between physical activity and brain health has been demonstrated across the life span and is particularly important in the population over the age of 65 where there is an increasing prevalence of cognitive decline and dementia. Additional information in this area can be found in Chapter 11.

3.6 PHYSICAL ACTIVITY IN YOUTH

Physical activity results in multiple benefits for children. In the 2008 Physical Activity Guidelines for Americans (2008 PAGA) (17), recommendations for 60 minutes of moderate intensity physical activity per day were made for children aged 6–17. This recommendation was expanded in the PAGA 2018 since enough data were available to indicate that there were also benefits for children 3–6 years of age (7). In children 3–6 years old, physical activity has been demonstrated to improve bone health and weight status. In children aged 6–17, regular physical activity improves both bone health and weight status and also improves muscular fitness, cognitive function, and cardiorespiratory fitness. More detailed information concerning these links can be found in Chapter 14.

3.7 PHYSICAL ACTIVITY IN OLDER ADULTS

Increased physical activity plays an important role for older adults in multiple areas (18). These individuals are particularly susceptible to cognitive decline and dementia—both of which have been shown to be reduced in individuals who participate in regular physical activity. Regular physical activity has also been demonstrated to result in a decreased likelihood of falls and fall-related injuries. Aerobic physical activities and musculoskeletal strength building as well as balance and flexibility exercises are also important. The recommendations from PAGA 2018 of doing 150 minutes of moderate-intensity physical activity and two sessions of strength training per week also apply for individuals aged above 65, although it may be necessary to modify these levels slightly, depending on the current level of fitness in these individuals.

3.8 PHYSICAL ACTIVITY IN INDIVIDUALS
WITH CHRONIC CONDITIONS

Regular physical activity has been associated with reduced risk of a variety of chronic conditions, including some cancers (e.g., breast cancer, colorectal cancer, prostate cancer), as well as improved quality of life and function in individuals with osteoarthritis (19). The roles of increased physical activity in individuals with chronic conditions are discussed in multiple chapters throughout this book.

3.9 OVERCOMING SEDENTARY BEHAVIOR

In the past decade, there has been increased scientific interest in data-related sedentary behavior and chronic disease (20). It is estimated that children and adults spend approximately 7.7 hours per day (55% of waking time) in sedentary pursuits.

Sedentary behavior has been associated with increased risk of CVD, T2DM, obesity, and metabolic syndrome. The highest risk of CVD occurs in individuals who are the least active and who also get the least amount of physical activity. Individuals who participate in higher levels of physical activity can largely ameliorate the health risks of sedentary behavior.

3.10   THE ROLE OF PHYSICIANS IN PROMOTING INCREASED PHYSICAL ACTIVITY

Physician counseling has been shown in multiple studies to play an important role in many positive lifestyle behaviors (21). This includes physical activity, weight management, proper diet, and avoidance of tobacco. Unfortunately, less than 40% of physicians routinely discuss these issues with their patients. It has also been shown that physicians who are involved in regular physical activity and other health-promoting behaviors in their own lives are much more likely to discuss these issues with their patients.

3.11   EVALUATING PATIENTS FOR INCREASED PHYSICAL ACTIVITY AND PRESCRIBING INCREASING PHYSICAL ACTIVITY FOR HEALTHY INDIVIDUALS AND SPECIAL POPULATIONS

A variety of resources are available from ACSM to assist physicians in evaluating individuals prior to recommending increased physical activity and providing exercise prescriptions for both the healthy population and those with chronic disease, or for special populations (22). To increase moderate intensity physical activity, a prior examination by a physician is often not necessary. This is what is recommended in PAGA 2018; however, there are some instances where examination by a physician who has knowledge of physical activities will be helpful for both safety and benefit of patients.

My research team at Rippe Lifestyle Institute (RLI) has been routinely prescribing physical activity for our patients and research subjects for over 25 years. In this chapter, we will also provide some background information on how we approach this important topic.

3.12   PRE-PARTICIPATION SCREENING

Both the PAGA 2008 and the reiterated PAGA 2018 state that in the area of physical activity, "some is better than none." Both these guidelines and the ACSM recommend that clinicians must have a discussion about physical activity with every patient and make it as easy as possible for individuals to become physically active.

Pre-participation screening at its most fundamental level may involve simply inquiring of individuals how much physical activity they currently perform and then working with them to increase their level of physical activity. As already indicated, the PAGA 2018 recommends accumulating 150 minutes of moderate to vigorous physical activity on a weekly basis and in addition, two strength training sessions per week. It was noted in the PAGA 2018, however, that formerly inactive individuals who acquire even 30 minutes per week gain significant reduction in risk factors for morbidity and all-cause mortality.

A good way of starting a conversation about physical activity uses the recommendation which is supported by the U.S. National Physical Activity Plan and the Exercise Is Medicine® (EIM) initiative (23). Tools to inaugurate discussion were developed at Stanford University, and involve asking the following two questions:

- On average how many days per week do you engage in moderate or strenuous physical activity (like a brisk walk)?
- On average how many minutes do you engage in exercise at this level?

Answers to these questions should give a clinician a good place to start to help individuals gradually increase their physical activity and ultimately achieve guidelines from the PAGA 2018 Scientific Report.

Other tests are available which can help estimate where a person should start on their physical activity program. One that was developed at my research laboratory, Rippe Lifestyle Institute (RLI), is the One-Mile Walk Test (24). Details about how to take this test and score it can be found at https://www.verywellfit.com/rockport-fit ness-walking-test-calculator-3952696. This test simply involves walking a mile at a brisk pace and taking your heart rate at the end of the mile. Equations and tables can then be utilized based on these parameters. Age and gender can be utilized to estimate maximum aerobic fitness (Vo_2 max) and serve as the basis for starting an exercise program.

3.13 PRINCIPLES OF EXERCISE PRESCRIPTION

The fundamental underlying principle to develop an exercise prescription for sedentary individuals is simply to get more activity in their lives. The typical way that exercise and physical activity are prescribed by exercise physiologists utilizes the principles endorsed by organizations such as ACSM. This typically would not be necessary for individuals who have been sedentary and simply want to obtain more physical activity in their lives. For clinicians who want to be more precise with regard to exercise and physical activity, the prescription framework recommended by ACSM goes by the acronym "FITT," which stands for the following (22):

- Frequency
- Intensity
- Time
- Type

These parameters are very straightforward and simply provide a framework for the amount of physical activity that the clinician is recommending.

3.14 AEROBIC PHYSICAL ACTIVITY/EXERCISE PRESCRIPTION

Aerobic activities are defined as those that require oxygen to provide energy. These activities involve large muscle groups which are used in a repeated or rhythmic fashion. While many forms of physical activity can certainly be included under the rubric of "aerobic" activity, walking is the most common form of this type of activity. Recent advances in technology have given us the ability to prescribe this type of physical activity with more precision than we had in the past. The PAGA 2018 Scientific Report recommends individuals participate in 150 minutes of aerobic physical activity per week. Individuals who have been sedentary will want to start at a lower level and work up to this level slowly.

Walking is the most popular form of physical activity. When physicians are asked about what kind of physical activity they would recommend for their patients, over 90% say walking. My laboratory at RLI has been a leading source of walking research for the past 25 years. In fact, we coined the term "fitness walking" with the publication of our first book of that name back in the early 1980s. We also developed the first "field test" of walking (The One-Mile Walk Test), which allows people to estimate their aerobic capacity by simply walking 1 mile and taking some measurements such as time to walk the mile and heart rate at the end.

While there are many benefits of walking, one of the key issues is that it is low impact. That is because when walking, one foot is always in contact with the ground; thus, each footstep lands with 1–1.5 times body weight in contrast to running since an individual literally leaps off the ground with each stride. Thus, in running, the impact on landing is approximately three times body weight. Activities which require even higher leaping such as basketball may generate six times body weight upon landing.

My team and I at RLI have written five books on walking. These are available through my amazon.com book page (25). Of course, there are many other forms of aerobic activities, such as stationary cycling or swimming. The PAGA 2018 recommends activities that are low impact and less likely to cause injuries such as contact sports.

3.15 MUSCULAR FITNESS

Muscular fitness is also an important component of physical activity for a variety of reasons. Improved muscle fitness can reduce the risk of injury during activities of daily living as well as maintaining balance and the ability to safely perform all types of physical activities.

Two concepts of muscular fitness are interrelated. One is muscular strength. This is the maximum amount of force a muscle group can produce. Strength is typically utilized in single-effort activities such as moving a heavy box, lifting a young child or grandchild, etc. The second concept, namely, muscular endurance, is the ability of a muscle or muscle group to exert force repeatedly. Both components of muscular fitness are important. Muscular fitness is also important to lower the age-related loss of muscle. Individuals typically begin to lose muscle after the age of 40, and this can result in 10% loss of muscle per year, accelerating to 10–15% loss of mean muscle per decade. Muscle loss can lower strength and endurance and slow metabolism and contribute to a variety of chronic conditions. Muscular fitness has been shown in multiple studies to lower the risk of various metabolic conditions such as CVD or T2DM.

To improve muscular fitness, a good place to start is to recommend a patient seek professional guidance, which may be available from a fitness trainer at a health club or YMCA. The highest levels of fitness trainers also carry fitness training certification from the ACSM. When working for muscular fitness, it is important to include exercise involving all the major muscle groups including the following:

Quadriceps (front of thigh), hamstring (back of thigh), hips, abdomen, biceps, triceps, and chest.

At RLI, we always recommend that individuals utilize a 5–7-minute warm-up and cool down to help avoid injuries and lower the amount of muscular soreness following strength training sessions.

3.16 FLEXIBILITY

Flexibility is the ability of a joint to move through its whole range of motion. This is an important component of an overall comprehensive program for physical activity. Flexibility is particularly important in the aging population since lack of use and the aging process itself can lower this parameter. We at RLI typically recommend flexibility programs for all individuals who we see either in our clinic or in research trials.

Flexibility was also highlighted in multiple ACSM publications and the PAGA Scientific Report 2018. We often recommend to individuals that they utilize their stretching program to also focus on mind/body issues.

There are two important concepts related to regular stretching. One is called "static stretching." This is the most common method to improve flexibility and involves moving the joint to the point where the individual begins to feel tension in the muscles being stretched and then hold at that position for 10–30 seconds. The other type of flexibility exercise is "dynamic stretching," which involves moving body parts through a full range of motion while gradually increasing the reach and speed of the movement in a controlled manner. An example of this would be arm circles where the individual begins with small circles and gradually progresses to larger, faster circles. It is important to emphasize to individuals not to engage in "ballistic" stretching, where an individual bounces up and down in a stretch which may cause injury. Multiple programs are available in stretching and can be found in any of the exercise books generated through ACSM.

3.17 DURATION OF WORKOUT

For many years it was thought that the duration of a bout of physical activity needed to be at least 10 minutes in order to yield important health benefits. This was incorporated in the original guidance from the ACSM and the American

Medical Association in 1995. I was pleased to have been one of the coauthors on these recommendations. As knowledge in physical activity has advanced at the time of publication of PAGA 2018, research has supported that any duration of physical activity could yield important benefits. This is important to emphasize to patients who have been sedentary. The mantra emphasized in PAGA 2018 is "some is better than none."

3.18   BALANCE

Balance is a very important part of an overall plan for physical activity and should be a component of any exercise prescription. This is particularly important for older individuals. Improved balance can be built either by utilizing specific balance exercises or by increasing physical activity and muscular fitness. A wide variety of balance exercises are also available through the various ACSM publications.

3.19   MIND/BODY APPROACHES

There has been increasing emphasis in exercise physiology on recognizing the interactions between mind and body. This is also a powerful way of helping people understand the multiple health and fitness benefits of increased physical activity. We typically recommend to individuals that they focus on relaxation strategies during warm-up and cool down. It should also be noted that regular physical activity is a very powerful stress reducer. In fact, many regular exercisers report that stress reduction is a major reason why they are engaging in regular physical activity. Regular physical activity also lowers the likelihood of depression and anxiety, which could also be components of stress.

3.20   EXERCISE ADHERENCE

While some benefits of physical activity occur immediately following each session, most of the long-term benefits, particularly reduction and the risk of chronic disease, accrue to individuals who stay with their exercise program for a lifetime. At the end of this chapter, you will find recommendations that we typically give at RLI as a means of increasing the likelihood of staying with an exercise program.

3.21   SPECIAL POPULATIONS

Some modifications for physical activity programs may be necessary in special populations. The general guidance from the PAGA 2018, however, remains for individuals to attempt to accumulate 150 minutes of moderate intensity physical activity and two sessions of strength training on a weekly basis. Specific population groups where physical activity may play an important role include the following: pregnant women, cancer survivors, older individuals, overweight individuals, and many other populations. Each of these will be handled in separate chapters in this book.

3.22 TIPS FOR STARTING AND STAYING WITH A PROGRAM OF REGULAR PHYSICAL ACTIVITY

As already indicated, our team at RLI has recommended physical activity programs for thousands of patients and research subjects. Over this period of time, we have developed a variety of tips to help people get started and stay with an exercise program. These were often developed in conjunction with our walking research and clinical programs, but apply equally to other forms of physical activity. Here are some of the tips that we have developed to help clinicians encourage their patients to start and stay with a physical activity program (26).

- *Exercise with others*: Having other individuals to exercise with can make it into a more enjoyable social experience. This may involve taking group exercise classes at a fitness facility or simply finding friends to exercise with.
- *Establish a time and place*: Make physical activity a priority. If you leave your physical activity program as a nebulous part of your life and do not establish a specific time and place within your calendar to block off for physical activity, it is less likely that you will participate in it.
- *Find an activity you enjoy*: Having an enjoyable experience in physical activity is key to looking forward to it every day.
- *Keep a journal*: Writing down your progress is a habit that many regular exercisers have adopted throughout their life. Journaling allows you to see how much progress you have made and also note parts of your physical activity program that you want to remember.
- *Elicit the support of family and friends*: Having other people who care about you know that you are working on your health through a physical activity program can be very motivational.
- *Set realistic goals*: Many times people falter by choosing the wrong type of physical activity or engaging in too much right away or progressing too rapidly. This applies to walking or running programs or any other type of physical activity.
- *Purchase appropriate equipment*: This may be as simple as getting a good pair of walking shoes and also all-weather gear if you are going to walk or run outside. Other forms of physical activity are made more enjoyable if you have the right equipment. For example, for swimming get a good swimsuit and a pair of good goggles that do not leak water.
- *Vary your exercise routines*: In walking, this may be accomplished by taking different walking routes or it may be accomplished by blending different types of physical activity such as walking three times a week and stationary cycling three times a week.
- *Avoid injury*: The key to avoiding injury is to choose the types of activities that are lowest in injury potential such as walking, swimming, or stationary cycling and also not progressing too rapidly, which can lead to injuries and excessive soreness.

- *Upgrade your fitness program as you progress*: As you continue with your physical activity program, be sure to have slow progression so that you gain all the benefits of increased physical activity. For individuals who have been very sedentary in the past, even small amounts of physical activity can yield enormous benefits, but ultimately the goal is to slowly progress to the recommended 150 minutes of moderate or vigorous physical activity per week.
- *Reward yourself*: By choosing to be more physically active, you have made one of the most important health-related decisions possible in your life. Allow yourself to celebrate and reward your progress and your commitment. Not only are you improving your health and lowering your risk of chronic disease but you are also improving your mental outlook and building more endurance. You will also simply look and feel better by engaging in regular physical activity.

3.23 PUBLIC HEALTH CONSIDERATIONS

Various factors impact on the likelihood of increasing physical activity. Some of the issues involve recommending physical activity on an individual level, such as a specific exercise program involving older adults, youth, or healthy adults. Some options may involve community resources, while others may involve environmental or policy decisions, such as the built environment, which can either inhibit or facilitate such aspects as parks and other exercise facilities, or such parameters as transportation to or from school. New technologies such as wearable activity monitors and web-based internet programs can also enhance the likelihood of increasing physical activity. All of these factors are discussed in Chapter 20.

3.24 STEPS IN PROMOTING REGULAR PHYSICAL ACTIVITY

A number of factors also have been utilized and shown to positively or negatively influence the likelihood of adopting higher levels of physical activity. These are also discussed in Chapter 20.

3.25 CONCLUSIONS

Physical activity plays a critically important role in enhancing the health of individuals in the United States and other countries. The multiple benefits of physical activity are applicable throughout the entire age range and involve healthy individuals as well as individuals with chronic conditions. Increased physical activity is one of the most powerful mechanisms that all physicians can utilize to improve the health of their patients.

3.26 CLINICAL APPLICATIONS

- Physicians should recommend increased physical activity to all patients.
- Physical activity plays an important role in decreasing the risk of chronic diseases, and it serves as an adjunct to their treatment.

- Increased physical activity plays an important role in improving the quality of life of individuals.
- Counseling on physical activity and its benefits should be a routine part of every physician encounter with patients.

REFERENCES

1. Rippe JM. *Lifestyle Medicine* (3rd edition). CRC Press (Boca Raton), 2019.
2. Lloyd-Jones D, Hong Y, Labarthe D, et al. Defining and Setting National Goals for Cardiovascular Health Promotion and Disease Reduction: The American Heart Association's Strategic Impact Goal through 2020 and Beyond. *Circulation.* 2010;121:586–613.
3. American Academy of Pediatrics. Guidelines for Healthy Child Care. https://www.aap.org/en-us/advocacy-and-policy/aap-health-initiatives/healthy-child-care/Pages/default.aspx. Accessed July 1, 2020.
4. American Diabetes Association. Practice Guidelines Resources. https://professional.diabetes.org/content-page/practice-guidelines-resources. Accessed June 26, 2020.
5. Office of Disease Prevention and Health Promotion. Healthy People 2020. https://www.healthypeople.gov/. Accessed June 26, 2020.
6. Office of Disease Prevention and Health Promotion. Development of Healthy People 2030. https://www.healthypeople.gov/2020/About-Healthy-People/Development-Healthy-People-2030. Accessed June 26, 2020.
7. Physical Activity Guidelines Advisory Committee. *2018 Physical Activity Guidelines Advisory Committee. 2018 Physical Activity Guidelines Advisory Committee Scientific Report.* US. Department of Health and Human Services (Washington, DC), 2018.
8. American College of Sports Medicine. https://www.acsm.org/. Accessed June 26, 2020.
9. American College of Lifestyle Medicine. https://www.lifestylemedicine.org/. Accessed June 26, 2020.
10. Evert A, Dennison M, Gardner C, et al. Nutrition Therapy for Adults with Diabetes or Prediabetes: A Consensus Report. *Diabetes Care.* 2019;42:731–754.
11. Centers for Disease Control and Prevention. National Diabetes Prevention Program. https://www.cdc.gov/diabetes/prevention/index.html. Accessed June 26, 2020.
12. Pan X, Li G, Hu Y, et al. Effects of Diet and Exercise in Preventing NIDDM in People with Impaired Glucose Tolerance. The Da Qing IGT and Diabetes Study. *Diabetes Care.* 1997;20:537–544.
13. Lindström J, Louheranta A, Mannelin M, et al. The Finnish Diabetes Prevention Study (DPS). Lifestyle Intervention and 3-Year Results on Diet and Physical Activity. *Diabetes Care* 2003 Dec.;26(12):3230–3236.
14. Jakicic J, Rogers R, Collins KA. Exercise Management for the Obese Patient. In: Rippe JM, ed., *Lifestyle Medicine* (3rd edition). CRC Press (Boca Raton), 2019.
15. Birsner M, Gyamfi-Bannerman C. Physical Activity and Exercise during Pregnancy and the Postpartum Period: ACOG Committee Opinion Summary, number 804. *Obstetrics & Gynecology.* 2020;135:991–993.
16. Gorelick P, Furie K, Iadecola C, et al. Defining Optimal Brain Health in Adults: A Presidential Advisory from the American Heart Association/American Stroke Association. *Stroke.* 2017;48:e284–e303.
17. U.S. Department of Health and Human Services. OCTOBER 2008 Physical Activity Guidelines for Americans. https://health.gov/sites/default/files/2019-09/paguide.pdf
18. 2018 Physical Activity Guidelines Advisory Committee. *Older Adults. Part F, Chapter 9.* Page F9-1–F9-52, 2018.

19. 2018 Physical Activity Guidelines Advisory Committee. *Individuals with Chronic Conditions. Part F, Chapter 10.* Page F10-2–F10-117.
20. 2018 Physical Activity Guidelines Advisory Committee. *Sedentary Behavior. Part F, Chapter 2.* Page F2-1–F2-42.
21. Edshteyn I. *Lifestyle Medicine Clinical Processes in Rippe J: Lifestyle Medicine* (3rd edition). CRC Press (Boca Raton), 2019.
22. *ACSM Resource Manual for Exercise Testing and Prescription.* American College of Sports Medicine Lippincott Williams & Wilkins, 2017.
23. *Exercise is Medicine.* https://exerciseismedicine.org/ (Accessed July 1, 2020).
24. Kline GM, Porcari JP, Hintermeister R, et al. Estimation of VO_2 Max from a One-Mile Track Walk, Gender, Age, and Body Weight. *Medicine & Science in Sports & Exercise* 1987;19:253–59.
25. Rippe JM, MD amazon.com page. https://www.amazon.com/James-M.-Rippe/e/B001I LHH2O%3Fref=dbs_a_mng_rwt_scns_share (Accessed July 1, 2020).
26. Rippe JM. *The Exercise Exchange Program.* Simon & Schuster (New York), 1992.

4 Behavioral Change

KEY POINTS

- Most of the key modalities in lifestyle medicine involve making changes in behavior.
- Numerous behavior change frameworks are available which can demonstrate efficacy in helping people make positive lifestyle changes.
- Clinicians should become knowledgeable about motivational interviewing and positive psychology since both of these areas can enhance the likelihood that people will adopt new, more healthy behaviors.

4.1 INTRODUCTION

Behavioral change is a fundamental tool that is utilized in lifestyle medicine (1). For this reason, health care providers should become well acquainted with behavioral change techniques that help their patients improve self-efficacy for change. These techniques also allow physicians to cultivate a therapeutic relationship to empower the change process. While there are many different frameworks for behavioral change, all of them include goal-setting, problem-solving, self-monitoring, and follow-up with the health care provider.

The purpose of the current chapter is to provide a basic framework for the various research-proven behavioral change constructs. The goal is to provide health care workers with a summary of the variety of techniques and situations in which they are most effective. It is important to note that these techniques are also very valuable for health care providers who are experiencing their own process of change.

Medical schools have not taught behavior change in the past, and currently behavior change theories and techniques are not a routine part of medical training. The closest information to incorporating behavioral change theories in medicine came when the medical college admission test (MCAT) included a section on psychology which, in turn, provided information on behavioral change.

The National Institutes of Health have been interested in behavior change for years and a number of high-level academicians have made major contributors to this area. The major models that these investigators have developed are summarized in this chapter. In addition, this chapter will also explore how behavioral change models can be employed in nutrition and diet counseling, obesity, and physical activity.

All of the behavioral change techniques involve establishing realistic goals. An acronym that many people find helpful in this area is called SMART goals (2). This stands for goals that are "Specific, Measurable, Action-Oriented, Realistic and Time sensitive."

Several techniques have arisen which offer great promise in the area of behavioral change. One technique is motivational interviewing. This is a topic that many people are now exploring as a means of creating a more effective dialogue between health care providers and their patients. Another relatively new option in the area of behavior change is coaching. This technique has become increasingly prominent in the lifestyle medicine world and can offer options for health care providers to access people who have performed in-depth study in coaching techniques and are certified by one of the national organizations in this area.

Another area that has seen increasing prominence over the last decade is the impact of positive psychology. A section of this chapter will also be focused on this technique. This chapter will also explore advances in digital health technologies and how they are increasingly being employed in behavior change.

Finally, some attention in this chapter will be paid to an interesting area that has gained increasing prominence in lifestyle medicine, which is called the "Intention Behavior Gap." This area is an exploration of how to bridge the gap between what people know they should be doing and what they actually are doing when it comes to positive behavior change.

4.2 APPLYING PSYCHOLOGICAL THEORIES TO PROMOTE HEALTHY LIFESTYLES

Many of the psychological frameworks for behavior change focus on individuals; however, some are interpersonal and others are ecological. We will separate these theories into the following three levels of emphasis in this section.

4.2.1 INDIVIDUAL LEVEL

The most robust data currently available on effective ways of promoting behavior change come from initiatives designed to encourage these changes in individuals. This is also true for children but particularly for the adult population and older adults.

Typical formats for individual change involve either one-on-one sessions or group-delivered programs where educational approaches have also been employed to teach individuals how to make behavioral changes.

Individual approaches provide the most flexible way of dealing with behavioral change by supporting how individuals meet their needs and preferences. A downside, however, is that they require a high level of involvement from health care providers themselves and can result in significant costs over the long run. Benefits of many individual behavioral change programs are enhanced when they are incorporated into family settings. In general, good data are now available to suggest that a variety of theory-based interventions carry some efficacy to help people make behavior change in their daily lives. There are some behavioral change models that have been shown to be efficacious.

4.2.1.1 The Health Belief Model (HBM)

This model has been around since the 1950s and is based on attempting explain why many individuals are not participating in preventive health services (3–5). This model proposes that the likelihood that individuals will participate in a given health behavior largely depends their perceptions of the following three issues:

- Severity of illness(es) or issues
- Benefits of engaging in the behavior
- Barriers to engaging in the behavior

According to the HBM, individuals are more likely to adopt a health behavior if they believe it is likely to lower their risk of potential illnesses and carry benefits from engaging in the action. Many factors may prompt these actions such as media campaigns, physician reminders, etc.

Self-efficacy, which has been described as self-confidence in a specific behavior, was subsequently added to the HBM model to increase the model's ability to actively predict health behavior. The concept of self-efficacy permeates many of these behavior change models.

The HBM model has been applied to a variety of long-term health behaviors, including healthy nutrition, weight control, and physical activity. The HBM model has been used in health behavior research. It has been criticized, however, because some of the constructs such as "reasoned actions" are difficult to empirically test. In addition, other models have subsequently shown stronger predictive ability for health behavior change than HBM. The HMB model, however, might be quite useful in the hands of physicians, particularly, as they initiate a program for behavior change.

4.2.1.2   Theory of Reasoned Action, Planned Behavior, and Integrated Behavior Model

The Theory of Reasoned Action (TRA) model arises from premises found in cognitive and social psychology (6,7). The TRA model proposes that an individual's likelihood of engaging in particular health behavior can be predicted by the strength of their intention to engage in that behavior. These intentions represent a combination of individuals' attitudes about behavior and the "social norms."

The TRA model was subsequently extended to the "Theory of Planned Behavior (TPB)." TPB is based on the concept of perceived facilitators and barriers to behavior (7). Finally, the Integrated Behavior Model (IBM) further extended the TRA and the TPB models by adding the importance of evaluating the intention to engage in a behavior. These models have been demonstrated to be efficacious in various behaviors, including healthy nutrition, physical activity, and weight management.

4.2.1.3   Trans Theoretical Model

The Trans Theoretical Model (TTM) is a model of behavior change including many different psychological theories (8,9). Prochaska and colleagues first described this model by noting that people vary in terms of motivational readiness to make behavioral change. Initially, this was applied to smoking cessation and now is utilized in many other behaviors. The model is based on people progressing through a series of changes called "stages of change." The model outlines moving from the pre-contemplation stage to the contemplation stage, followed by the action stage, and finally the maintenance phase. The TTM model been widely adopted throughout behavioral medicine and is applied to many aspects of behavior.

4.2.1.4   Social Cognitive Theory

The Social Cognitive Theory (SCT) is a robust behavioral change theory which evolved from Social Learning Theory (10,11). It is focused on individuals' responses to watching others' behavior (this also referred to as "modelling"). Self-efficacy is a central construct for SCT. This can be increased through mass experiences, social modeling, improving physical and emotional states, and verbal persuasion. This theory has been widely used and tested in a variety of different populations and has been applied to increases in physical activity, nutrition, and weight management.

4.2.1.5   Positive Psychology

A recent interest has emerged in the science of positive psychology and its impact on behavioral change. Positive psychology is defined as the scientific study of "conditions and processes that contribute to the flourishing or optimal functioning of people, groups and institutions." Since this is an emerging and central component of lifestyle medicine, a separate section of this chapter will be devoted to positive psychology.

4.2.2   ECOLOGICAL LEVEL

In the last decade, psychological theories and models have been increasingly incorporated into broader context that effect health behaviors. This approach recognizes that these external factors are often as influential as internal factors. Ecological models are based on four fundamental principles that are central to understanding health behavior change (12–14). They are the following:

1. Environmental and personal factors that influence health behavior dynamically interact with each other.
2. Environments are multidimensional and complex.
3. People are multidimensional and complex. Intervention studies should consider both the individual and the groups (20) with which the individual is affiliated.
4. People–environment interactions exert multiple levels of influence.

These principles suggest that health behavior change strategies should consider not only individual behavior changes but also person-focused environmental changes in health behavior (see Figure 4.1).

4.3   THEORY-BASED HEALTHY LIFESTYLE INTERVENTION IN RESEARCH AND PRACTICE

The use of psychological models to better understand and predict behavior change is now widely accepted in the scientific literature. Thus, these models have been applied in the design of health promotion interventions—for both research and practice.

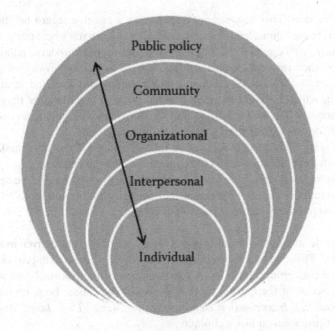

FIGURE 4.1 Socioeconomic model. Factors that impact behavioral changes.

These resulted in behavior constructs related to translating intention into behavior and most frequently constructs used are goal-setting, action and coping planning, and self-monitoring. These constructs recognize the importance of acknowledging goals and improving self-efficacy.

Implementation of intention models is a planning strategy that helps an individual specify their plans by putting them in an "if-then" format that makes an explicit link to an anticipated behavior and specific response to the "then" part of the plan.

4.4 MOTIVATIONAL INTERVIEWING AND LIFESTYLE CHANGE

Motivational interviewing (MI) has emerged as a significant strategy for helping people make changes in behavior (15). MI started out in the addiction field and specifically deals with the language of change. The goal is to get the clinician and the patient on the same page, recognizing that change is difficult. MI has been utilized in a wide variety of behavioral change settings (16–19). There is a strong body of information suggesting that it is very helpful. The basis of MI is to create a nonjudgmental partnership between the clinician and the individual who is seeking behavior change. It is based on the following parameters:

- *Partnership*: MI establishes a collaboration between clinician and patient instead of a relationship where the clinician is viewed as an expert and the patient is viewed as the recipient of getting advice from a more learned individual.

- *Compassion*: This involves not only having a positive regard for the individual being counseled but also prioritizing this person's best interest.
- *Evocation*: The goal of MI is to help the patient better understand and recognize their own reasons for making changes to their behavior.
- *Acceptance*: This is divided into four components. The first is absolute worth, which is based on unconditional positive regard rather than being judgmental. The next is affirmation. This involves recognizing an individual's efforts as well as their positive attributes.
- *Autonomy*: This concept is based on full acceptance of the individual. Their attitudes and decisions need to be appreciated and respected.
- *Accurate empathy*: This involves clinicians prioritizing the perspective individual seeking to change and purposefully asking questions to better understand their interests, views, and beliefs.

A considerable amount of training is necessary to effectively deliver motivational interviewing. This can be learned and delivered by any health care provider as long as they have background training. A full depiction of motivational interviewing is beyond the scope of the current chapter; however, the classic book on this is entitled *"Motivational Interviewing: Helping People Change Their Lives"* and offers a wealth of information on this technique.

4.5 THE IMPACT OF POSITIVE PSYCHOLOGY ON BEHAVIORAL CHANGE AND HEALTHY LIFESTYLE CHOICE

Positive psychology is defined as a science that focuses on human strengths to increase well-being and flourishing in individuals and groups. It is linked to positive health—the concept that subjective well-being is a "health asset" that protects against risk of physical illness (20).

There is a considerable body of evidence that connects positive emotions, optimism, and subjective well-being with better health and longevity outcomes (21–24). Positive Psychology Interventions (PPIs) have been demonstrated in a variety of research settings to be an effective way of improving positive emotions and assisting in behavior change. A number of PPI techniques have been demonstrated in various research settings to be effective:

- *Gratitude visit*
     In this setting, an individual delivers a letter of gratitude to a person who has been especially kind to them but that have not properly thanked.
- *Gratitude list (Counting blessings)*
     Individuals are asked to write down three to five things in their lives each day that they are grateful for.
- *Three good things*
     Individuals are instructed to write three things that went well for them each day.

- *Using signature strengths*
  Individuals are instructed to write down and utilize their "signature strengths."
- *Best possible self*
  Individuals are instructed to think about their life in the future and imagine everything has gone as well as it possibly could.
- *Acts of kindness*
  Individuals are instructed to perform five acts of kindness on a daily basis for six weeks.
- *Mindfulness meditation*
  In some research studies on PPIs, mindfulness interventions which cultivate nonjudgmental awareness of the present moment have proven beneficial.

All of these factors can play a very significant role in behavior change and lifestyle medicine. This is an emerging area with enormous potential.

4.6   INTENTION–BEHAVIOR GAP

The vast majority of individuals know that certain lifestyle habits such as proper nutrition and regular physical activity yield health benefits, yet there is still a very low adoption of these behaviors. Thus, the major issue is how to move from the knowledge and intention to change to actually foster change. This has given rise to the study which has been called the "Intention-Behavior Gap" (24). Intention alone has not been found to be a reliable predictor of behavior change in areas such as physical activity or dietary behavior even if the intention is high. The clinician should, therefore, consider factors that have been shown to impact on how this intention is turned into behavior. These include action and coping planning, self-efficacy, and capacity (executive function). By utilizing these components, clinicians can help bridge the gap between intention and behavior and increase the likelihood of behavior change.

4.7   COGNITIVE AND BEHAVIORAL APPROACHES TO ENHANCING PHYSICAL ACTIVITY PARTICIPATION AND DECREASING SEDENTARY BEHAVIOR

Regular physical activity has been demonstrated to yield multiple benefits for a wide variety of conditions (26). This includes lowering the risk of such conditions as cardiovascular disease (CVD), type 2 diabetes (T2DM), metabolic syndrome, many cancers, and weight gain and obesity. In addition, regular physical activity plays a very significant role in improving brain health and lowering the risk of dementia. In addition, regular physical activity helps in the therapy of a wide variety of conditions such as osteoarthritis and high blood pressure. Regular physical activity plays important roles at every life stage, including youth, adulthood, and in older adults. For all these reasons, the positive behavior of physical activity is of extreme importance. Despite all the known benefits of physical activity, it is estimated that only 20% of the adult population in the United States engages in regular physical activity at the levels recommended by the Centers for Disease Control and the Physical Activity Guidelines for Americans 2018 Scientific Report. In addition, the American society has been increasingly sedentary, which also carries multiple health risks.

For all of these reasons, it is important to find effective techniques for encouraging adaption of increased physical activity. A more in-depth exploration of physical activity and health is found in Chapter 2.

Multiple frameworks exist which have been demonstrated to effectively help individuals make behavior change to increase physical activity (25). Some of these involve behavioral frameworks which have been discussed previously in this chapter. Various levels of clinical research have been shown to effectively increase physical activity which have involved individual interventions, community interventions, and broader ecological interventions—all of these are discussed in more detail in Chapter 2.

Physicians should be aware of the behavioral medicine literature since the multiple benefits of physical activity are critically important. Finding effective ways of helping people incorporate this behavior into their daily lives should be a mandate for clinicians at every visit and patient encounter.

4.8   ENHANCING THE NUTRITION PRESCRIPTION USING BEHAVIORAL APPROACHES (27)

Proper nutrition is a key to healthy living. In fact, nutritional practices play a significant role in seven out of the ten chronic diseases worldwide. Guidelines for nutritional strategies are very similar across multiple organizations, including recommendations from the American Heart Association (AHA), the Dietary Guidelines for Americans 2015–2020 (28), the US Healthy Eating Pattern from the CDC, and Dietary Recommendations from the Academy of Nutrition and Dietetics (29). All of these recommendations include increasing the consumption of fruits and vegetables and whole grains, as well as matching calories consumed to calories expended to avoid weight gain and obesity. All of these issues are handled in detail in Chapter 3. Despite abundant and consistent knowledge about the health benefits of consuming sound nutrition, the American public is falling woefully short. For example, less than 30% of Americans consume the recommended amount of fruits and vegetables. The current consumption of whole grains and fiber in the diet is about 50% of the recommended amounts. Given the difference between the recommendations from various prestigious organizations and what Americans are actually doing, it is important to develop behavioral approaches to encourage people to follow more healthy nutritional habits.

Thus, nutrition prescription is one of the most important components of the lifestyle intervention. It is also important for clinicians to take into account the various cultural and social factors involved in dietary habits. A coaching approach can help promote positive dietary change when it comes to nutrition. It is also important for patients to possess fundamental culinary skills so they can prepare health-promoting meals at home. A number of research studies have shown that home cooking improves the likelihood of following a healthy dietary pattern.

The psychological theories which were described previously in this chapter are all applicable to the nutrition prescription. Also, motivational interviewing and positive psychology play important roles in helping people to adopt more positive nutritional practices.

In addition, practical culinary skills can be helpful to promote behavioral change. This involves learning the basic tools and skills as well as putting healthy foods in the pantry and emphasizing consumption of seasonal foods and vegetables to help increase the amount of fruit and vegetable consumption.

4.9 BEHAVIORAL APPROACHES TO MANAGE STRESS

Stress is endemic in our modern, fast-paced society. It has been estimated that over one-third of all adults experience enough stress in their daily lives to hamper their performance either at home or at work. Thus, finding ways of helping people to manage stress is extremely important).

Multiple programs have been demonstrated to be efficacious to manage stress. One of these is the relaxation response, which involves being in the present tense to lower the physiologic and biochemical response to stress. One of the most prominent investigators in this area was Dr. Herbert Benson, who developed a practice which was called the Relaxation Response (30). There are also multiple mind/body therapies which can play a significant role in lowering stress. These include meditation, breath awareness, body scanning, guided imagery, contemplation, and prayer and love and kindness. One of the most prominent investigators in this area has been Dr. Jon Kabat-Zinn (31). A number of movement practices also can result in lowering levels of stress. Most prominent in this area are yoga and Thai chi.

Recently, some elements of positive psychology have been utilized in lowering stress. Components of these therapies involve practicing gratitude and building a positive response. It is also important to help patients develop positive adaptive coping strategies. An effective strategy in this area is cognitive reappraisal as a component of cognitive therapy. This helps patients identify negative thoughts and behavior patterns and then change the negative and underlying beliefs to reflect more positivity while dealing with emotional stress.

A centerpiece for helping individuals is to reframe negative patterns away from situations that they feel stressful. This can be achieved by helping patients identify negative emotions linked to underlying beliefs of how this stressful situation will affect them.

A number of other lifestyle modifications can also help lower stress. Following nutritional practices, including avoiding stress and eating and seeking highly palatable foods, is also an effective way of reducing stress. One strategy to assist in this process is mindful eating. In addition, following a good sleep routine can also help lower stress. Oftentimes, people find that stress creates lack of sleep, which can further impact in negative ways.

4.10 HEALTH COACHING AND BEHAVIOR CHANGE

Despite the enormous evidence-based literature on the benefits of various lifestyle behaviors, such as sound nutrition and regular exercise, individuals often struggle to achieve those things on their own. Information alone typically does not result in significant or sustainable health behavior change. It is important for people to have reliable support, encouragement, empowerment, and accountability. All of these can be provided by health coaches (32).

The profession of health coaching has increased dramatically over the past decade. It is important for clinicians either to become knowledgeable about coaching techniques or to refer patients who are having trouble making behavior change to certified coaches. A number of coaching organizations have arisen that provide in-depth education for individuals who seek to include coaching as part of their clinical experience. These organizations have worked very hard to establish national standards for the techniques used in coaching and definitions of coaching. The one I can highly recommend is the National Consortium of Credentialing Health and Wellness Coaches (NCCHWC). This organization, which can be accessed via the internet, can provide introductions to local certified health and wellness coaches in virtually every market in the United States.

It is important to draw distinction between health coaching and therapy. Therapy is typically reserved for individuals with mental health conditions such as depression, anxiety, or addiction. Health coaches, however, use techniques to focus not on the pathology but on behavior change. There are multiple interactions between a therapist and health coaches, which will continue to evolve over the years to come.

4.11   DIGITAL HEALTH TECHNOLOGIES AND BEHAVIOR CHANGE

A wide variety of digital health technologies have been developed to promote healthy behavior change, including mobile health (mHealth), health information technology (IT) wearable devices, telehealth and telemedicine, and personalized medicine (33). Digital health can be broadly defined as the use of digital techniques for healthy living, health care, and society. These technologies continue to evolve. It is important for health care practitioners to evaluate what is available in various digital technologies and assist their patients in utilizing the most appropriate ones for their individual situation. It is important to recognize that to utilize these digital technologies a patient needs to be motivated to acquire and use the device. Second, devices must be able to accurately track the target behavior. A good example is the use of digital physical activity platforms to increase one's physical activity.

Finally, and perhaps most importantly, information which is displayed must help stimulate a user in a way that motivates lifestyle changes for health.

4.12   CONCLUSIONS

As physicians focus on lifestyle changes to improve health, it is important that there is a firm understanding that behavior change is difficult, but can be accomplished. Numerous psychological theories have been developed which can assist in behavior change as outlined in this chapter. In addition, some emerging techniques such as motivational interviewing and positive psychology can also play very important roles in helping people make the transition to more positive health behaviors. Most of the literature that is available currently in this area has to do with how behavioral approaches can be utilized to enhance physical activity and nutrition as well as manage stress. The profession of health coaching has also emerged and can be very helpful for selected patients to provide support and ongoing counseling in the process of making behavior change.

4.13   CLINICAL APPLICATIONS

- It is important for clinicians to recognize that information alone is not typically adequate for making behavior change.
- Framing information into proven psychological theories for behavior change can increase the likelihood that patients will adopt new behaviors and stick with them.
- Emerging information in the area of motivational interviewing and positive psychology can help clinicians create the framework for helping people make behavior change.
- Clinicians should become knowledgeable about behavior change theories and utilize them to increase the likelihood that their patients will stick with new, healthier behaviors.
- Behavioral therapies have been shown to increase the likelihood of physical activity and sound nutrition as well as helping to manage stress.
- Health coaching has become an important element of helping people start and stick with behavior change and should be utilized in patients who need this extra support.

REFERENCES

1. Frates B. Behavioral Medicine Section. In: Rippe JM, ed., *Lifestyle Medicine* (3rd edition). CRC Press (Boca Raton), 2019.
2. Frates B, Eubanks J. Behavioral Change. In Rippe JM (ed): *Lifestyle Medicine* (3rd edition). CRC Press (Boca Raton), 2019.
3. Becker M, Maiman L. Sociobehavioral Determinants of Compliance with Health Care and Medical Care Recommendations. *Medical Care.* 1975;13:10–24.
4. Rosenstock I. Why People Use Health Services. *Milbank Memorial Fund Quarterly.* 1966;44(3):94–127.
5. Rosenstock I. Historical Origins of the Health Belief Model. *Health Education Monographs.* 1974;2(4):328–335.
6. Fishbein M., Ajzen I. *Belief, Attitude, Intention and Behavior: An Introduction to Theory and Research.* Addison-Wesley (Reading, MA), 1975.
7. Ajzen I. From Intentions to Actions: A Theory of Planned Behavior. In: J Kuhl and J Beckmann, eds., *Action-Control: From Cognition to Behavior.* Springer (Heidelberg), 1985.
8. Pekmezi D, Barbera B, Marcus B. Using the Transtheoretical Model to Promote Physical Activity. *ACSM's Health & Fitness Journal.* 2010;14(4):8–13.
9. Prochaska J, Redding C, Evers K. The Transtheoretical Model and Stages of Change. In: K Glanz, BK Rimer, K Viswanath, eds., *Health Behavior and Health Education.* Jossey-Bass (San Francisco, CA), 2008.

10. Glanz K, Rimer B, National Cancer Institute (U.S.). Theory at a Glance: A Guide for Health Promotion Practice. *NIH Publication* 97–3896. US Dept. of Health and Human Services, Public Health Service, National Institutes of Health, National Cancer Institute (Bethesda, MD), 1997, 48 p.

11. McAlister A, Perry C, Parcel G. How Individuals, Environments, and Health Behaviors Interact: Social Cognitive Therapy. In: Glanz K, Rimer B, Viswanath K, eds., *Health Behavior and Health Education*. Jossey-Bass (San Francisco, CA), 2008.

12. Baranowski T., Cullen C. Nicklas T, et al. Are Current Health Behavioral Change Models Helpful in Guiding Prevention of Weight Gain Efforts? *Obesity.* 2003;11(S10).

13. Grzywacz J, Fuqua J. The Social Ecology of Health: Leverage Points and Linkages. *Behavioral Medicine.* 2000;26(3):101–115.

14. King A., Stokols D, Talen E. et al., Theoretical Approaches to the Promotion of Physical Activity: Forging a Transdisciplinary Paradigm. *American Journal of Preventive Medicine.* 2002;23(2)Supplement:15–25.

15. Fifield P. Motivational Interviewing and Lifestyle Change. In: Rippe JM, ed., *Lifestyle Medicine* (3rd edition). CRC Press (Boca Raton), 2019.

16. Rollnick S, Miller W. What is Motivational Interviewing? *Behavioural and Cognitive Psychotherapy.* 1995;23(4):325–334.

17. Alperstein D., Sharpe L. The Efficacy of Motivational Interviewing in Adults with Chronic Pain: A Meta-Analysis and Systematic Review. *Journal of Pain.* 2016;17(4):393–403.

18. Barnes R., Ivezaj V. A Systematic Review of Motivational Interviewing for Weight Loss among Adults in Primary Care. *Obesity Reviews.* 2015;16(4):304–318. doi: 10.1111/obr.12264.

19. Barnes R, Ivezaj V. A Systematic Review of Motivational Interviewing for Weight Loss among Adults in Primary Care. *Obesity Reviews.* 2015;16(4):304–318.

20. Seligman M. *Flourish: A Visionary New Understanding of Happiness and Well-Being.* Free Press (New York), 2011.

21. Fredrickson B. Positive Emotions Broaden and Build. *Advances in Experimental Social Psychology.* 2013;47(1):53.

22. Tugade M, Barbara L. Resilient Individuals Use Positive Emotions to Bounce Back from Negative Emotional Experiences. *Journal of Personality and Social Psychology.* 2004;86(2):320–333.

23. Fredrickson B. The Role of Positive Emotions in Positive Psychology: The Roaden-and-Build Theory of Positive Emotions. *American Psychologist.* 2001;56:218–226.

24. Faries M. The Intention-Behavioral Gap. In: Rippe JM, ed., *Lifestyle Medicine* (3rd edition). CRC Press (Boca Raton), 2019.

25. Stetson B. Cognitive and Behavioral Approaches to Enhancing Physical Activity Participation and Decreasing Sedentary Behavior. In: Rippe JM, ed., *Lifestyle Medicine* (3rd edition). CRC Press (Boca Raton), 2019.

26. Sokolof J, Vasques M, Lee J, et al. Enhancing the Nutrition Prescription Using Behavioral Approaches. In: Rippe JM, ed., *Lifestyle Medicine* (3rd edition). CRC Press (Boca Raton), 2019.

27. US Department of Health and Human Services and US Department of Agriculture. *2015–2020 Dietary Guidelines for Americans* (5th ed). Washington, DC, 2015.

28. The Academy of Nutrition and Dietetics. https://www.eatright.org/. Accessed: June 29, 2020.

29. Loiselle E, Mehta D, Proszynski J. Behavioral Approaches to Manage Stress. In: Rippe JM, ed., *Lifestyle Medicine* (3rd edition). CRC Press (Boca Raton), 2019.

30. Benson H. The Relaxation Response. Avon Publishers. *Reissue Edition* (August 1, 1976).

31. Kabat-Zinn J. *Full Catastrophe Living (Revised edition): Using the Wisdom of Your Body and Mind to Face Stress, Pain, and Illness.* Bantaon Books (New York), 2013.
32. Lawson K, Moore M, Clark M, et al. Health Coaching and Behavior Change. In: Rippe JM, ed., *Lifestyle Medicine* (3rd edition). CRC Press (Boca Raton), 2019.
33. Krauss J, Zheng P, Stewart C, et al. Digital Health Technology for Behavior Change. In: Rippe JM, ed., *Lifestyle Medicine* (3rd edition). CRC Press (Boca Raton), 2019.

5 Lifestyle Medicine and Cardiovascular Disease

KEY POINTS

- Cardiovascular disease remains the leading cause of morbidity and mortality in the United States and other developed countries.
- Lifestyle measures such as increased physical activity, proper nutrition and weight management, and avoidance of tobacco products all powerfully lower the risk of cardiovascular disease.
- Despite the abundant knowledge of how lifestyle lowers the risk of cardiovascular disease, fewer than 40% of physicians counsel patients on these lifestyle factors.
- It is incumbent on physicians to stress these lifestyle factors as an important way of lowering the leading cause of morbidity and mortality in the United States.

5.1 INTRODUCTION

Daily habits and actions profoundly affect a variety of metabolic diseases, in general, and cardiovascular disease (CVD), in particular (1). Thousands of studies support the concept that regular physical activity, maintenance of a proper body weight, sound nutritional practices, and avoiding tobacco products all significantly reduce the risk of CVD (2). The strength of this literature has been underscored by the inclusion of these principles in numerous documents and guidelines from both the American Heart Association (AHA) and the American College of Cardiology (ACC) (3–6).

Despite the overwhelming evidence that positive lifestyle measures lower the risk of CVD, it has been difficult to translate this information into the habits and actions of individuals. Improvements in lifestyle measures have been cited as the major reason for reduction in CVD in the past 20 years. However, major challenges remain. For example, between 1980 and 2000, the mortality rates from coronary heart disease (CHD) in the United States fell by 40% (7). Almost half of the reduction in CHD between 1980 and 2000 was attributed to improvement in such lifestyle risk factors as smoking cessation, increased physical activity, and better control of cholesterol and blood pressure. It is important to note, however, that increase in obesity and inadequate glucose level have the potential to wipe out the gains achieved in other lifestyle-related risk factors.

Despite significant progress in lifestyle measures and CVD, it still remains the leading cause of mortality in the United States with more than 37% of annual deaths resulting from CVD. The biggest challenge that remains is helping individuals incorporate current knowledge into their daily lives. This is the biggest gap when it comes to reducing CVD, in general, and CHD, in particular. For example, as noted in the AHA Strategic Plan 2020, only 5% of individuals achieve "ideal cardiovascular health" (3), which encompasses a series of lifestyle factors such as regular physical activity, sound nutrition, weight management, and avoidance of tobacco, as well as some other cardiovascular health-related factors such as control of cholesterol, blood pressure, and glucose.

The AHA and ACC have been leaders in promoting the power of lifestyle habits, particularly over the past decade. For example, the AHA Strategic Plan 2020 introduced the concept of "primordial" prevention, which is defined as preventing risk factors from occurring in the first place. In addition, the Strategic Plan added the concept of "ideal cardiovascular health" to the health-related lexicon.

Numerous studies have been published related to lifestyle factors and health. It appears likely, however, that the discipline will coalesce under the concept of "lifestyle medicine." For example, the AHA and ACC in 2013 issued "Guidelines for Lifestyle Management to Reduce Cardiovascular Disease" (4). Positive lifestyle was also listed as the major factor in the Joint Recommendations for Blood Cholesterol issued by the AHA, ACC, and multiple other groups. Various lifestyle measures were also listed as key components of controlling blood pressure in the ACC/AHA 2017 Guidelines for Prevention, Detection, Evaluation and Management of High Blood Pressure in Adults (5). Of note, the Council within the AHA, which had previously been called the "Council of Nutrition, Physical Activity and Metabolism," in 2013 changed its name to the "Council on Lifestyle and Cardiometabolic Health" (8). All of these initiatives underscore the power of utilizing lifestyle factors and practices to lower the risk of heart disease. They are also consistent with the Dietary Guidelines for Americans 2015–2020 (9) and the Physical Activity Guidelines for Americans 2018 (PAGA 2018) (10). Thus, the role of lifestyle is continuing to emerge as a cornerstone of the prevention of heart disease.

As a cardiologist and researcher in the area of lifestyle medicine, I have found these trends deeply gratifying. I had the privilege of naming the field "lifestyle medicine" in the academic literature with the publication of my first, multiauthored textbook in this area in 1999 (*Lifestyle Medicine*, Blackwell Science, 1999) (11). The 3rd edition of this book was published in 2019 (12). This is a 1,500 page textbook with over 200 contributors who are experts in various areas of lifestyle medicine and health.

This chapter will attempt to summarize recent scientific literature related to how lifestyle habits and practices can be utilized to lower the risk of CVD and will frame this literature as a major component of "lifestyle medicine."

5.2   DEFINING CARDIOVASCULAR HEALTH

As more emphasis has been placed by AHA and ACC on lifestyle measures, the definition of cardiovascular health has matured and is moving more toward emphasizing to individuals how their daily habits and actions impact on their likelihood of developing CVD. In the Strategic Plan for 2020 from the AHA, the goal was articulated that "by 2020 to improve the cardiovascular health of all Americans by 20% by reducing deaths from CVD and stroke by 20%" (3). To accomplish these goals, a series of steps were outlined by AHA, many of which depend on lifestyle modalities. Three pillars were articulated as the key foundation for these goals:

(a) Primordial prevention
(b) Evidence that risk factors for CVD develop early in life
(c) Balancing individualized risk with related population-level approaches

The Strategic Plan 2020 also introduced the important concept of "primordial prevention," which involves avoiding the development of cardiovascular risk factors in the first place. The Strategic Plan 2020 also outlined the concept of "ideal cardiovascular health" and defined it as a series of seven health behaviors and health factors, including not smoking, maintaining a healthy body mass index (BMI >18.5 kg/m^2 and <25 kg/m^2), achieving appropriate levels of physical activity, consuming a healthy diet, maintaining total cholesterol of <200 mg/dL, maintaining a blood pressure <120/80 mmHg, and maintaining fasting glucose of <100 mg/dL. The health factors such as cholesterol, blood pressure, and glucose were all defined as "untreated" values. In addition to the major emphasis on the benefits of lifestyle factors themselves, it is clear that lifestyle factors also strongly interact with other health parameters such as cholesterol, blood pressure, and glucose control.

5.3   THE CONCEPT OF RISK FACTORS

The concept of risk factors is relatively new to the history of medicine. In fact, the initial construct of risk factors was based on data from the Framingham Study, published in the 1960s. Before that, the concept of risk factors for CVD did not formally exist (1).

Framingham data showed that factors such as diabetes, dyslipidemia, high blood pressure, and cigarette smoking each independently and significantly increased the risk of CVD. The concept of CVD risk factors has been expanded by the AHA to include physical inactivity and obesity. It should be noted that Framingham data also demonstrated that risk factors act synergistically and tend to cluster with each other. Thus, the presence of two risk factors in an individual quadruples the chances for developing CVD compared to individuals with no risk factors. Individuals who have three risk factors increase their risk of developing CHD by 8–20-fold compared to individuals with no risk factors.

Other risk factors for CVD are currently under investigation and include an elevated c-reactive protein (CRP), hemostatic factors, and alcohol consumption. It is possible that stress and other psychological factors, such as depression, may also increase the risk of CVD, although much less data are available in this area.

In addition to the risk factors that can be modified by positive lifestyle behaviors, there are also non-modifiable risk factors, including age, gender, and family history. While all of these may contribute in substantial ways to the risk of CVD, it is important to note that in each of these categories of non-modifiable risk factors, lifestyle strategies can still decrease the CVD risk.

Numerous studies have demonstrated that reducing risk factors for CVD can significantly decrease its likelihood. Lifestyle measures are a particularly powerful and effective way of lowering risk factors. In addition, these measures are of low risk and many of them simultaneously affect multiple risk factors.

5.4 LIFESTYLE STRATEGIES FOR CARDIOVASCULAR HEALTH

PHYSICAL ACTIVITY

Of all the lifestyle-related factors that impact on risk factors for CVD, regular physical activity is the most powerful (10,13). Physical inactivity represents a significant risk factor for CHD and is a more powerful predictor of CHD than either cigarette smoking or hypertension. Unfortunately, fewer than half of adults in the United States meet the minimum recommendations for regular physical activity. Young people are even less likely to meet recommended standards, with fewer than 20% of adolescents performing the 60 minutes or more of daily physical activity recommended by the Physical Activity Guidelines for Americans 2018 Scientific Report.

When sedentary individuals are compared to those who are very physically active, the risk of CHD in sedentary individuals is 150–240% higher. Only 25% of all Americans engage in the minimum standards from the Centers for Disease Control and Prevention and the Physical Activity Guidelines for Americans 2018 Scientific Report which recommends at least 150 minutes per week of moderate intensity physical activity or 75 minutes of vigorous activity and muscle strengthening activities at least two days per week (10).

Even levels significantly lower than these will yield very substantial benefits. As demonstrated in Figure 5.1, the greatest benefit with regard to reduction of risk of CHD comes from those engaged in 150–300 minutes per week of moderate intensity physical activity (10). However, as emphasized in Figure 5.1, there is no lower threshold for benefits and even individuals who engage in only 30 minutes of regular physical activity on a weekly basis lower their risk of all-cause mortality and CVD mortality by approximately 20%. These data strongly suggest that even small increases in physical activity could result in a significant decrease in CVD for a large portion of the American population. As demonstrated in Figure 5.1, approximately 75% of the maximum benefit comes to individuals who meet the guidelines from the PAGA 2018. Additional benefits come for individuals who exceed this amount of regular physical activity, although as illustrated in Figure 5.1, the reduction of the risk curve flattened out considerably at the highest levels of physical activity.

The PAGA 2018 also emphasizes that physical activity significantly lowers the risk of adult weight gain, helps control blood pressure, and lowers the risk of hypertension, in the first place. In addition, physical activity also lowers the risk of stroke and heart failure in a dose-dependent manner.

In general, the impact of physical activity on lipids is modest, although regular physical activity has been repeatedly shown to increase HDL cholesterol and lower triglycerides. Regular physical activity has minimal effects on low density lipoprotein (LDL) cholesterol.

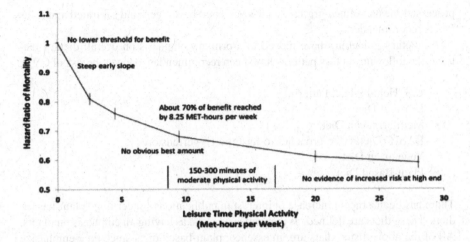

FIGURE 5.1 Relationships of moderate-to-vigorous physical activity to all-cause mortality, with highlighted characteristics common to studies of this type. *Source:* From the 2018 Physical Activity Guidelines Advisory Committee. 2018 Physical Activity Guidelines Advisory Committee Scientific Report. Washington DC: US Department of Health and Human Services; 2018.

Despite the well-known benefits of physical activity, many physicians are not encouraging their patients to exercise. Studies have demonstrated that less than 40% of physicians routinely recommend physical activity in patient encounters. In one survey of 175 primary care physicians, only 12% were aware of the recommendations from the American College of Sports Medicine for regular amounts of physical activity (14). Of note, physicians who engage in physical activity in their own lives are more likely to counsel patients about this than those who do not. (See also Chapter 3 for more details.)

DIET

Nutritional factors play an important role in lowering the risk of CVD and CHD. Multiple documents from the AHA and ACC as well as the DGA 2015–2020 all recommend dietary intervention to lower the risk of CVD (3–7,9). The recommendations are quite similar. They emphasize diets that contain more fruits and vegetables, fish (particularly oily fish), whole grains, and fiber, and maintaining a caloric balance to prevent weight gain and lower the risk of obesity, all of which will lower the risk of CVD.

All of these consensus statements now focus on the overall diet patterns rather than individual foods in the diet. These dietary patterns contain the above-mentioned recommendations for more fruits, vegetables, and whole grains. In addition, non-fat dairy, seafood, legumes, and nuts are also included in all of the consensus statements. Besides, these guidelines recommend that those who consume alcohol (among adults) must do so in moderation, and also lower consumption of red and processed meats, refined grains, sugar-sweetened beverages, and saturated and trans fats is recommended.

As dietary guidelines have moved to a primary emphasis on overall dietary patterns, the following dietary patterns have been recommended to lower the risk of CVD:

- U.S. Healthy Diet Pattern
- Low-Fat Diet
- Mediterranean Diet
- DASH (Dietary Approaches to Systolic Hypertension)
- Vegetarian Diet
- Plant-Based Diet

There has been a recent increase in interest in publications concerning "plant-based" diets. These diets are defined, as the name suggests, as having an emphasis on plants. All of the above-listed diets are, in essence, plant-based diets since they emphasize fruits, vegetables, legumes, and nuts, and limit the amount of red meat, processed meat, sweets, and oils.

There has also been some question about what actually constitutes a "plant-based" diet. A recent publication drew a distinction between a "healthy" plant-based diet and an "unhealthy" plant-based diet (15). This publication included an index for the healthy plant-based diet (hPBDI) where healthy foods such as whole grains, fruits, vegetables, nuts, legumes, oils, tea, and coffee received positive scores and less healthy plant foods (uPBDI), juices/sweetened beverages, refined grains, potatoes/French fries, sweets, and animal foods received adverse scores. In an analysis of over 90,000 women in the U.S. Nurses' Health Study, those who scored high on the hPBDI category had substantially lowered their CHD risk; whereas individuals who consumed more foods in the uPBDI had higher CHD risk. This type of analysis offers an opportunity to make specific recommendations about components of plant-based diets and their impact on CVD. (See Chapter 2 for more details on healthy nutrition.)

WEIGHT

Overweight and obesity are extremely prevalent in the United States. Recent data suggest that approximately 70% of individuals in the United States are either overweight, with BMI >25–30 kg/m^2 or BMI >30 kg/m^2 (16,17). The prevalence of overweight for women in the United States is 30% and adult men 40%. Estimates for obesity (BMI ≥30 kg/m^2) are currently 40% for women and 35% for men. Both overweight and obesity represent significant risk factors for CVD. AHA lists obesity as a major risk factor for CVD not only because of its association with other risk factors (e.g., diabetes, dyslipidemias, elevated blood pressure, metabolic syndrome), but also because it serves as an independent risk factor.

Distribution of body fat also adds additional risk since abdominal obesity is an independent risk factor for CHD (18). It is thought that the accumulation of abdominal fat promotes insulin resistance which can lead to glucose intolerance, elevated triglycerides, and low HDL, as well as hypertension.

To combat overweight and obesity, guidelines were published in 2013 by the AHA, the ACC, and The Obesity Society (TOS) (19). These guidelines contain the following five recommendations:

- Use BMI as the first step in establishing criteria to judge potential health risks.
- Counsel patients that lifestyle changes can produce modest and sustained weight loss and achieve meaningful health benefits, while greater weight loss produces greater benefits.
- Multiple dietary therapy approaches to weight loss are acceptable for weight loss. However, diets should be prescribed to achieve reduced caloric intake.
- Overweight or obese patients should be enrolled in comprehensive lifestyle interventions for weight loss delivered in programs of six months or longer.
- Advice should be provided to patients who might be contemplating bariatric surgery (BMI $\geq$40 kg/m^2 or BMI $\geq$30 kgm^2 with obesity-related comorbid conditions).

It is important to recognize that all of these recommendations carry a significant lifestyle component.

SMOKING AND TOBACCO PRODUCTS

Overwhelming evidence from multiple sources demonstrates that cigarette smoking significantly increases the risk of heart disease and stroke. This evidence has been extensively summarized elsewhere and is incorporated in virtually every risk factor reduction document from the AHA and other health-promoting documents (20, 21).

Unfortunately, cigarette smoking in men remains at approximately 18% and in women 14%. Thus, the overall percentage of cigarette smoking for adults over the age of 18 is slightly more than 15% (21). Sadly, the rate of discontinuing cigarette smoking has slowed down in the last decade. The good news is that substantial benefits accrue in terms of reduction of CVD in individuals who stop smoking. These benefits occur over a very brief period of time. It should be noted, however, that secondhand smoke also substantially increases the risk of CVD.

PSYCHOLOGICAL FACTORS AND STRESS

A number of psychological factors may impact on risk factors for CVD. The most prevalent chronic psychological condition in the United States is anxiety with a prevalence of more than 31% (22). Major depression has a lifetime incidence of approximately 10% (23). Depression may increase the risk of heart disease by making individuals less likely to adhere to programs that lower the risk of heart disease.

It has also been estimated that over one-third of individuals in the United States have enough stress in their daily lives to impair their life either at home or at work. There is some suggestion that chronic levels of stress may increase the risk of sudden cardiac death, although this literature is not as well developed as other risk factors.

Lifestyle factors can play a significant role in helping to ameliorate psychological issues and also to reduce stress.

BLOOD PRESSURE

Elevated blood pressure is a significant risk factor for CVD and the leading risk factor for stroke. According to the Joint National Commission VII (JNC VII) (24), normal blood pressure was defined as <120/<80 mmHg, while 80–89 mmHg diastolic and 120–139 mmHg systolic were defined as prehypertension and >140 mmHg systolic and >90 mmHg were classified as "hypertension." These were the criteria also incorporated in the AHA Strategic Plan 2020.

In 2017, the ACC/AHA issued Guidelines for the Prevention, Detection, Evaluation, and Management of High Blood Pressure in Adults, which were similar to the JNC VII Guidelines (5). However, these guidelines defined normal blood pressure as systolic <120 mmHg and diastolic <80 mmHg. The systolic value of 120–129 mmHg and the diastolic value of >80 mmHg were considered as elevated blood pressure. Stage one hypertension in people was defined as blood pressure 130–139 mmHg or 80–89 mmHg, while stage two hypertension was defined as systolic blood pressure >140 mmHg or diastolic >90 mmHg.

These more stringent blood pressure criteria were based largely on the results of the Systolic Blood Pressure Intervention Trial (SPRINT), which showed that these lower numbers of blood pressure control significantly reduced both all-cause mortality and mortality from CVD (25). In order to reach these lower levels of blood pressure in the SPRINT Trial, however, it was often necessary to utilize three blood pressure medicines. This highlights the importance of lifestyle modalities which can help lower blood pressure.

In the 2013 AHA/ACC Lifestyle Management Guidelines (4), the following lifestyle management recommendations were listed for blood pressure control:

- Consuming a diet high in vegetables, fruits, and whole grains, as well as low-fat dairy products, poultry, fish, legumes and non-tropical vegetable oils and nuts, while limiting sweets, sugar-sweetened beverages, and red meat.
- Consuming no more than 2,300 mg of sodium per day.
- Engaging in aerobic physical activity three to four sessions per week, each session lasting on average 40 minutes of moderate-to-vigorous intensity physical activity.

More information concerning the role of physical activity and diet in blood pressure control may be found in Chapters 2 and 3.

LIPIDS

Dietary management of blood lipids has been a cornerstone, along with pharmaceutical therapy, for risk factor reduction in cardiovascular disease for many years

(26, 27). In the 2013 AHA/ACC Lifestyle Medicine Guidelines, proper nutrition is listed as an important component for managing blood lipids. These guidelines advocate a diet consisting of vegetables, fruits, and whole grains, including low-fat dairy products, poultry, fish, legumes, non-tropical oils, and nuts, and limiting sweets, sugar-sweetened beverages, and red meat. This is the same dietary pattern which is advocated for helping to control blood pressure. These guidelines also advise managing caloric intake to prevent weight gain. Food patterns recommended include the DASH Dietary Pattern, the U.S. Department of Agriculture's Healthy Food Pattern, and the AHA Diet.

BLOOD GLUCOSE: PREDIABETES AND DIABETES

Diabetes is a significant risk factor for CHD (28). CHD is the leading cause of morbidity and mortality among individuals with diabetes. In fact, over two-thirds of all individuals with diabetes will die of CVD. Lifestyle therapies, including proper nutrition, regular physical activity, and weight management, are key lifestyle-related modalities to reduce the risk of CHD in individuals with diabetes. Dietary patterns for treatment of diabetes are categorized as Medical Nutrition Therapies (MNT) (29).

In addition, the same levels of physical activity that are recommended for other chronic conditions by the PAGA 2018 Scientific Report, including 150 minutes of moderate-to-vigorous physical activity on a weekly basis, are also highly appropriate for individuals with diabetes. Other lifestyle factors such as smoking cessation, counseling, psychosocial care, and self-management education support are also highly relevant. Finally, reducing the amount of sedentary time also plays an important role in lowering the risk of diabetes. These issues are discussed in more detail in Chapter 6.

METABOLIC SYNDROME

The metabolic syndrome is a cluster of metabolic abnormalities that significantly increases the risk of CVD. It includes the following:

- Blood pressure >130/85 mmHg
- Triglycerides >150 mg/dL
- Blood glucose >100 mg/dL
- Abdominal circumference >40 inches in men and >35 inches in women
- HDL <40 mg/dL

The most common criterion utilized to define metabolic syndrome, which was developed by the National Cholesterol Education Program, states that individuals who have at least three of these five conditions are considered to have metabolic syndrome (30). It has been estimated that 36–38% of the adult population in the United States have metabolic syndrome by these criteria (31).

Individuals who have metabolic syndrome should be treated as though they already have CVD. Therapies for metabolic syndrome are similar to those for

CVD, including regular physical activity, sound nutrition, and weight management. Recommendations for treatments of lipid and blood pressure in individuals with the metabolic syndrome are comparable to those with diabetes.

BRAIN HEALTH

The issue of brain health has become increasingly important, particularly as the population in the United States and other industrialized countries continues to age. Many of the same strategies employed to lower the risk of CVD are highly relevant to preserve or enhance brain health.

For this reason, the AHA and the American Stroke Association (ASA) joined forces to issue a Presidential Advisory on "Optimal Brain Health." (32) This concept is designed to help physicians understand the lifestyle measures that contribute to optimizing brain health. This includes regular physical activity, proper nutrition, and blood pressure control. Optimal brain health involves not only lowering the risk of stroke but also improving the likelihood of maintaining cognition throughout the lifetime and lowering the risk of dementia.

The Optimal Brain Health Initiative involved the utilization of seven metrics, which are very similar to those in the AHA Strategic Plan 2020, including non-smoking, physical activity at goal levels, a healthy diet consisting of current AHA guidelines, regular physical activity, and a body mass index of <25 kg/m^2. Ideal health measurements for untreated blood pressure, untreated cholesterol, and fasting blood glucose are identical to those listed in the AHA Strategic Plan 2020, as indicated earlier in this chapter.

5.5   BEHAVIORAL STRATEGIES AND ADHERENCE

Given the power of lifestyle factors to lower the risk of CVD, it is important to adopt strategies that optimize changes in these behaviors (33). A detailed science of behavioral change has arisen, along with various frameworks that have been shown to help individuals change behavior and maintain that change. This topic is so important that a whole, separate chapter in this manual has been devoted to it (Chapter 4).

5.6   REDUCTION OF CARDIOVASCULAR DISEASE
IN CHILDREN AND ADOLESCENTS

It is well known that the roots of many cardiovascular diseases and many other metabolic diseases are found in childhood. While most of this manual is devoted to issues related to lifestyle and health in adults, it is important to at least address some of the key risk factors which are increasingly present in children and adolescents (34–36). A large body of information on physical activity and children can be found in the recently released Physical Activity Guidelines for Americans 2018 (10). Nutritional guidance for children is also available in the Dietary Guidelines for Americans 2015–2020 (9). An entire chapter in the manual will be devoted to strategies for improving the health and lowering the risk of CVD and other chronic disease in children (Chapter 16).

5.7 PRACTICAL STRATEGIES FOR INCREASING LIFESTYLE MEDICINE IN CARDIOVASCULAR PRACTICE

Given the power of lifestyle medicine decisions in reducing the risk factors for cardiovascular disease, it is very important that physicians counsel every patient on these issues during every office visit. A key way to start is to simply recognize and counsel patients that what they do in their daily lives profoundly impacts on their likelihood of developing cardiovascular disease. Specific ways of doing this involve the following:

Physical Activity

Utilize the information from the Exercise is Medicine Initiative from the American College of Sports Medicine (37). There are multiple, user-friendly documents to help initiate a conversation on the positive role of physical activity. (More on Exercise is Medicine can be found in Chapter 3.)

Proper Nutrition

The guidelines for proper nutrition are found throughout this chapter. Initiate a discussion with individuals about the importance of following a diet that has increased amounts of fruits and vegetables, whole grains, and low-fat fish, while maintaining proper calorie balance to prevent weight gain or help with weight loss, if that is needed.

Weight Management

Obtain a BMI on all patients and discuss the implications of this with an emphasis on why it is important to maintain a healthy body weight. Utilize the guidance from the AHA/ACC TOS to frame the discussion on proper weight management.

Avoid Tobacco Products

Counsel people to avoid tobacco products or help with smoking cessation for individuals who are already smoking cigarettes.

5.8 CONCLUSIONS

The role of positive lifestyle measures is important in every disease, probably none more important than reducing the risk of CVD. Abundant evidence is available to show that regular physical activity, proper nutrition, weight management, and avoidance of tobacco products all significantly lower the risk of cardiovascular disease. Practical ways of discussing all of these factors are laid out in this chapter, and in subsequent chapters such issues as physical activity, proper nutrition, and weight management will be discussed.

5.9 CLINICAL APPLICATIONS

- Utilize the structures as outlined in this chapter to initiate conversation with every patient on ways that positive lifestyle factors can lower the risk for cardiovascular disease.

- Utilize materials from the Exercise is Medicine Initiative from the American College of Sports Medicine to frame a discussion of increased physical activity.
- Utilize multiple documents from the American Heart Association to discuss components of a healthy diet. Good places to start are the DASH Diet, Mediterranean Diet, and the U.S. Healthy Eating Plan.
- Utilize materials available from the AHA/ACC/TOS to frame discussions of healthy weight management, particularly in individuals who are overweight or obese.

REFERENCES

1. Rippe JM., Angelopoulos TJ. Lifestyle Strategies for Risk Factor Reduction, Prevention and Treatment of Cardiovascular Disease. In: Rippe JM, ed., *Lifestyle Medicine* (3rd edition). CRC Press (Boca Raton), 2019.
2. Rippe JM. Lifestyle Strategies for Risk Reduction, Prevention and Treatment of Cardiovascular Disease. *American Journal of Lifestyle Medicine.* 2018;13(2):204–212.
3. Lloyd-Jones DM, Hong Y, Labarthe D, et al. Defining and Setting National Goals for Cardiovascular Health Promotion and Disease Reduction: The American Heart Association's Strategic Impact Goal through 2020 and Beyond. *Circulation.* 2010;121:586–613.
4. Goff C, Lloyd-Jones D, Bennett G, et al. 2013 ACC/AHA Guideline on the Assessment of Cardiovascular Risk. A Report of the American College of Cardiology/American Heart Association Task Force on Practice Guidelines. *Circulation.* 2014;129:S49–S73.
5. Whelton PK, Carey RM, Aronow WS, et al. 2017 ACC/AHA/ABC/ACPM/AGS/ APHA/ASH/ASPC/NMA/PCNA Guideline for the Prevention, Detection, Evaluation, and Management of High Blood Pressure in Adults: A Report of the American College of Cardiology/American Heart Association Task Force on Clinical Practice Guidelines. *Hyperten.* 2018;71(6):E13–E115.
6. US Department of Health and Human Service National Heart Lung and Blood Institute. National Institutes of Health. Third Report of the Expert Panel on Detection, Evaluation, and Treatment of High Blood Cholesterol in Adults (Adult Treatment Panel III), Washington, DC, 2004. *Circulation.* 2002;106(25):3143–421.
7. Ford ES, Ajani UA, Croft JB, et al. Explaining the Decrease in U.S. Deaths from Coronary Disease, 1980–2000. *New England Journal of Medicine.* 2007;356:2388–2398.
8. American Heart Association. Council on Lifestyle and Cardiometabolic Health. https ://professional.heart.org/professional/MembershipCouncils/ScientificCouncils/UCM _322856_Council-on-Lifestyle-and-Cardiometabolic-Health.jsp. Accessed June 30, 2020.
9. U.S. Department of Health and Human Services and U.S. Department of Agriculture. *2015–2020 Dietary Guidelines for Americans* (8th edition). December 2015. Available at http://health.Gov/dietaryguidelines/2015/guidelines/.
10. Physical Activity Guidelines Advisory Committee. *2018 Physical Activity Guidelines Advisory Committee Scientific Report.* U.S. Department of Health and Human Services (Washington DC), 2018.
11. Rippe JM. *Lifestyle Medicine.* Blackwell Science, Inc. (London), 1999.
12. Rippe JM. *Lifestyle Medicine* (3rd edition). CRC Press (Boca Raton), 2019.
13. Zoeller R. *Physical Activity and Fitness in the Prevention of Cardiovascular Disease. Lifestyle Medicine* (3rd edition). CRC Press (Boca Raton), 2019.

14. Walsh JM, Swangard DM, Davis T, McPhee SJ. Exercise Counseling by Primary Care Physicians in the Era of Managed Care. *American Journal of Preventive Medicine* 1999;16(4):307–313.

15. Satija A, Bhupathiraju SN, Spiegelman D, et al. Healthful and Unhealthful Plant-Based Diets and the Risk of Coronary Heart Disease in U.S. Adults. *Journal of the American College of Cardiology*. 2017;70(4):411–422.

16. Flegal KM, Kruszon-Moran D, Carroll MD, Fryar CD, Ogden CL. Trends in Obesity among Adults in the United States, 2005 to 2014. *JAMA*. 2016;315(21):2284–2291.

17. National Center for Health Statistics. *Health, United States, 2016: With Chartbook on Long-Term Trends in Healthy*. Hyattsville, MD, 2017.

18. Despres JP. Abdominal Obesity as Important Component of Insulin-Resistance Syndrome. *Nutrition*. 1993;9:452–459.

19. Jensen MD, Ryan DH, Apovian CM, et al. 2013 AHA/ACC/TOS Guideline for the Management of Overweight and Obesity in Adults: A Report of the American College of Cardiology/American Heart Association Task Force on Practice Guidelines and The Obesity Society. *Journal of the American College of Cardiology*. 2014;63:2985–3023.

20. *The Health Consequences of Smoking: A Report of the Surgeon General*. US Department of Health and Human Services, Centers for Disease Control and Prevention, National Center for Chronic Disease Prevention and Health Promotion, Office on Smoking and Health (Atlanta), 2004.

21. Centers for Disease Control and Prevention. Current Cigarette Smoking among Adults in the United States. Accessed June 30, 2020. https://www.cdc.gov/tobacco/data_statist ics/fact_sheets/adult_data/cig_smoking/index.htm. Accessed June 30, 2020.

22. Kessler RC, Petukhova M, Sampson NA, Zaslavsky AM, Wittchen HU. Twelve-Month and Lifetime Prevalence and Lifetime Morbid risk of Anxiety and Mood Disorders in the United States. *International Journal of Methods in Psychiatric Research*. 2012;21(3):169–184.

23. National Institute of Mental Health. Major Depression. February 2019 https://www.nim h.nih.gov/health/statistics/index.shtml. Accessed June 30, 2020.

24. Chobanian AV, Bakris GL, Black HR, et al. National Heart Lung, and Blood Institute Joint National Committee on Prevention, Detection, Evaluation and Treatment of High Blood Pressure; National High Blood Pressure Education Program Coordinating Committee. The Seventh Report of the Joint National Committee on Prevention, Detection, Evaluation, and Treatment of High Blood pressure: The JNC 7 Report. *JAMA*. 2003;289:2560–2572.

25. SPRINT Research Group, Wright J, Williamson J, et al. A Randomized Trial of Intensive versus Standard Blood-Pressure Control. *New England Journal of Medicine*. 2015;373:2103–2116.

26. American Heart Association Nutrition Committee; Lichtenstein AH, Appel LJ, et al. Diet and Lifestyle Recommendations Revision 2006: A Scientific Statement From the American Heart Association Nutrition Committee. *Circulation*. 2006;114:82–96.

27. Stone NJ, Robinson J, Lichtenstein AH, et al. 2013 ACC/AHA Guideline on the Treatment of Blood Cholesterol to Reduce Atherosclerotic Cardiovascular Risk in Adults: A Report of the American College of Cardiology/American Heart Association Task Force on Practice Guidelines. *Circulation*. 2014;129(25 suppl 2):S1–S45.

28. American Diabetes Association (ADA) Position Statement. Cardiovascular Disease and Risk Management. *Diabetes Care*. 2017;40(Supplement 1):S75–S87.

29. American Diabetes Association (ADA) Position Statement. Lifestyle Management: *Standards of Medical Care in Diabetes—2018*. *Diabetes Care*. 2018;41(Supplement 1):S38–S50.

30. Grundy SM, Cleeman JI, Daniels SR, et al. Diagnosis and Management of the Metabolic Syndrome: An American Heart Association/National Heart, Lung, and Blood Institute Scientific Statement. *Current Opinion in Cardiology*. 2006;21(1):1–6.

31. Ford ES, Giles WH, Dietz WH. Prevalence of the Metabolic Syndrome among US Adults: Findings from the third National Health and Nutrition Examination Survey. *JAMA*. 2002;287:356–359.

32. American Heart Association and American Stroke Association. AHA/ASA Presidential Advisory. http://www.heart.org/HEARTORG/Professional/FocusonQuality/e-Communications/AHAASA-Presidential-Advisory_UCM_460822_Article.jsp?appName=MobileApp. Accessed June 30, 2020.

33. Linke SE, Robinson CJ, Pekmezi D. Applying Psychological Theories to Promote Healthy Lifestyles. *AJLM*. 2014;8:4–14.

34. Gidding SS, Lichtenstein AH, Faith MS, et al. Implementing American Heart Association Pediatric and Adult Nutrition Guidelines. A Scientific Statement from the American Heart Association Nutrition Committee of the Council on Nutrition, Physical Activity and Metabolism, Council on Cardiovascular Disease in the Young, Council on Arteriosclerosis, Thrombosis and Vascular Biology, Council on Cardiovascular Nursing, Council on Epidemiology and Prevention, and Council for High Blood Pressure Research. *Circulation*. 2009;119:1161–1175.

35. Kavey RE, Daniels SR, Lauer RM, et al. American Heart Association Guidelines for Primary Prevention of Atherosclerotic Cardiovascular Disease Beginning in Childhood. *Journal of Pediatrics*. 2003;142:368–372.

36. Kavey RE, Allada V, Daniels SR, et al. Cardiovascular Risk Reduction in High-Risk Pediatric Patients: A Scientific Statement from the American Heart Association Expert Panel on Population and Prevention Science; the Councils on Cardiovascular Disease in the Young, Epidemiology and Prevention, Nutrition, Physical Activity and Metabolism, High Blood Pressure Research, Cardiovascular Nursing, and the Kidney in Heart Disease; and the Interdisciplinary Working Group on Quality of Care and Outcomes Research. *Journal of Cardiovascular Nursing* 2007;22(3):218–253.

37. Exercise is Medicine. https://www.exerciseismedicine.org/Accessed August 7, 2020.

6 Diabetes, Prediabetes, and Metabolic Syndrome

KEY POINTS

- The prevalence of diabetes has grown substantially in the last 30 years.
- Over 9% of the population in the United States currently has diabetes.
- Lifestyle interventions, including weight loss (if necessary), medical nutrition therapy (MNT), and increased physical activity have all been shown to assist not only in the treatment of individuals with diabetes, but also in the prevention of diabetes and in lowering the risk of prediabetes being converted to diabetes.
- Lifestyle interventions can also lower the risk of the metabolic syndrome and play a central role in its treatment.

6.1 INTRODUCTION

In the United States, the prevalence of diabetes has increased dramatically over the past 30 years. As of 2015, the Centers for Disease Control and Prevention recorded that more than 100 million U.S. adults were living with diabetes and prediabetes (1). Of these, 30.3 million U.S. residents (9.4% of the population) had diabetes and another 84.1 million had prediabetes (33.9% of adults). Nearly one in four adults (7.2 million Americans) do not know that they have diabetes and these are included in the 110 million figure (2). Of the individuals over the age of 65, over 25% have diabetes. In children and adolescents, approximately 193,000 have either type 1 diabetes (T1DM) or type 2 diabetes (T2DM). The number of adults with diabetes increased to 422 million in 2014, with the number of adults who have diabetes increasing fastest in low- and middle-income countries (3).

The lifestyle therapies, including MNT, physical activity, and/or education/counseling and support, play critically important roles in both the prevention and management of diabetes (4,5). Multiple studies have shown that lifestyle interventions implemented in individuals with prediabetes can effectively prevent or delay T2DM, in some instances by up to 15–20 years (6). Lifestyle interventions are effective throughout the disease process and have their greatest impact early in the course of the disease (7).

6.2 LIFESTYLE MEDICINE THERAPIES FOR THE MANAGEMENT OF DIABETES

- Introduction

Among lifestyle interventions, preventing obesity, increasing physical activity, and following healthy nutrition are priorities in the prevention of prediabetes and diabetes (T2DM) as well as other chronic diseases such as cardiovascular disease (CVD). The goal of MNT in diabetes is to support healthy eating patterns and obtain individualized glycemic blood pressure and lipid goals. As diabetes progresses, the goal of MNT is to delay or prevent and help manage any potential complications. MNT needs to be evidence based and support healthy eating patterns. In addition, MNT must address individual needs, health literacy, access to health and food choices, and the willingness for the person to make behavioral changes.

- Diagnosis of Diabetes

Diabetes is typically diagnosed based on blood glucose criteria—either fasting blood glucose (FPG) or two hour glucose tolerance test (2-hPG) after a 75 g oral glucose load. A random plasma glucose of ≥200 mg/dl in the presence of symptoms is also sufficient to make the diagnosis of diabetes. Health care professionals will typically want to know the hemoglobin A1C (HbA1C) to determine how long the patient has had hypoglycemia. Testing for T2DM in asymptomatic persons should be considered in adults of any age who are overweight or obese and who have at least one other additional risk factor for diabetes. Testing for all individuals should begin at age 45. Unfortunately, in the last decade, the prevalence of T2DM in adolescents has increased dramatically. Therefore, screening the T2DM in asymptomatic youth who are overweight and have an additional two risk factors is recommended (see also Chapter 14).

6.3   TYPE 1 DIABETES

T1DM accounts for only 5% of diagnosed diabetes. T1DM is thought to be due to a destruction of insulin-producing pancreatic beta cells by a beta cell-specific autoimmune process leading to an absolute insulin deficiency. The rate of beta cell destruction varies considerably in individuals. T1DM commonly occurs in childhood and adolescence, but can occur in any age, even into the eighth or ninth decade of life. Children and adolescents may present with ketoacidosis as the first symptom of this disease, while adults may retain enough beta cell function to prevent ketoacidosis, but eventually these individuals become dependent on insulin for survival and are also at risk for ketoacidosis.

- Treatment of T1DM

Insulin and blood glucose monitoring: Persons with T1DM must be treated with multiple, daily subcutaneous injections (MDI) of basal insulin and rapid acting insulin after meals or continuous subcutaneous insulin (CSI) infusion. Typically, their physicians will need to decide which format for insulin therapy is best. The Diabetes Control and Complications Trial (DCCT) (9) clearly showed that intensive therapy with MDI or CSI delivered by multidisciplinary teams of physicians, registered dietician nutritionists (RDNs), nurses and behavioral scientists, among others, improved

TABLE 6.1

Lifestyle Therapies for the Management of Diabetes

A1C	Preprandial capillary PG[a]	Peak postprandial capillary PG	Bedtime/ overnight
Adults			
ADA: <7.0% (53 mmol/mol)[b]	80–130 mg/dL	<180 mg/dL (10.0	
AACE/ACE: ≤6.5%[c]	(4.4–7.2 mmol/L)[b]	mmol/L)[b,d]	
Children and Adolescents with Type 1 Diabetes[b,e]			
<7.5% (58 mmol/mol)	90–130 mg/dL		90–150 mg/dL
	(5.0–7.2 mmol/L)		(5.0–8.3 mmol/L)

Source: Franz M. Lifestyle Therapies for the Management of Diabetes, in: Rippe J. *Lifestyle Medicine*, 3rd edition, CRC Press, Boca Raton, 2019. Used with permission.

* See references (8, 12).

[a] Plasma glucose.

[b] More or less stringent glycemic goals may be appropriate for individual persons. Blood glucose goals should be modified in children with frequent hypoglycemia or hypoglycemia unawareness.

[c] Goal if it can be achieved safely.

[d] Postprandial PG may be used if A1C goals are not met despite reaching preprandial PG goals.

[e] In children and adolescents, postprandial PG values should be measured when there is a discrepancy between preprandial PG values and A1C levels and to assess pre- prandial insulin doses in those on basal-bolus or CSII regimens.

glycemia and reduced complication risk, while improving long-term outcome. Individuals with T1DM must perform self-monitoring of blood glucose. Recommended targets for blood glucose are found in Table 6.1.

• Lifestyle interventions for T1DM

Medical nutrition therapy: There is a large body of evidence that MNT using carbohydrate counting and insulin-to-carbohydrate ratios contributes to significant decreases in HbA1C and significant improvement in quality of life (10). MNT is optimally delivered with continued encounters with RDNs and patient use of carbohydrate counting to guide mealtime insulin dosage. Approximately half of insulin needs are for basal glucose control and half for prandial requirements. It is important to emphasize to individuals that carbohydrate, protein, and fat all require insulin at some point in their metabolism. Carbohydrate intake is the primary determinant of bolus insulin needs, but if a meal contains more protein and fat than usual, bolus insulin doses may be needed to compensate for delayed prandial glucose excursion.

Physical activity/exercise: As outlined in the Physical Activity Guidelines for Americans (PAGA) 2018 Scientific Report, youth with T1DM are recommended to engage in 60 minutes or more of daily moderate or vigorous physical activity and muscle-strengthening exercise at least two days a week (11). Adults are recommended by the PAGA 2018 to engage in 150 minutes or more of moderate to vigorous intensity physical activity a week.

Prevention of hypoglycemia with exercise is a major concern and individuals may need to adjust having carbohydrates if pre-exercise glucose levels are <100 mg/dl (12).

Education/counseling: It is very important that individuals with diabetes in their family receive diabetes self-management education and support (DSMES) (7). This allows for supporting the individual's empowerment to help self-control T1DM by providing tools to make informed management decisions.

Psychosocial care: Clinically significant emotional disorders such as anxiety, depression, and disordered eating behaviors are common in people with diabetes and require screening and referrals for treatment (7,13). Deliberate insulin omission causing glycosuria in order to lose weight is the most common recorded disorder eating behavior for individuals with T1DM. Other eating disorders in individuals with T1DM include anorexia nervosa, bulimia nervosa, and binge-eating disorders. The management of these conditions requires a multidisciplinary team.

6.4   TYPE 2 DIABETES

T2DM is responsible for 90–95% of all diabetes (1,7). Many of the people who have T2DM are obese, since obesity itself causes some degree of insulin resistance. Individuals who are not obese by BMI criteria may have an increased percentage of body fat which may be disproportionately distributed in the abdominal region which also causes insulin resistance. It is important to note that many obese individuals never develop T2DM. It appears that obesity combined with a genetic predisposition may be necessary for T2DM to develop.

T2DM is characterized by a combination of insulin resistance and β-cell failure. Insulin resistance is present in a number of target tissues, mainly muscle (14, 15), liver, and adipose cells. Insulin levels may be normal, low, or elevated and are not able to overcome the concomitant insulin resistance. Therefore, insulin production rates are not sufficient relative to glucose level and frank hyperglycemia and T2DM develop. Hyperglycemia typically is first exhibited in elevations of postprandial blood glucose, but ultimately elevated fasting glucose concentrations also occur. Insulin resistance at the adipocyte level also leads to elevated free fatty acids, which further increases insulin resistance.

T2DM is a progressive disease which will ultimately require increased dosages of either oral hypoglycemic agents or, eventually, insulin. The leading cause of morbidity and mortality in individuals with diabetes is CVD. Hypertension and dyslipidemia are also common in individuals with T2DM and are additional risk factors for CVD, although diabetes itself confers an independent risk.

- Medical Nutrition Therapy

    MNT is a vital component of the medical management of diabetes. Diabetes educators, such as RDNs, should be utilized to deliver MNT, which should include carbohydrate counting alone or within the context of meal plans (5). Reduced energy intake should also be established. This may cause either weight loss or, in some, weight gain. A summary of the MNT interventions for adults with diabetes is found in Table 6.2.

- Physical Activity

    There is a significant role of physical activity across the spectrum of diabetes. In addition to its role in reducing the risk of developing diabetes, regular physical activity can also play an important role in the management of diabetes in people who already have the condition (12). These facts are recognized in both the position statement from the American Diabetes Association on Physical Activity/Exercise in Diabetes and the PAGA 2018 Scientific Report (11) and the ADA Lifestyle Management Standards for Medical Care in Diabetes (16).

    In addition to lowering the risk or preventing or delaying T2DM, regular physical activity conveys health benefits for people with both T2DM and T1DM. Aerobic activity such as walking, cycling, jogging, or swimming has been shown to lower the risk of diabetes and assist in its treatment. Resistance exercise has also been demonstrated to convey multiple benefits for individuals with diabetes. The recommendations from ACSM and the PAGA 2018 as well as the ADA Standards for Medical Management in Diabetes (16) all recommend 150 minutes of moderate intensity physical activity per week as well as two episodes of strength training per week.

- Education/Counseling and Support

    Every person with diabetes should be actively involved in education, self-management, and management planning along with his/her health care team, including both individualized physical activity and eating plans (8). The emphasis on healthy eating involves consuming nutrient-dense foods with reduced energy intake. The Mediterranean diet (17) as well as the DASH diet (18) and plant-based diets are all examples of healthy eating patterns. Metabolic outcomes should also be monitored to determine levels of medication. The overall objective of education is to help patients with diabetes make informed decisions and participate in self-care behaviors in active collaboration with the health care team to improve clinical outcomes (19).

- Psychosocial Care

    Individuals with T2DM can also benefit from psychosocial care, particularly because the disease can cause increased stress, avoidance of care, mistrust of doctors, and poor adherence to diabetes care recommendations (20, 21). This is particularly true of individuals who have obesity because, unfortunately, some health care providers may have negative attitudes or stereotypes of people with obesity.

6.5   LIFESTYLE MEDICINE AND THE MANAGEMENT OF PREDIABETES

Prediabetes is the state where hyperglycemia is present, but blood glucose levels are lower than diabetes thresholds. There is compelling evidence that lifestyle

TABLE 6.2

Academy of Nutrition and Dietetics Evidence-Based Nutrition Therapy Intervention Recommendations for Type 1 and Type Diabetes in Adults*

Topic	Recommendations	Rating
Nutrition prescription	Individualize in collaboration with the adult; a variety of eating patterns are acceptable based on the individual's preferences	Fair
Energy intake	• For overweight or obese adult: a reduced energy, healthful eating plan with goal of weight loss, weight maintenance, and/or prevention of weight gain • For appropriate-weight adults: a healthful eating plan with goal of weight maintenance and/or prevention of weight gain	Strong Consensus
Macronutrient composition	An individualized, healthful eating plan within appropriate energy intake. Differing amounts of carbohydrate (39–57%) and fat (27–40%) report no significant effects on A1C or insulin levels, independent of weight loss	Fair
Carbohydrate management strategies	• Adults on MDI or CSII: educate on carbohydrate counting using insulin-to-carbohydrate ratios • Adults on fixed insulin doses or on insulin secretagogues: educate on carbohydrate consistency (timing and amount) • Adults on MNT alone or on diabetes medication (other than insulin secretagogues): educate on carbohydrate management strategy • All recommendations are based on the individual's abilities, preferences, and management goals. Monitoring carbohydrate intake is a key strategy for achieving glycemic goals	Strong Fair Fair Fair
Fiber intake	Encourage consumption of dietary fiber from foods, such as fruits, vegetables, whole grains, legumes, at the levels recommended by the Dietary Reference Intakes of U.S. Department of Agriculture due to the overall health benefits of dietary fiber	Fair
Glycemic index (GI) and glycemic load (GL)	Lowering GI or GL may or may not have a significant effect on glycemic control. Studies longer than 12 weeks report no significant influence of GI or GL, independent of weight loss, on A1C levels	Fair
Nutritive sweeteners	• Nutritive sweeteners when substituted isocalorically for other carbohydrates, will not have a significant effect on A1C or insulin levels • Advise against excessive intake of nutritive sweeteners to avoid excessive calorie and carbohydrate intake	Fair Fair
Non-nutritive sweeteners (NNS)	• Intake of FDA-approved NNS within the recommended daily intake levels established by the FDA does not have a significant influence on glycemic control • Substituting foods and beverages containing FDA-approved NNS within the recommended daily intake can reduce overall calorie and carbohydrate intake; however, the other sources of calories and carbohydrates in these foods and beverages need to be considered	Weak Fair

(Continued)

TABLE 6.2 (CONTINUED)
Academy of Nutrition and Dietetics Evidence-Based Nutrition Therapy Intervention Recommendations for Type 1 and Type Diabetes in Adults*

Topic	Recommendations	Rating
Protein intake	• Adding protein to meals and/or snacks does not prevent or assist in the treatment of hypoglycemia. Ingested protein appears to increase the insulin response without increasing plasma glucose concentrations; therefore, protein should not be used to treat or prevent hypoglycemia	Fair Strong Weak
	• Adults with diabetes and diabetic kidney disease do not need protein restriction; there is no significant influence of protein intake	
	• Type of protein (vegetable-based vs. animal-based) does not have a significant effect on glomerular filtration rate	
Cardioprotective eating patterns	• Encourage consumption of a cardioprotective eating pattern within the recommended energy intake	Strong Fair
	• Encourage an individualized reduction in sodium intake. Less than 2000 mg sodium per day is appropriate; for adults with both diabetes and hypertension, further reduction in sodium should be individualized	
Nutrient adequacy: vitamin, mineral, and/or herbal supplements	If proposed as a diabetes management strategy, advise that there is no clear benefit from supplementation in people who do not have deficiencies	Fair
Alcohol	When adults choose to drink alcohol, they should do so in moderation (up to one drink/day for women and up to two drinks/day for men). Alcohol consumption may place adults using insulin or insulin secretagogues at increased risk for delayed hypoglycemia	Weak
Physical activity	Encourage an individualized physical activity plan, unless medically contraindicated, to gradually achieve the following:	Strong
	• Accumulating 150 minutes or more of physical activity per week	
	• Moderate intensity aerobic exercise spread over at least three days/week with no more than two consecutive days without exercise	
	• Resistance training at least twice per week	
	• Reduce sedentary time by breaking up extended amounts of time (more than 90 minutes) spent sitting	
Glucose monitoring	Ensure that adults are educated about glucose monitoring and using data to adjust therapy	Fair

MacLeod J, Franz MJ, Handu D, et al. Academy of Nutrition and Dietetics Nutrition Practice Guideline for Type 1 and Type 2 Diabetes in Adults: Nutrition Intervention Evidence Reviews and Recommendations. J Acad Nutr Diet. 2017;117:1637–1658.

interventions that focus on achieving and maintaining a healthy body weight, improving dietary patterns, and increasing physical activity can prevent or reverse prediabetes. Prediabetes is diagnosed when there is a high fasting blood sugar (high FG). The American Diabetes Association defines high FG as a fasting blood sugar (FBG) between 100 and 125 mg/dl. High FBG reflects primarily hepatic insulin resistance and impaired early phase of insulin secretion. In addition, high FBG reflects muscle insulin resistance and impaired, late-phase insulin secretion. In the United States, approximately 34% of adults aged 18–64 had prediabetes and 48% aged 65 or older had prediabetes in 2015. Prediabetes prevalence is higher in men (36.6%) than women (29.3%).

- Role of Lifestyle Factors in the Development of Prediabetes

    Prediabetes has the common characteristics of impaired insulin secretion, insulin resistance, and subclinical insulin production disproportionate to body fat distribution or a combination of these factors (22, 23). Excessive calorie intake and physical inactivity lead to overweight/obesity and increases in the insulin resistance, thereby increasing prediabetes risk. Insulin resistance has also been shown to increase with age. Smoking has also been found to be associated with a 78% increased risk of impaired glucose intolerance (IGT). Reducing body weight and increasing exercise are key lifestyle factors to counter the effects of obesity on hyperglycemia (24). It is particularly important to emphasize lifestyle change to restore normal glycemia early in the history of prediabetes since lifestyle change alone is less likely to restore normal glycemia later in the natural history of glucose intolerance.

    Individuals with prediabetes can be particularly benefitted by some modification of activities. These include diet and physical activity modifications, which can improve glucose regulation and reduce cardiovascular risk factors. In the Diabetes Prevention Program (DPP), overweight participants who had both IGT and IFT were randomized to a placebo arm, Metformin (850 mg twice a day), or intensive lifestyle interventions (25). The intensive lifestyle modification program included 16 weekly educational sessions, followed by 8 monthly sessions, all focusing on reducing body weight by 7% and increasing moderate intensity physical activity to ≥150 minutes per week. At the end of a 2.8-year follow-up period, the lifestyle intervention program proved superior to either Metformin or the placebo group and lowered the risk of advancing to diabetes by 58%. Other studies have shown similar results.

- Components of Effective Lifestyle Interventions in Prediabetes

    Weight loss programs improve glucose regulation and help reestablish normal glycemia. In the Finnish Diabetes Prevention Study (FDPS) (26), weight loss of 7% improved insulin sensitivity and beta cell function and significantly reduced the incidence of T2DM. This was primarily due to weight loss. The most successful lifestyle modification programs implement strategies in promoting weight loss, improving diet, and increasing physical activity.

6.6 PREVENTING AND MANAGING PREDIABETES IN THE REAL WORLD

The research studies already discussed in this chapter are labor intensive. However, a number of translational T2DM programs have been tested worldwide and have demonstrated positive results (27, 28). These studies have routinely supported the effectiveness of the benefits of T2DM prevention programs using a variety of delivery formats, including individual and group sessions as well as different individuals delivering the program (e.g., health care professionals and community members) and in diverse settings (clinics, churches, and fitness centers). With this in mind, these programs are highly likely to be beneficial to individuals with prediabetes.

6.7 CONCLUSIONS

Lifestyle interventions are important and highly effective in the management of both T1DM and T2DM. These include MNT, increased physical activity, and education. These same modalities are highly effective in prediabetes where they can significantly reduce the likelihood of progression to diabetes. These types of programs should be discussed and prescribed to all individuals with T1DM, T2DM, or prediabetes.

6.8 PRACTICAL APPLICATIONS

- Lifestyle therapies are central to the treatment and prevention of T1D and T2DM.
- Lifestyle modalities such as weight loss (if necessary) and MNT and increased physical activity are cornerstones for effective treatment of diabetes and assist in substantially lowering the risk of prediabetes developing into diabetes.
- Similar programs are highly effective in reducing the risk of the metabolic syndrome and in treating it if already present.

REFERENCES

1. Centers for Disease Control and Prevention. *National Diabetes Statistics Report, 2017.* Centers for Disease Control and Prevention, U.S. Department of Health and Human Services (Atlanta, GA), 2017.
2. Gregg EW, Li Y, Wang J, et al. Changes in Diabetes-Related Complications in the United States, 1990–2010. *New England Journal of Medicine.* 2014;370:1514–1523.
3. NCD Risk Factor Collaboration (NCD-RisC). Worldwide Trends in Diabetes since 1980: A Pooled Analysis of 751 Population-Based Studies with 4.4 Million Participants. *Lancet.* 2016;387:1513–1530.
4. Knowler WC, Fowler SE, Hamman RF, et al. 10-Year Follow-Up of Diabetes Incidence and Weight Loss in the Diabetes Prevention Program Outcomes Study. *Lancet.* 2009;374:1677–1686.
5. Franz MJ, MacLeod J, Evert A, et al. Academy of Nutrition and Dietetics Nutrition Practice Guideline for Type 1 and Type 2 Diabetes in Adults: Systematic Review of Evidence for Medical Nutrition Therapy Effectiveness and Recommendations for

Integration into the Nutrition Care Process. *Journal of the Academy of Nutrition and Dietetics.* 2017;117:1659–1679.

6. Holman RR, Paul SK, Bethel MA, Matthews DR, Neil HA. 10-Year Follow-Up of Intensive Glucose Control in Type 2 Diabetes. *New England Journal of Medicine.* 2008;359:1577–1589.

7. American Diabetes Association. Standards of Medical Care in Diabetes—2017. *Diabetes Care.* 2017;40(Suppl 1):S1–S127.

8. Handelsman Y, Bloomgarden ZT, Grunberger G, et al. American Association of Clinical Endocrinologists and American College of Endocrinology – Clinical Practice Guidelines for Developing a Diabetes Mellitus Comprehensive Care Plan – 2015. *Endocrine Practice.* 2015;21(Suppl 1):1–87.

9. Diabetes Control and Complications Trial (DCCT)/Epidemiology of Diabetes Interventions and Complications (EDIC) Study Research Group. Mortality in Type 1 Diabetes in the DCCT/EDIC versus the General Population. *Diabetes Care.* 2016;39:1378–1383.

10. Chamberlain JJ, Kalyani RR, Leal S, et al. Treatment of Type 1 Diabetes: Synopsis of the 2017 American Diabetes Association Standards of Medical Care in Diabetes. *Annals of Internal Medicine.* 2017;167:493–498.

11. Physical Activity Guidelines Advisory Committee. *2018 Physical Activity Guidelines Advisory Committee. 2018 Physical Activity Guidelines Advisory Committee Scientific Report.* U.S. Department of Health and Human Services (Washington, DC), 2018.

12. Colberg SR, Sigal RJ, Yardley JE, et al. Physical Activity/Exercise and Diabetes: A Position Statement of the American Diabetes Association. *Diabetes Care.* 2016;39:2065–2079.

13. Larrañaga A, Docet MF, Garcia-Mayor RV. Disordered Eating Behaviors in Type 1 Diabetic Patients. *World Journal of Diabetes.* 2011;2:189–195.

14. Inzucchi S, Bergenstal R, Buse J, et al. Management of Hyperglycemia in Type 2 Diabetes, 2015: A Patient-Centered Approach: Update to a Position Paper of the American Diabetes Association and the European Association for the Study of Diabetes. *Diabetes Care.* 2015;38:140–149.

15. Garber A, Abrahamson M, Barzilary J, et al. Consensus Statement by the American Association of Clinical Endocrinologists and American College of Endocrinology on the Comprehensive Type 2 Diabetes Management Algorithm–2016 Executive Summary. *Endocrine Practice.* 2016;22:84–113.

16. Colberg S, Sigal R, Yardley J, et al. Physical Activity/Exercise and Diabetes: A Position Statement of the American Diabetes Association. *Diabetes Care.* 2016;39:2065–2079.

17. Estruch R, Ros E, Salas-Salvadó J, et al. Primary Prevention of Cardiovascular Disease with a Mediterranean Diet. *New England Journal of Medicine.* 2013;368:1279–1290.

18. Obarzanek E, Sacks FM, Vollmer WM, et al. Effects on Blood Lipids of a Blood Pressure-Lowering Diet: The Dietary Approaches to Stop Hypertension (DASH) Trial. *American Journal of Clinical Nutrition.* 2001;74:80–89.

19. Powers M, Bardsley J, Cypress M, et al. Diabetes Self-Management Education and Support in Type 2 Diabetes: A Joint Position Statement of the American Diabetes Association, the American Association of Diabetes Educators, and the Academy of Nutrition and Dietetics. *Journal of the Academy of Nutrition and Dietetics.* 2015;115:1323–1334.

20. Phelan S, Burgess D, Yeazel M, et al. Impact of Weight Bias and Stigma on Quality of Care and Outcomes for Patients with Obesity. *Obesity Review.* 2015;16:319–326.

21. Ochner C, Tsai A, Kushner R, et al. Treating Obesity Seriously: When Recommendations for Lifestyle Confront Biological Adaptations. *Lancet Diabetes Endocrinology.* 2015;3:232–234.

22. World Health Organization. About Diabetes. Intermediate States of Hyperglycemia. https://www.who.int/news-room/fact-sheets/detail/diabetes. Accessed July 1, 2020.
23. Nathan D, Davidson M, DeFronzo R, et al. American Diabetes Association. Impaired Fasting Glucose and Impaired Glucose Tolerance: Implications for Care. *Diabetes Care.* 2007;30(3):753–759.
24. Garber A, Abrahamson M, Barzilay J, et al. Consensus Statement by the American Association of Clinical Endocrinologists and American College of Endocrinology on the Comprehensive Type 2 Diabetes Management Algorithm–2017 Executive Summary. *Endocrine Practice.* 2017;23(2):207–238.
25. Berger S, Huggins G, McCaffery J, Lichtenstein AH. Comparison among Criteria to Define Successful Weight-Loss Maintainers and Regainers in the Action for Health in Diabetes (Look AHEAD) and Diabetes Prevention Program Trials. *American Journal of Clinical Nutrition.* 2017;106:1337–134.
26. Lindström J, Louheranta A, Mannelin M, et al., The Finnish Diabetes Prevention Study (DPS). Lifestyle Intervention and 3-Year Results on Diet and Physical Activity. 2003;26:3230–3236.
27. Flay B. Efficacy and Effectiveness Trials (and Other Phases of Research) in the Development of Health Promotion Programs. *Preventive Medicine.* 1986;15(5):451–474.
28. Ackermann R, Finch E, Brizendine E, et al. Translating the Diabetes Prevention Program into the Community: The DEPLOY Pilot Study. *American Journal of Preventive Medicine.* 2008;35(4):357–363.

7 Cancer Prevention and Treatment

KEY POINTS

- Regular physical activity is a powerful mechanism for primary prevention of cancer as well as an adjunct to its treatment.
- The goals outlined by the Physical Activity Guidelines for Americans 2018 Scientific Report (PAGA 2018) for 150 minutes of moderate intensity physical activity and two strength training sessions per week are highly appropriate for primary prevention of cancer and may be utilized in secondary and tertiary prevention with modifications made by the clinician.
- Healthy nutrition, physical activity, and weight management are all important lifestyle modalities at all stages of cancer prevention or treatment.

7.1 INTRODUCTION

Lifestyle measures play significant roles in both the prevention and treatment of cancer. In addition, lifestyle measures play an important role in the ongoing health of cancer survivors. These facts are underscored by the Joint Statement issued by the American Cancer Society (ACS), the American Diabetes Association (ADA), and the American Heart Association (AHA) on preventing cancer, cardiovascular disease (CVD), and diabetes (T2DM) (1).

Cancer is a generic term that represents more than 100 diseases, each of which has a different etiology. Nonetheless, lifestyle measures can play a critically important role in virtually every form of cancer. In 2016, it was estimated that 1,685,210 new cases of cancer were diagnosed in the United States and 595,690 people died from the disease. Worldwide, it has been estimated that the number of new cancers could rise by as much as 70% over the next two decades. Approximately 70% of all deaths from cancer will occur in low- and middle-income countries (2).

Cancer is no longer viewed as an inevitable consequence of aging. In fact, only 5–10% of cancers are classified as familial (2). Thus, most cancers are associated with multiple lifestyle factors and other environmental factors. For example, the importance of nutrition has been known for 35 years, following the work of Dal and Petro who estimated that 35% (10–70% of all cancers) in the United States could be attributable to dietary factors (3). The World Cancer Research Fund and the American Institute for Cancer Research (WCRF/AICR) in 2007 evaluated 7000 studies and concluded that diet and physical activity were major determinants of cancer risk. Thus, it has been estimated that on a global scale 3–4 million cancer cases could be prevented each year from more positive lifestyle habits and actions (4).

The relationship of obesity with cancer is also very strong. The AICR and IARC have concluded that sufficient evidence exists to link 13 malignancies to excess body fat. Obesity is now the second leading preventable cause of cancer, behind only cigarette smoking (5).

In this chapter, we will explore issues related to various lifestyle measures, including diet and nutrition, obesity, and physical activity as they relate to both prevention and treatment of cancer.

7.2   DIET AND CANCER PREVENTION

Consumption of various foods has been either shown to increase or decrease cancer risk. In general, individuals should eat a healthy diet rather than relying on supplements to protect against cancer. Foods associated with increased cancer risk such as red meat (e.g., beef, pork, and lamb), processed meats (e.g., ham and bacon), alcoholic drinks, and salt-preserved foods should be decreased in the diet (6).

TOTAL FRUITS AND VEGETABLES

Evidence that consumption of fruits and vegetables provides increased protection against cancer is typically based on epidemiological studies, although support also comes from animal and cell culture studies. Vegetables and fruits are typically low in energy density and high in fiber, vitamins, minerals, and other biological compounds (phytochemicals). The recommendations to include increased fruit and vegetable consumption typically exclude starchy vegetables such as potatoes, yams, sweet potatoes, and casaba. Examples of non-starchy vegetables that have been shown to decrease risk of cancer include broccoli, cabbage, spinach, kale, cauliflower, carrots, lettuce, cucumber, tomato, leeks, rutabaga, and turnips. These vegetables seem to protect against cancers of the mouth, pharynx, and larynx and those of the esophagus and stomach (4).

Fruits also seem to predominately protect from cancers of the mouth, pharynx, and larynx and those of the esophagus, lungs, and stomach. There is some evidence that fruits may also protect against cancers of the nasal, pharynx, pancreas, liver, and colorectal area.

There is also some recent evidence that fruits and vegetables may lower the risk of lung cancer. This effect is only significant in current smokers and not former or never smokers. There is conflicting evidence about fruit and vegetable intake and breast cancer survival (7).

Fruits and vegetables contain as many as 100,000 unique bioactive components, including both essential micronutrients (e.g., vitamins C and D and folic acid) and minerals such as selenium, zinc, iodine, and calcium. It should be noted that the magnitude of response to fruit and vegetable consumption, as well as other dietary components, may be influenced by many other factors, including an individual's genetic background and a host of environmental factors.

The World Cancer Research Fund has made a number of personal and public health recommendations regarding the consumption of fruits and vegetables for cancer prevention. Their recommendations include that individuals should eat at least five portions or servings (at least 400 g or 14 ounces) of a variety of non-starchy vegetables or fruits every day, featuring different colors, including red, green, yellow, white, purple, and orange. Also included are tomato-based products and allium vegetables, such as garlic (8).

SPECIFIC MICRONUTRIENTS AND PHYTOCHEMICALS

The micronutrients present in fruits and vegetables can also yield a large number of biological responses that can also modify the initiation of cancer. Here are a couple of examples of many micronutrients (6):

- **Garlic and allium vegetables:** The allium vegetables contain over 500 species, including garlic, onions, leeks, chives, and scallions. Allium vegetables are used throughout the world, both for flavorings and also for possible health benefits. The health benefits of allium vegetables are attributed to sulfur-containing compounds. They may also involve other components. The WCRS/AICR Report indicates that garlic may protect against colorectal cancer. Other studies support that there may be a protective effect of allium vegetables, particularly garlic, against gastric, colorectal, and upper G.I. tract cancers. These effects are only for garlic itself and not garlic supplements.
- **Folate**: Folate is a water-soluble vitamin B and derives its name because it is abundant in foliage (e.g., green, leafy vegetables). It can also be used to fortify flour and cereal products, grains, and breads. A recent meta-analysis suggests that a high dietary intake of folate is protective against upper G.I. cancers, including esophageal, gastric, and pancreatic cancers. Recent studies have suggested that 50–100 genes are directly or indirectly involved with folate metabolism. Thus, there are considerable human genetic differences which may determine biological responses to folate.
- **Carotenoids:** Carotenoids are common in green, yellow/red, and yellow/orange vegetables. Some epidemiological studies have suggested that high-beta carotene-rich fruits and vegetables reduce the risk of lung cancer. A leading source of carotenoids in the human diet is tomatoes. Some studies have suggested that supplements with high levels of carotenoids in them may actually have the adverse effect of increasing the risk of cancers.

Dietary fiber: Dietary fiber encompasses mostly non-digestible, plant cell compounds and has variable effects on diet physiology. The major classification for fiber includes soluble fiber which means that it dissolves in water, and insoluble fiber which means that it does not dissolve in water. Soluble fiber is found in oats, barley, beans, and various fruits and vegetables. Insoluble fiber is found in whole grains, legumes, seeds, nuts, and dark green leafy vegetables. Fiber slows digestion, which helps lower blood sugar and which may also dilute harmful substances in the colon and prevent constipation.

Current recommendations from various health organizations involve eating 25 g of fiber each day for women and 38 g for men. This should be divided throughout the day. The current fiber consumption in the United States is only about half of this recommendation. Multiple studies include in the WCRS/AICR Continuous Update Project, where foods containing dietary fiber showed a decrease of colorectal cancer related to dietary fiber. This project concluded that there were probable protective effects of fiber for lowering the risk of colorectal cancer. However, studies results linking dietary fiber in colon cancer remain somewhat inconclusive.

The effects of dietary fiber on mammary and prostate cancer risk has also been inconsistent. Some studies suggest that there is a 32% decreased risk of breast cancer per 10 g of increase in dietary fiber. However, some studies have suggested that dietary fiber can lower the risk of breast cancer, but others have not. One confounding factor related to fiber and cancer risk is that high-fiber diets also typically contain folate and phytochemicals found in high-fiber foods.

Meat intake: Consumption of meat is typically defined as either red meat (beef, pork, lamb, and goat) or poultry (which typically has more white than red muscle fibers). The term "processed" meat refers to meats that have been preserved by salting, smoking, curing, or adding chemical preservatives. Examples of processed meats include ham, bacon, pastrami, salami, hot dogs, and sausages.

The WCRF/AICR Report suggested that there was probable evidence that red meat and convincing evidence that processed meat are related to increased risk of colon cancer (4). The Agency for Research on Cancer (IARC) further classified red meat as a probable cause of cancer and processed meat as a definite cause of cancer (9). However, to put these results in perspective, the lifetime risk of an individual developing colon cancer is 5% and the increase from eating the amount of processed meat or red meat in the IARC Report (50 g/day) raises the average lifetime risk to 6%. A variety of other cancers are also increased by anywhere from 4% to 20% from consuming 50 g/day of processed meat. These include prostate cancer (4%), breast cancer (9%), colorectal cancer (18%), and pancreatic cancer (19%).

Increased cancer risk may not be a function of the meat per se, but may reflect high-fat intake or other carcinogens generated through various cooking and processing methods. Moreover, meat consumption is positively associated with weight gain in large cohort studies. It is also important to recognize that meat can be a valuable source of many nutrients, including protein, iron, zinc, selenium, and vitamins B6 and B12. Iron deficiency is the most common and widespread nutritional deficiency in the world. Therefore, it seems prudent to limit red meat consumption rather than to totally avoid it. The WCRF recommends that population average consumption of red meat be no more than 300 g (11 ounces) per week, very little of which should be processed. It is also important to consider the consumption of meat in the context of the entire diet, particularly fruit and vegetable consumption.

Alcohol: Alcohol is the common name for ethanol which is found in beer, wine, and liquor. Alcohol is acknowledged and classified by the IACR as a human carcinogen, and the WCRF/AICR Panel reported that there was convincing evidence that alcoholic drinks increased mouth, pharynx, esophagus, colorectal (men), and breast cancer (4). Alcoholic drinks probably also are a cause of liver cancer and colorectal cancer in women.

A number of potential mechanisms have been identified whereby alcohol may contribute to the increased risk of cancer. First, ethanol is mainly oxidized in the liver by alcohol dehydrogenase (ADH) into the acid aldehyde, which is a toxic metabolite and a probable human carcinogen. Second, the generation of reactive oxygens generated during ethanol metabolism can damage DNA, lipids, and proteins and activate molecules involved in inflammation and angiogenesis. Third, intake of ethanol may also increase the composition of enteric bacteria. Further, chronic alcohol consumption can result in decreased absorption of a variety of nutrients associated with cancer risk, including folate.

While ethanol consumption has been linked to several types of cancers, recommendations are complicated by the fact that low to moderate alcohol intake has been linked with a lower risk of heart disease. The WCRF/AIRC recommends that if alcoholic drinks are to be consumed, consumption should be limited to two drinks per day for men and one drink per day for women.

7.3   OBESITY AND CANCER

Overweight and obesity are accompanied by an increased risk and worse prognosis for multiple malignancies (10). For individuals who are overweight or obese, intentional weight loss lowers cancer risk and improves survival. Patients who already have cancer should avoid weight gain and, if already overweight or obese, should lose weight to improve prognosis.

The public and medical profession is aware that there is significant relationship between obesity and heart disease, stroke, and diabetes. However, a report from the American Institute for Cancer Research (AICR) indicated that only 50% of Americans are aware that obesity stimulates cancer growth.

The relationship between excess adipose tissue in obesity plays an important role in the linkage between obesity and cancer. Adipose tissue was once considered a storage depot of little metabolic import. However, it has now been conclusively shown that adipose tissue is intensely metabolic and participates in multiple physiologic functions which may impact on its relationship to cancer.

Mechanisms of obesity impact on cancer: There are multiple mechanisms by which obesity effects cancer. Obesity is not thought to initiate the carcinogenic process, but rather to promote cancer progression (11). One mechanism by which obesity interacts with cancer is its stimulation of pro-inflammatory factors which include cytokines, IL-6, IL-1, and TNF-α. These inflammatory factors promote cellular and humoral growth, which leads to insulin resistance. Levels of insulin and insulin-like growth factor (IGF-1) are often increased in obesity and may contribute to tumor growth. Elevated levels of insulin stimulate cellular uptake in normal cells, but may also promote tumor cell growth and cancer progression. Obesity may also promote epigenetic processes which can contribute to tumor growth as well. These alterations may include methylation of DNA which alters its structure and function. Obesity may also change metabolic and hormonal factors in addition to its pro-inflammatory effects. While all of these factors may be important in cancer growth, the elimination of obesity and restoration of normal body weight is desirable at any time of life and may also reverse cancer-promoting consequences of obesity.

Dietary composition in obese individuals may also further contribute to tumor growth. Different dietary fats may have different effects on the potential relationship to cancer. In general, tumor-promoting dietary fats include medium-chain saturated fatty acids such as lauric and myristic acids and long-chain fatty acids, including palmitic and stearic acids. In contrast, unsaturated fatty acids may have anti-inflammatory properties and function as tumor suppressors. In addition, high carbohydrate diets may lead to hyperglycemia and insulin resistance, particularly in obese or diabetic individuals and may contribute to cancer progression and its adverse effects.

Strategies to disrupt the obesity cancer linkage: The most effective way to prevent increased cancer risk associated with obesity is to maintain a lean body mass throughout life utilizing lifestyle practices such as dietary regulation and regular physical activity. In individuals who are overweight or obese, these same lifestyle factors should be utilized to lose weight and restore normal body mass. There are still conflicting data about the long-term outcomes from intentional weight loss in overweight or obese individuals with cancer. However, beneficial consequences of intentional weight loss with regard to cancer have been successfully demonstrated in bariatric surgery. A large study from Swedish Obesity Subjects (SOS) investigators compared the outcomes of 210 bariatric surgery-treated patients to 236 controls. Bariatric surgery was associated with a 40% reduction in risk of cancer at 29 years of follow-up. Another study from Utah, which was retrospective in nature, of 7925 patients who underwent bariatric bypass surgery, a 60% decrease in cancer mortality was found in comparison to 7955 controls.

Thus, dietary interventions which result in modest weight loss improve cancer biomarkers and may decrease the incidence of several cancers or improve overall extended survival. In contrast, bariatric surgery has produced greater and more sustained weight loss and a greater reduction in cancer risk.

Recommendations for lifestyle modifications for primary cancer prevention: A number of guidelines for physical activity and diet in cancer prevention are available, including those from the American Cancer Society, the American Institute for Cancer Research, the National Heart, Lung and Blood Institute, the U.S. Department of Health and Human Services, and the President's Council on Physical Fitness and Sports. These guidelines are consistent in recommending the following guidelines for disrupting the obesity/cancer link:

- Achieve and maintain a lean weight across the lifespan.
- Avoid high-calorie foods and sugary drinks.
- Prioritize healthy-eating patterns rich in whole foods and plant-based elements.
- Increase physical activity.
- Maintain good sleep hygiene.
- Lose weight if you are overweight or obese.
- Follow cancer screening guidelines.

7.4 TYPE 2 DIABETES MELLITUS (T2DM) AND CANCER RISK

T2DM and obesity are closely linked to each other (12). T2DM is defined by resistance to insulin, which leads to sustained hyperinsulinemia and hyperglycemia. T2DM has been associated with an increased risk of a number of malignancies, including pancreatic, colon, endometrial, breast, and hepatobiliary cancers. One hypothesis for the increased cancer risk in T2DM is the cancer-promoting effects of insulin and IGF-1. Levels of these two hormones are typically increased in obese individuals. There is some controversy regarding the association between insulin use in patients with T2DM and possible increased risk of cancer and decreased survival. For this reason, individuals with both cancer and T2DM should be sure that their T2DM is managed by a physician knowledgeable about these potential interactions.

7.5 PHYSICAL ACTIVITY IN THE PREVENTION AND TREATMENT OF CANCER

Physical activity plays a key role in the risk of cancer (13). Although specific biological mechanisms linking physical activity to cancer reduction remain unknown, there is a large body of evidence supporting the role of physical activity in various cancer diagnoses. According to the World Cancer Research Fund, 20% of cancers in the United States could be prevented through physical activity, weight control, and consumption of a healthy diet (14). A pooled analysis of 12 prospective cohort studies involving 1.4 million participants in the United States and Europe demonstrated an association between higher levels of leisure time physical activity and risk reduction for 13 different cancer types (15).

Among those cancers linked to activity, colon, breast, and endometrial cancers are the most studied. Links between physical activity and breast cancer may be through reducing levels of sex hormones and increasing concentrations of sex hormone binding globulin proteins.

The relationship between exercise and decreased endometrial cancer risk may be through similar mechanisms. The relationship between physical activity and decreased colon cancer risk may be due to immune function modulation, reduction in intestinal transit time, reduction in hyperinsulinemia, and inflammation. Despite these postulated underlying factors, biological links between physical activity and reduced colon cancer are not completely understood.

Multiple physical activity guidelines have been issued which have summarized the risk of cancer and also may be utilized as a treatment tool for cancer survivors. Guidelines for physical activity and cancer have been issued by both the American Cancer Society and the AICR.

The role of physical activity in primary cancer prevention: The most studied cancers are colon, breast, and endometrial cancer. In breast cancer, exercise lowers the risk in both premenopausal and postmenopausal women. As already indicated, the relationship between exercise and endometrial cancer seems to be through similar mechanisms. Even the low intensity physical activity of walking may decrease one's predisposition to endometrial cancer. With regard to colon cancer, a recent study showed a 20% reduced risk of colon cancer comparing active people to inactive people.

The role of physical activity in secondary cancer prevention: In addition to its role in primary cancer prevention, physical activity may also have a role in secondary cancer prevention. Physical activity also lowers side effects from cancer treatment such as fatigue, anxiety, depression, and reduced sexual activity. In addition, patients who have physical activity as part of their secondary cancer prevention program can also improve health status and long-term health outcomes. In one study of breast cancer patients, after diagnosis physical activity decreased mortality by 39% and overall mortality declined by 46%, when comparing most to least physically active women after diagnosis.

Unfortunately, after the diagnosis of cancer, not enough cancer patients are consistently physically active. Once study suggested that breast carcinoma patients decreased physical activity by two hours per week between pre- and post-diagnosis.

As already indicated, inactivity can have deleterious disease-specific and nonspecific effects on cancer and non-cancer patients. Therefore, clinicians should include physical activity as an important secondary treatment tool, while being conscious of patients' physical and psychological well-being and capacity to exercise post-diagnosis.

Physical activity and tertiary cancer prevention: Physical activity can also play a valuable role in rehabilitation and chronic disease management in cancer patients. One meta-analysis of 26 prospective cohort studies of colorectal and prostate cancer showed a 37% pooled risk reduction in cancer-specific mortality when comparing the most active to least active individuals (16). Of course, other modifiable risk factors such as smoking, diet, and alcohol intake can also play a role; however, physical activity has been shown to have the strongest effect of attenuating the risk of breast cancer reoccurrence and reducing mortality (17).

Long-term cancer survivors should also incorporate regular physical activity and exercise into their daily routine. Up to 52% of adult survivors of childhood cancer are sedentary (18). This suggests that clinicians are not placing sufficient emphasis on physical activity in previously diagnosed cancer populations who are currently cancer-free.

Perhaps the biggest factor distinguishing physical activity from other cancer therapies is the lack of treatment-specific adverse side effects. No studies have shown that physical activity adversely affects cancer outcomes. Since protracted cancer treatment may hamper physical function, it is important that clinicians take into account such limitations when prescribing physical activity to cancer survivors in order to personalize prescriptions.

7.6 DEFINING HEALTH-ENHANCING PHYSICAL ACTIVITY

Over the past two decades, the role of physical activity in health has evolved. Most recently, the PAGA 2018 emphasized that even small amounts of physical activity lower the risk of many chronic diseases, including CVD, T2DM, metabolic syndrome,

TABLE 7.1
Clinical Recommendations for Physical Activity

Organization	Target Population	Stage in Cancer Care Continuum	Recommendation
American Cancer Society	Adults	Prevention	150 min moderate intensity, 75 min vigorous intensity, or equivalent combination of the two each week [44]
American Cancer Society	Children	Prevention	60 min moderate or vigorous intensity each day; at least three days with vigorous intensity activity [44]
American Cancer Society	Non-specific	Survivorship	150 min exercise with strength training activities at least twice per week [49]
American College of Sports Medicine	Adults	Prevention	30 min moderate to vigorous activity five times per week; at least two days of strength training each week [42]
American Institute for Cancer Research	Non-specific	Prevention	30 min moderate activity every day; limit sedentary habits [43]
American Institute for Cancer Research	Non-specific	Survivorship	30 min moderate intensity activity each day; at least two days of strength training each week [50]
Oncology Nursing Society	Non-specific	Survivorship	150 min moderate intensity or 75 min vigorous intensity aerobic activity [51]
National Comprehensive Cancer Network	Non-specific	Treatment	30 min aerobic activity at least five times per week [52]

Source: Rippe JM. *Lifestyle Medicine*, 3rd edition. CRC Press, Boca Raton, 2019. Used with permission.

cancer, osteoarthritis, and many others. A large amount of evidence affirms the value of physical activity in cancer risk reduction and symptom management.

Clinicians should consider exercise as an integral strategy across the cancer prevention and treatment spectrum. Multiple, different organizations have issued guidelines for prevention of cancer as well as for a component of treatment for cancer survivors. A list of these recommendations is found in Table 7.1.

These recommendations are generally consistent with each other and also consistent with the recently released PAGA 2018 document.

More information on the multiple roles of physical activity in promoting good health is found in Chapter 3. Unfortunately, neither most healthy individuals nor cancer survivors heed recommendations for regular physical activity levels. The National Health Interview Survey suggested that only 20.9% of Americans under the age of 18 years meet the PAGA 2018 recommendations for 150 minutes of moderate to vigorous intensity physical activity and two strength training sessions per week.

This raises great concern about the cancer inactivity nexus. Physical activity should be a central tenet of any cancer prevention or treatment strategy.

7.7 PHYSICAL ACTIVITY AND BEHAVIOR CHANGE

Making changes either in nutrition or in physical activity requires, for many individuals, new behaviors. Behavior change is not easy, but it is possible. A number of studies have shown that various frameworks help people make changes in their behavior. This is such an important area that we have devoted a whole chapter to it (see Chapter 4).

Cancer can compromise quality of life and restrict physical capabilities. Treatment, such as chemotherapy, can compound the problem. Physical activity among cancer patients can be undercut by fatigue and side effects from various therapies, including chemotherapy and radiation. Some factors, however, do predict positive exercise adherence to regular physical activity. Among them are baseline physical activity, pretreatment fatigue, emotional disturbance, or trauma from treatment and medical status which have been shown to influence a patient's adherence to various behavior change regimens, including physical activity.

Physiological barriers such as pain and tiredness symptoms from treatment represent further obstacles which may undercut the ability of patients with cancer to exercise.

A further restriction is time. In fact, a study of adult cancer patients between the ages of 42 and 88 showed that time constraints were a primary barrier to exercise and poor health was the only negative more significant than time. In addition, many people feel that exercising around other severely ill patients makes them feel sicker, while others believe that maximizing sleep is the best way to counteract the side effects of chemotherapy.

With all of these potential restrictions, it is important that clinicians use various strategies to overcome these challenges and are aware of ways to counsel cancer patients about strategies for continuing to exercise at pretreatment levels.

7.8 STRATEGIES FOR PHYSICAL ACTIVITY INTERVENTIONS

Given how important physical activity is for improving outcomes at all levels of cancer treatment, clinicians need to adopt effective strategies for helping patients with exercise adherence. A number of studies have shown that self-efficacy is a key determinate of adhering to exercise regimens. It is important for clinicians to counsel patients and emphasize the vital benefits of physical activity. Referral to certified personal trainers with experience in cancer patients is also highly effective. It has been demonstrated that cancer survivors and those in treatment are highly responsive to counseling from health care providers. In one study of cancer survivors 40–44 year old, 78% were interested in participating in physical activity and 50% wanted to receive counseling from fitness experts at their cancer center (19). In addition, increasing rates of internet accessibility and smartphone ownership have made these modalities a powerful disease management and prevention technique.

One study showed that 80% of older cancer patients were willing to participate in online physical activity.

7.9 LIMITATIONS OF PHYSICAL ACTIVITY IN CANCER RESEARCH

Research investigating the correlations between physical activity and cancer risk and survivorship is still hampered by uncertainty concerning the underlying biological mechanisms involved in why physical activity improves various stages of cancer treatment as well as cancer prevention. Some basic issues may also confound research such as body mass index, dietary intake, and other intervening variables which may impact on the efficacy of physical activity.

7.10 NUTRITION THERAPY FOR THE CANCER PATIENT

Nutrition therapy is a key component of lifestyle strategies in managing cancer patient treatment and quality of life. The metabolic response to cancer and its treatment is varied and certain tumors cause more nutritional alterations than others. In particular, solid tumors such as lung, pancreas, head and neck, and gastrointestinal (G.I.) cancers are often associated with poor nutritional status and weight loss. G.I. and pancreatic cancers have the highest prevalence of weight loss at approximately 83% and 87%, respectively. In addition, cancer treatment often leads to symptoms that hinder dietary intake and digestion and may result in numerous side effects such as anorexia, nausea, vomiting, diarrhea, constipation, stomatitis, mucositis, dyspepsia, and alterations in taste and smell. In addition, many patients also experience emotional distress from the cancer diagnosis and treatment. Various counseling techniques as well as complementary medicine strategies may help manage behavior-related factors such as depression, fatigue, pain, and stress.

Malnutrition and cardiac cachexia: Up to 80% of cancer patients receiving multimodal cancer therapy experience unintentional weight loss. Individuals who experience weight loss receive lower doses of treatment and more severe dose-limiting toxicities and also poorer overall outcomes and survival. Both malnutrition and cachexia are very common in cancer patients. Depending on the type of cancer, a large percentage of patients, perhaps 50–80%, of advanced cancer experience cachexia as their disease progresses. This cachexia is responsible for an estimated 24% of total deaths in cancer patients.

An International Consensus Conference defined cachexia as a multifactorial syndrome of ongoing loss of skeletal muscle mass with or without loss of fat mass that cannot be fully reversed by conventional nutritional support and leads to progressive functional impairment. The diagnostic criteria for cachexia is weight loss of >5% or weight loss from baseline weight of >2% in individuals showing depletion of body weight of <20 kg/m^2. Cachexia is marked by loss of appetite, impaired glucose tolerance, and involuntary weight loss. Cachexia may ultimately be manifested by loss of subcutaneous fat, muscle mass, and an inability to maintain weight. Significant muscle loss has also been called sarcopenia and may be difficult to determine in previously overweight or obese individuals.

Metabolic alterations in cancer: Weight loss, anorexia, and metabolic dysfunction are common in cancer patients. These may result in higher resting energy expenditure and may play a role in the progression in cancer cachexia. Although the underlying mechanism of cachexia is not well understood, systemic inflammation is thought to occur. The Academy of Nutrition and Dietetics recommends assessing markers of inflammation such as elevated CRP and other signs of wasting to help determine the acuteness of weight loss in cancer patients. Metabolic abnormalities in cancer may include altered carbohydrate metabolism and altered fat metabolism.

7.11 NUTRITION SCREENING

Nutrition status impacts on cancer treatment plans and poor nutrition status is associated with decreased tolerance for chemotherapy and radiation. There are several screening tools which have been validated for use in oncology patients, including the Patient Generated Subjective Global Assessment (PG-SGA), the Malnutrition Screening Tool (MST), the Malnutrition Screening Tool for Cancer Patients (MSTCP), and the Malnutrition Universal Screening Tool (MUST). These tools are simple to use and can be utilized by the patient or the health care professional. These tools determine whether the patient is at risk for malnutrition and requires further nutritional evaluation.

The nutrition care process utilizes a systemic approach to nutrition and consists of nutrition status, diagnosis, and intervention to detect the root cause of the nutritional problem, monitoring, and evaluation. Medical Nutrition Therapy (MNT) is a specific application of the nutritional care process in clinical settings and involves in-depth, individualized nutrition assessments to manage the disease. A detailed description of MNT is beyond the scope of this chapter, but information is available in multiple publications from the American Cancer Society to provide specific information about MNT. These issues are discussed in considerable detail also in the chapter on nutrition therapy for the cancer patient in the 3rd edition of *Lifestyle Medicine* textbook which I have edited.

7.12 CANCER TREATMENT AND SIDE EFFECT MANAGEMENT

Multiple anticancer therapies, including chemotherapy, hormone therapy, radiation therapy, biotherapy, and surgery, can significantly impact on nutritional status. Depending on the anticancer treatment, early satiety, and decreased desire to eat, changing to smaller amounts of food and other nutritional symptoms may impact cancer patients and managing these symptoms may prevent a decline in nutritional status.

Nutritional components of the cancer treatment experience can be influenced by being prepared as much as possible with meal planning and eating healthful and appealing foods which can diminish side effects. The approach to this is found in Table 7.2.

TABLE 7.2

Lifestyle Strategies when Eating during Treatment

	SUGGESTIONS
General approaches	• Plan meals ahead, i.e., month, week, and day
	• Plan to eat five to six small meals/day that have protein and are nutrient-dense with vitamins, minerals, and phytonutrients
	• Engage in light physical activity to stimulate appetite, if possible
	• Maximize quality and quantity of food intake when most hungry
Specific approaches	Two days before chemotherapy:
	• Eat as well as possible to give your body "the extra boost and hopefully minimize side effects." Also, avoid favorite foods to minimize developing a food aversion associated with nausea/vomiting during chemotherapy. Lastly, avoid greasy, fried, or high-fat foods
	During the week of treatment (chemotherapy or radiation):
	• Try eating something every hour or so, *even* if not hungry. *Nausea* is worse if the stomach is *empty*
	• Bare minimum menu if no appetite: try to consume homemade broths, two servings of smoothies with protein powder, two cups of healing tea, e.g., ginger tea
	• If any sort of appetite, try easy-to-digest nourishing soups that are full of vitamins, minerals, and phytonutrients. Be sure to add veggies when possible and protein-building foods
	• If hungry, eat well! Add in protein-building foods, such as chicken and rice, eggs as in egg salad to poached eggs. Continue with tonics and elixirs, i.e., ginger lemonade and mango coconut smoothies. Anytime foods may include oatmeal, hummus, and quinoa pilaf
	A week after chemotherapy:
	• When taste buds are back, add favorite foods that jump-start the appetite
	Between treatments:
	• When appetite is normal, focus on plant-based foods that offer phytonutrients, i.e., cancer-fighting nutrients

Source: Rippe JM. *Lifestyle Medicine*, 3rd edition. CRC Press, Boca Raton, 2019. Used with permission.

Katz R, Edelson M. *The Cancer Fighting Kitchen.* 2009, Crown Publishing Group, New York, 217.

7.13 COMPLEMENTARY AND RESTORATIVE TREATMENT OF CANCER

Complementary therapy is typically not included in normal allopathic medicine. However, the National Institute of Health Center for Complementary and Integrative Health can provide useful information on this approach to therapy which may include dietary supplements and Mind/Body Interventions (MBI). Many patients undergoing therapy for cancer will find these therapies useful. The reader is referred to the National Institute of Health Center for Complementary and Integrative Health Modalities for further information.

7.14   GUIDELINES FOR SECONDARY PREVENTION IN CANCER SURVIVORS

Cancer survivorship is defined by life after diagnosis of cancer. Goals for treatment should focus on both treatment for curative measures and lengthening survival as well as decreasing and treating complications to therapy and preventing or detecting new cancer survivors. The number of cancer survivors has increased substantially in the past few decades. There are currently more than 15.5 million cancer survivors in the United States. Some guidelines from various cancer research organizations have been developed. These are somewhat similar to primary prevention. Here is a listing of recommendations:

- Avoid weight gain after the cancer diagnosis.
- Continue to use exercise as a tool to decrease weight gain and obesity.
- Use exercise to increase survival odds.
- Make dietary changes to achieve weight loss, if overweight or obese.
- Invest in sleep hygiene.

7.15   CONCLUSIONS

Some therapies are very important in both the prevention and treatment of cancer. These include avoiding obesity, paying close attention to a variety of issues in the diet and overall nutrition, and engaging in regular physical activity. The recommendations from the recently released PAGA 2018 include participation in 150 minutes of moderate intensity physical activity on a weekly basis and two strength training sessions per week. These are highly appropriate as modalities for primary prevention of cancer and also goals to try to accomplish during secondary and tertiary prevention. Once cancer has been diagnosed, the clinician may need to make some modifications in order to properly use nutrition, weight management, and physical activity as components of therapy for cancer.

7.16   CLINICAL APPLICATIONS

- Clinicians should discuss and counsel patients on roles and importance of physical activity both as primary prevention and secondary and tertiary prevention.
- Clinicians should emphasize to patients the importance of weight management for reduction of risk of cancer and weight loss for individuals who are overweight or obese.
- Healthful nutrition with increased fruit and vegetables and whole grains as well as reduced consumption of red meat and processed meats and alcohol should be recommended.
- All of these issues should be discussed with individuals for both primary prevention and treatment of cancer in individuals who already have been diagnosed with cancer.

REFERENCES

1. Clark AM, Raine K, Raphael D. The American Cancer Society, American Diabetes Association, and American Heart Association. Joint Statement on Preventing Cancer, Cardiovascular Disease, and Diabetes: Where Are the Social Determinants? *Diabetes Care.* 2004;27:3024.
2. World Health Organization. The Top 10 Causes of Death, 2020. http://www.who.int/mediacentre/factsheets/fs310/en/. Accessed July 1, 2020.
3. United States Census Bureau. QuickFacts: United States, 2016. https://www.census.gov/quickfacts/fact/table/US/PST045219. Accessed July 1, 2020.
4. Global Burden of Disease Cancer Collaboration. Global, Regional, and National Cancer Incidence, Mortality, Years of Life Lost, Years Lived with Disability, and Disability-Adjusted Life-Years for 29 Cancer Groups, 1990 to 2017: A Systematic Analysis for the Global Burden of Disease Study. *JAMA Oncology.* 2019;5(12):1749–1768. doi:10.1001/jamaoncol.2019.2996
5. Lauby-Secretan B, Scoccianti C, Loomis D. et al. Body Fatness and Cancer — Viewpoint of the IARC Working Group. *New England Journal of Medicine.* 2016;375(8):794–798.
6. Davis C, Ross S. Diet and Cancer Prevention. In Rippe J, ed., *Lifestyle Medicine* (3rd edition). CRC Press (Boca Raton), 2019.
7. Al-Amri A. Prevention of Breast Cancer. *Journal of Family and Community Medicine.* 2005;12(2):71–74.
8. World Cancer Research Fund International. Cancer Preventability Estimates for Diet, Nutrition, Body Fatness, and Physical Activity. https://www.wcrf.org/dietandcancer/recommendations. Accessed July 1, 2018.
9. Rock C, Doyle C. Demark-Wanefried W, et al. Nutrition and Physical Activity Guidelines for Cancer Survivors. *Cancer Journal for Clinicians.* 2012;62(4):243–274.
10. Bruno D, Berger N. *Lifestyle Approaches Targeting Obesity to Reduce Cancer Risk, Progression & Recurrence in Rippe J: Lifestyle Medicine* (3rd edition). CRC Press (Boca Raton), 2019.
11. Berger N. Obesity and Cancer Pathogenesis. *Annals of the New York Academy of Sciences* 2014;1311:57–76.
12. Tsilidis KK, Kasimis JC, Lopez DS, et al. Type 2 Diabetes and Cancer: Umbrella Review of Meta-Analyses of Observational Studies. *BMJ.* 2015;350:g7607.
13. Keltner C, Bowles H. Physical Activity and the Prevention and Treatment of Cancer. in Rippe J, ed., *Lifestyle Medicine* (3rd edition). CRC Press (Boca Raton), 2019.
14. World Cancer Research Fund International. Cancer Preventability Estimates for Diet, Nutrition, Body Fatness, and Physical Activity. http://wcrf.org/int/cancer-facts-figures/preventability-estimates/cancer-preventability-estimates-diet-nutrition. Accessed July 1, 2020.
15. Moore SC, Lee IM, Weiderpass E, et al. Association of Leisure-Time Physical Activity with Risk of 26 Types of Cancer in 1.44 Million Adults. *JAMA Internal Medicine.* 2016;176(6):816–825.
16. Brown J, Winters-Stone K, Lee A. Cancer, Physical Activity, and Exercise. *Comprehensive Physiology.* 2012;2(4):2775–2809.
17. Friedenreich CM, Neilson HK, Farris MS, Courneya KS. Physical Activity and Cancer Outcomes: A Precision Medicine Approach. *Clinical Cancer Research* 2016;22(19):4766–4775.
18. Demark-Wahnefried W, Werner C, Clipp EC, et al. Survivors of Childhood Cancer and Their Guardians. *Cancer.* 2005;103(10):2171–2180.
19. Belanger LJ, Plotnikoff RC, Clark A, Courneya KS. A Survey of Physical Activity Programming and Counseling Preferences in Young-Adult Cancer Survivors. *Cancer Nursing.* 2012;35(1):48–54.

8 Obesity and Weight Management

KEY POINTS

- Overweight and obesity are very prevalent in the United States and around the world.
- Worldwide it is estimated that over 2.1 billion people are obese.
- In the United States it is estimated that over 70% of the adult population is either overweight or obese.
- Obesity is associated with multiple chronic diseases such as cardiovascular disease (CVD), type 2 diabetes (T2DM), many different cancers, osteoarthritis, and multiple other medical conditions.
- A weight gain of as little as 10–12 pounds increases the risk of multiple chronic diseases.
- Both regular physical activity and attention to proper nutrition are key lifestyle modalities for treating obesity and preventing weight gain.
- Obesity results from an increase in adipose tissue. There are multiple techniques available to determine obesity and more advanced techniques to measure adiposity.

8.1 INTRODUCTION

Obesity is a pandemic representing one of the most significant public health challenges to world health in recent history. It is currently estimated that 2.1 billion people in the world are obese. In many ways, obesity represents the quintessential lifestyle disease (1).

Obesity is the result of energy imbalance since energy expenditure and energy intake are key factors in the energy balance equation. Thus, both nutrition and physical activity are components of lifestyle interventions, which are critically important to both short-term weight loss and also long-term maintenance of a healthy body weight.

Obesity significantly contributes to morbidity and mortality around the world. In 2013, obesity was recognized by the American Medical Association as a disease. Research supports that obesity increases the risk for many chronic diseases, including CVD, T2DM, cancer, chronic kidney disease, the metabolic syndrome, and many musculo/skeletal conditions (2). It has been estimated that in 2000, there were over 100,000 deaths in the United States caused by obesity in individuals less than 70 years of age and 2.8 million deaths worldwide attributed to the disease (3,4).

Obesity is one of the leading, preventable causes of death and disease around the world. Unfortunately, rates of obesity continue to increase.

While it may seem simple that either decreased caloric intake or increased physical activity may contribute to weight loss, in fact, the process is complicated. The Consensus Statement on Metabolism from the American Society of Nutrition emphasizes that metabolism consists of multiple factors, including percent body fat and other issues related to a host of environmental factors (5).

At any given time, over 50% of obese Americans are actively trying to lose weight. Sustained weight loss of as little as 5–10% is considered clinically significant since it reduces risk factors for a variety of chronic diseases. Both the Diabetes Prevention Program (DPP) (6) and the Look AHEAD Trial (7) showed that weight loss of 7% in obese individuals resulted in significant improvement in risk factors for CVD and T2DM.

8.2 OBESITY AND ADIPOSITY

Obesity is a condition which is characterized by the accumulation of excess adipose tissue. Standards to define and classify obesity typically require an assessment of total body adiposity for highest accuracy. Unfortunately, the quantitative determination of body fat is difficult and costly to obtain. Techniques such as dual-energy X-ray absorptiometry (DEXA) has typically been the one that we use at our laboratory at Rippe Lifestyle Institute (RLI), although we have also used body mass index (BMI) on larger trials to estimate level of obesity. There are multiple ways of measuring the amount of fat in the body, which will be handled in the next section.

8.3 MEASUREMENT OF ADIPOSITY

A number of different methodologies are available for adiposity measure which either directly or indirectly measure body fat. Included in these are the following:

- *Hydrodensitometry:* This is typically done by a technique called under water weighing. While it is highly accurate, it is time- and labor-consuming and requires specialized training and individual discomfort since individuals must be fully immersed in water and hold their breath.
- *Air displacement plethysmography:* This technique was developed as an alternative to hydrodensitometry. This technique is similar, but determines body volume by measuring changes in chamber volume by placing an individual in a closed, air-filled chamber. The most commonly used air displacement plethysmograph apparatus is called a BOD POD. We have used this extensively over the years at RLI.
- *DEXA:* Another technique, as already indicated, is DEXA and requires individuals to remove metal accessories and lay in a supine position on a bed, while low-intensity X-ray passes through the bed. DEXA is quick and easy to perform and highly accurate. This is one of the reasons why we

have used it extensively. It does, however, require the purchase of relatively expensive DEXA equipment.

- *Other measurements:* These techniques are classified as "anthropometric" measurements. These techniques involve using computations based on making a few simple measurements. Included in these are BMI, where weight and height are measured and then equations used to determine BMI, which is the ratio of weight kilograms divided by the height in meters.[2] Many large-scale studies utilize this anthropometric measurement because of its simplicity. We have used BMI in thousands of patients over the years in our research laboratory.

While BMI is a reasonable way of classifying various levels of obesity, it does not separate lean tissue from fat. Most of the large-scale epidemiological studies utilize BMI to classify people either as normal weight or at various levels of obesity. How to classify a patient of overweight and obesity recommended by the NHLBI Guidelines is found in Table 8.1.

Other simple measurements include waist circumference and waist-to-hip ratio. Waist circumference criteria, according to NHLBI, are also found in Table 8.1.

Another anthropometric measurement is skinfolds thickness which uses a measurement of skinfold thickness to the nearest 0.1 mm on the right side of the body at the biceps, triceps, subscapular, and suprailiac regions. While it is simple and easy to

TABLE 8.1
Classification of Overweight and Obesity as Recommended by the NHLBI Guidelines

			Disease Risk* Relative to Normal Weight and Waist Circumference	
			Men <102 cm (<40 in)	>102 cm (>40 in)
	BMI(kg/m²)	Obesity Class	Women <88 cm (<35 in)	>88 cm (>35 in)
Underweight	<18.5		—	—
Normal†	18.5–24.9		—	—
Overweight	25.0–29.9		Increased	High
Obesity	30.0–34.9	I	High	Very High
	35.0–39.9	II	Very High	Very High
Extreme Obesity	≥40	III	Extremely High	Extremely High

Source: U.S. Department of Health and Human Services Public Health Service National Institutes of Health National Heart, Lung, and Blood Institute https://www.nhlbi.nih.gov/files/docs/guidelines/prctgd_c.pdf (accessed July 10, 2020).

* Disease risk for type 2 diabetes, hypertension, and CVD.

† Increased waist circumference can also be a marker for increased risk even in persons of normal weight.

perform, it does require a certain level of skills. We have used this extensively in our research laboratory, but typically only use it for large population-based studies. We insist that staff members must perform 1000 skinfold measurements under supervision before they are allowed to perform this on their own.

For more accurate scientific measurements of adiposity, we use DEXA scanning. Other techniques available include computerized tomography (CT), ultrasound, and magnetic resonance imaging (MRI), which we have also used in some studies. These are also quite accurate, but require expensive equipment and specialized facilities.

8.4 PREVALENCE OF OBESITY

Utilizing BMI as a proxy measure for obesity allows for standardized tracking and comparison of obesity among populations. The prevalence of obesity has been increasing for almost a hundred years in the United States. Since the 1960s, the National Health and Nutrition Examination Survey (NHANES) has been tracking obesity in the United States. The prevalence of obesity remained fairly constant between 1960 and 1980. However, utilizing NHANES data from 1988 to 1994, the prevalence of adult obesity increased by seven percentage points compared with 1980 (8).

Recent data suggest that from the interval of 2003–2010, obesity continued to increase. The current level of obesity in the United States is 37.7%, while 68.8% adults are considered overweight or obese (9). More men than women are considered overweight or obese with 72.9% versus 63.7%, respectively, in 2009–2010.

Obesity prevalence increased significantly from 1999 to 2014 in all age groups for both men and women. From a worldwide perspective, the prevalence of obesity among adults increased by 27.5% from 1980 to 2013. In 2013, it is estimated that 36.9% of men and 38% of women worldwide were obese. These figures differ substantially from country to country.

8.5 POTENTIAL CAUSES OF OBESITY

Multiple factors may contribute to causing obesity. The common underlying etiology is energy imbalance. As already indicated, this can be influenced by many factors. Two big contributors, however, are overconsumption of calories and inactivity. Other factors, including energy imbalance, will also be discussed in this section.

- *Energy imbalance:* At its most fundamental level, weight changes are associated with an imbalance between energy intake and energy expenditure. If energy intake exceeds energy expenditure, then the excess energy is stored as fat which leads to increased adiposity. Unfortunately, gaining weight is easier than losing it (10). Simply cutting down on calories will tip the energy balance equation in favor of weight loss, but may not result in steady weight loss because the body will adapt with physiological changes to decrease resting metabolism as well as energy consumed by physical activity (11).

Unfortunately, increased energy intake is hard to avoid. For example, the average size of portions in many common foods such as muffins, donuts, fruit drinks, French fries, hamburgers, and many other common foods have increased dramatically—in fact, in many instances almost doubling over the past 30 years (12). Energy density has also increased with inexpensive, convenient, and energy dense foods readily accessible throughout most of the day for most people.

Energy expenditure occurs from metabolism, thermoregulation, and daily physical activity. Metabolism and thermoregulation account for 60–70% of energy expenditure from daily physical activity, among predominantly sedentary individuals about 20–30% of total energy expenditure. Unfortunately, as will be discussed in detail in other chapters in this book, 75% of the adult population in the United States does not get enough physical activity to meet CDC guidelines. A further complicating matter is that technological conveniences have contributed to many labor-saving devices and further exacerbated the problem of inactivity. Most research in the area of obesity suggests that energy restriction and increased physical activity are required in combination with each other in order to lose weight and keep it off.

- *Genetics and epigenetics:* Although obesity is typically considered a consequence of prolonged energy imbalance, there is also increasing evidence that suggests inherited factors can also contribute in significant ways. It is now estimated that 30–50% of the variation in obesity can be explained by inherited genetic variations (12,13). In addition to genetic differences, epigenetic mechanisms may also contribute to molecular processes that result in differences in energy homeostasis (14). One particular area of recent interest has been in the area called DNA methylation that may result in inflammation, which may further result in changes in insulin signaling and lipid metabolism.
- *Infections:* Recent research has suggested that there may be a role for infections in the development of obesity. Ten different microorganisms have been linked in various research studies to obesity (15). This is an emerging field and much further work needs to be accomplished to provide compelling links between various viral infections and the likelihood of obesity.
- *Smoking:* Research has consistently shown that smokers weigh less than non-smokers. Furthermore, individuals who quit smoking have been shown to gain an average of 4.1 kg over five years compared to those who continue to smoke (16). Current smoking prevalence in the United States has declined from 20.9% in 2005 to 15.1% in 2015, while the prevalence of obesity has increased significantly. The decreased prevalence of smoking, therefore, may be associated with some of the rise in the prevalence of overweight and obesity. Clearly, continuing to smoke as a weight control measure is a bargain with the devil! Nonetheless, individuals who quit smoking need to be particularly vigilant to avoid weight gain.

- *Sleep:* A number of studies support an inverse relationship between the amount of sleep and obesity. This may be based on various endocrine factors, including decreased glucose tolerance and increased ghrelin levels, both of which have a role in obesity development by stimulating food intake and energy storage (17). As many as 30% of adults and 69% of teens do not get the recommended amount of sleep. This will be discussed in much more detail in Chapter 11.
- *Gut microbiota:* Bacteria in the gut play multiple roles in health and may also play a significant role in energy metabolism. Some of these bacteria such as Bacteroidetes may cause increased absorption of calories and contribute to obesity.
- *Other factors:* A variety of other factors are currently being researched with relationship to obesity risks, including pharmaceutical agents, temperature control, and endocrine disrupters. These are all under investigation without clear evidence at the current time.

8.6 IDENTIFICATION OF OBESITY

The implications of obesity on health have become clear definitions and the methods of measurements have also become more important in defining risk (18). It is important to have a clear framework and approach to identifying obesity. This information comes from a variety of sources.

First, there is information from the clinical interview. This includes how long the individual has been obese, whether there are other family members who are obese, history of medication use, and, perhaps most importantly, whether or not the individual is ready to put in the effort needed to lose weight and help the health care professional decide whether this is the right time to proceed with treatment.

The next step is the physical examination. This involves three important steps.

- Step #1: Weigh the individual.
- Step #2: Measure the individual's height.
- Step #3: Compute BMI.
- Step #4: Measure waist circumference.

The cut points for the establishment of obesity as defined by the National Heart, Lung, and Blood Institute Guidelines are found in Table 8.1.

The next step is to obtain laboratory values. Particularly important are plasma glucose, plasma lipids, thyroid-stimulating hormone (TSH), and possibly prostate-specific antigens (PSA). This latter measurement should be taken in males because of concerns related to cancer of the prostate, which is associated with obesity.

Once the basic tests have been done, other more advanced and specific tests for ascertaining the level of adiposity may also be ordered. These have been enumerated previously in the chapter. This may include DEXA scanning, MRI, or CT scanning. Each of these has specific indications, but all of them carry the disadvantage of greater expense both for equipment and conduct of the test.

Determination of the BMI may be obtained from charts, such as the one enclosed, which provides height and weight and allows the determination of BMI (Table 8.2).

TABLE 8.2
Body Mass Index Table

BMI	Normal						Overweight					Obese										Extreme Obesity														
	19	20	21	22	23	24	25	26	27	28	29	30	31	32	33	34	35	36	37	38	39	40	41	42	43	44	45	46	47	48	49	50	51	52	53	54
Height (inches)	Body Weight (pounds)																																			
58	91	96	100	105	110	115	119	124	129	134	138	143	148	153	158	162	167	172	177	181	186	191	196	201	205	210	215	220	224	229	234	239	244	248	253	258
59	94	99	104	109	114	119	124	128	133	138	143	148	153	158	163	168	173	178	183	188	193	198	203	208	212	217	222	227	232	237	242	247	252	257	262	267
60	97	102	107	112	118	123	128	133	138	143	148	153	158	163	168	174	179	184	189	194	199	204	209	215	220	225	230	235	240	245	250	255	261	266	271	276
61	100	106	111	116	122	127	132	137	143	148	153	158	164	169	174	180	185	190	195	201	206	211	217	222	227	232	238	243	248	254	259	264	269	275	280	285
62	104	109	115	120	126	131	136	142	147	153	158	164	169	175	180	186	191	196	202	207	213	218	224	229	235	240	246	251	256	262	267	273	278	284	289	295
63	107	113	118	124	130	135	141	146	152	158	163	169	175	180	186	191	197	203	208	214	220	225	231	237	242	248	254	259	265	270	278	282	287	293	299	304
64	110	116	122	128	134	140	145	151	157	163	169	174	180	186	192	197	204	209	215	221	227	232	238	244	250	256	262	267	273	279	285	291	296	302	308	314
65	114	120	126	132	138	144	150	156	162	168	174	180	186	192	198	204	210	216	222	228	234	240	246	252	258	264	270	276	282	288	294	300	306	312	318	324
66	118	124	130	136	142	148	155	161	167	173	179	186	192	198	204	210	216	223	229	235	241	247	253	260	266	272	278	284	291	297	303	309	315	322	328	334
67	121	127	134	140	146	153	159	166	172	178	185	191	198	204	211	217	223	230	236	242	249	255	261	268	274	280	287	293	299	306	312	319	325	331	338	344
68	125	131	138	144	151	158	164	171	177	184	190	197	203	210	216	223	230	236	243	249	256	262	269	276	282	289	295	302	308	315	322	328	335	341	348	354
69	128	135	142	149	155	162	169	176	182	189	196	203	209	216	223	230	236	243	250	257	263	270	277	284	291	297	304	311	318	324	331	338	345	351	358	365
70	132	139	146	153	160	167	174	181	188	195	202	209	216	222	229	236	243	250	257	264	271	278	285	292	299	306	313	320	327	334	341	348	355	362	369	376
71	136	143	150	157	165	172	179	186	193	200	208	215	222	229	236	243	250	257	265	272	279	286	293	301	308	315	322	329	338	343	351	358	365	372	379	386
72	140	147	154	162	169	177	184	191	199	206	213	221	228	235	242	250	258	265	272	279	287	294	302	309	316	324	331	338	346	353	361	368	375	383	390	397
73	144	151	159	166	174	182	189	197	204	212	219	227	235	242	250	257	265	272	280	288	295	302	310	318	325	333	340	348	355	363	371	378	386	393	401	408
74	148	155	163	171	179	186	194	202	210	218	225	233	241	249	256	264	272	280	287	295	303	311	319	326	334	342	350	358	365	373	381	389	396	404	412	420
75	152	160	168	176	184	192	200	208	216	224	232	240	248	256	264	272	279	287	295	303	311	319	327	335	343	351	359	367	375	383	391	399	407	415	423	431
76	156	164	172	180	189	197	205	213	221	230	238	246	254	263	271	279	287	295	304	312	320	328	336	344	353	361	369	377	385	394	402	410	418	426	435	443

Source: Adapted from Clinical Guidelines on the Identification, Evaluation, and Treatment of Overweight and Obesity in Adults The Evidence Report.

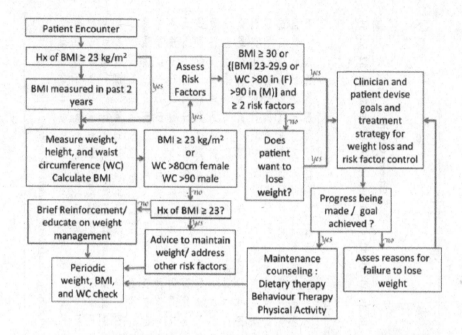

FIGURE 8.1 Treatment algorithm of overweight and obesity. The algorithm applies only to the assessment for overweight and obesity and subsequent decisions are based on that assessment. It does not reflect the initial general assessment for other cardiovascular risk factors that are indicated. *Source:* Adapted from NHLBI Obesity Education Initiative. *The Practical Guide: Identification, Evaluation, and Treatment of Overweight and Obesity in Adults.* National Institutes of Health, National Heart, Lung, and Blood Institute; October 2000. NIH Publication No. 00-4084.

8.7   GUIDELINES FOR TREATMENT

Once the workup for etiology and complicating factors of obesity is completed, the risk associated with elevated BMI, fat distribution, weight gain, and level of physical activity can be evaluated. A number of algorithms are available for this purpose, but the one most frequently used comes from the NHLBI and is found in Figure 8.1.

8.8   HEALTH CONSEQUENCES OF OBESITY

Obesity is associated with multiple morbidities and also increased overall mortality. Obesity is clearly associated with increased risk of CVD, T2DM, numerous cancers, asthma, osteoarthritis, gall bladder disease, pregnancy complications, and psychological disorders. Even small amounts of weight gain, as little as 10–12 pounds, are associated with increased risk of any of these conditions. A list of conditions where obesity is associated is found in Table 8.3 (19).

8.9   SEARCHING FOR SOLUTIONS

Given the complexity of underlying causes for the obesity epidemic, it is highly unlikely that one single solution will solve this problem. A comprehensive approach involving

TABLE 8.3
Medical Conditions Associated with Obesity

Metabolic Conditions
   Type 2 diabetes
   Metabolic syndrome
   Glucose intolerance
   Cardiovascular disease
   Coronary heart disease (CHD)
   Stroke
   Heart failure
   Deep venous thrombosis
CHD risk factors
   Dyslipidemia
   Hypertension
   Inflammation
   Hypercoagulability
Pulmonary disease
   Obstructive sleep apnea
   Hypoventilation syndrome
   Asthma
   Cancers
   Colorectal
   Esophageal
   Endometrial
   Breast (post-menopausal)
   Kidney
Gastrointestinal disease
   Non-alcoholic fatty liver disease
   Gallstones cholecystitis
   Gastroesophageal reflux
Other conditions
   Gout
   Kidney stones
   Osteoarthritis
   Psychological disorders
   Fertility and pregnancy complications
   Erectile dysfunction

Source: Bray G. Identification, Evaluation and Treatment of Overweight and Obesity, in: Rippe JM. *Obesity: Prevention and Treatment*. CRC Press, Boca Raton, 2012. Used with permission.

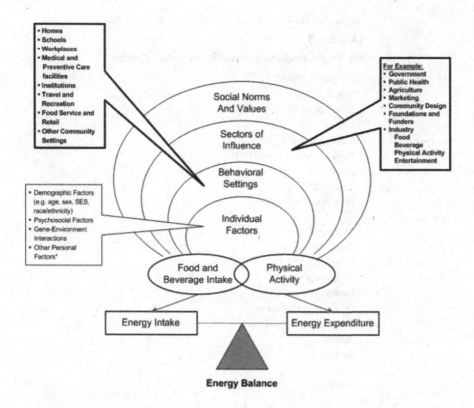

FIGURE 8.2 Community framework for addressing overweight and obesity. https://www
.michigan.gov/documents/mdch/Attachment_2__Nutrition_Physical_Activity_and_Obesity_P
revention_Program_Technical_Assistance_Manual_from_the_CDC__2008_261454_7.pdf

multiple levels of influencers and multiple areas of intervention appears most appropriate. One framework for approaching obesity and weight management has been proposed
by the Dietary Guidelines Advisory Committee (DGAC) (20). Figure 8.2 depicts the
socioeconomic framework offered by the DGAC for Guidelines for Americans 2010.

This framework stresses that issues related to maintaining proper energy balance
are complex and that factors influencing this issue are multiple and interconnected.
Many other frameworks have also been offered, but this one seems particularly
appropriate for providing a structure for thinking about potential, comprehensive
interventions for weight loss and weight management

8.10   ECONOMIC COSTS OF OBESITY IN THE UNITED STATES

Multiple factors impact on the economic costs associated with obesity in the United
States. These costs have continued to increase over the last several decades in both
the United States and worldwide. As already indicated, the global presence of obesity in 2014 was 2.1 billion people or approximately 30% of the global population.
The global economic impact of obesity alone was estimated to be $2 trillion or 2.8%

of the global domestic product (21). The economic costs associated with obesity involved both direct costs and indirect costs:

- *Direct costs:* Typically, direct costs for obesity involve the expenses related to the treatment services provided by a health care provider (e.g., physician or nurse practitioner) for office-based, outpatient, inpatient, or emergency room care, pharmaceuticals, and procedures (22). Since obesity as a condition is often not treated directly, direct costs are usually estimated based on treating comorbid conditions such as CVD, hypertension, T2DM, osteoarthritis, sleep apnea, etc., related to obesity. In the area of obesity, it has been estimated that the economic burden of treating obesity was annually around $49 billion in the United States. When obese individuals are compared with normal weight individuals, severely obese individuals have 1.5–3.9 times higher direct costs. When all of the comorbid conditions are included, it is very clear that obesity results in enormous individual and societal direct health care costs.
- *Indirect costs* (23): Indirect costs are typically regarded as the non-direct medical expenditures resulting in lost productivity. In the workforce, these include presenteeism, absenteeism, disability, and workmen's compensation claims as well as premature mortality. In the area of obesity, it has been estimated that indirect costs exceed those of direct costs. In fact, when indirect costs in obese individuals compared to normal individuals have been assessed, severely obese individuals have 1.7–8 times higher indirect costs. It has been further estimated that severely obese people represent 3% of the employed population, but 21% of the indirect costs.
- Some of these costs are involved in presenteeism and absenteeism. Presenteeism is defined as time and productivity lost to workers who are at work, but unable to perform in full capacity due to obesity-related health problems; whereas absenteeism results in loss of productivity associated with missed days of work or sick leave. When incremental average costs per worker for obese individuals, including absenteeism and presenteeism, have been evaluated, the additional annual expenses were estimated at $1962 and $5193 for absenteeism and presenteeism, respectively, for male workers; and $1736 and $5393 for these female workers.

In addition to issues related to absenteeism and presenteeism, disability and premature mortality also must be included in indirect costs. Several studies have concluded that obesity consistently predicts disability. In one study of obesity, in firefighters who were eligible for disability, each BMI unit increase was associated with a 5% increase in the likelihood that a firefighter would be disabled. In another study comparing normal weight employees to obese employees, disability costs were $349 more annually for obese employees. Premature mortality has also been quantified as years of life lost to obesity. It has been estimated that obesity results in a total loss of income of $468,333 and $376,667 for non-Hispanic, white men and women, respectively, due to lower life expectancies. Other studies have estimated that the annual cost of lost earnings in the United States due to obesity is approximately $30 billion.

8.11   EXERCISE MANAGEMENT OF THE OBESE PATIENT

It has been argued that physical activity alone is not a powerful tool for initial weight loss. Abundant evidence, however, supports the concept that regular physical activity is a key component of long-term maintenance of weight loss. Regular physical activity also plays an important role in preservation of lean body mass, which is a key component of maintaining adequate metabolism to support maintenance of weight loss. As discussed in detail in Chapter 3, regular physical activity also conveys a host of health-enhancing benefits in addition to its role in weight loss and weight management.

Physical activity also contributes to the prevention of weight gain and the incidence of obesity. Thus, health care providers and health and fitness professionals should work closely with patients to counsel them on the important role that physical activity can play on body weight regulation. Physical activity is also an important lifestyle behavior, even when the patient is receiving either medical-based forms of treatment (e.g., pharmaceutical therapy) or surgical treatment for obesity (e.g., bariatric surgery).

As already indicated, the level of cardiorespiratory fitness is associated with all-cause mortality. It has been argued that levels of fitness remain an important factor in reducing the risk of mortality, even in obese individuals. This appears to be independent of the influence of BMI or body fatness. It should be noted that even though fitness may reduce the risk of all-cause mortality, it does not reduce it to the level of normal weight individuals. Several studies have demonstrated that both fitness and BMI are associated with all-cause mortality.

Physical activity can contribute to short-term weight loss of 0.5–3 kg in trials lasting less than six months (24). However, physical activity is most effective when combined with a reduction in calories consumed, where physical activity can enhance weight loss by approximately 20% beyond the magnitude of weight loss achieved through a reduction in energy intake alone.

For all of these reasons, it is imperative that physicians and other health care workers include physical activity as part of the strategy to prevent weight gain and treat obesity.

8.12   DIETARY MANAGEMENT OF OVERWEIGHT AND OBESITY

Nutrition plays a critical role in the prevention and treatment of obesity. Typical nutritional interventions for weight loss in obese individuals involve sustaining an average daily caloric deficit of 500 kcals. It should be noted that energy consumption recommendations also include that caloric intake should not be lower than 1200/day for male or female adults in order to maintain adequate nutrient intake.

A variety of evidence-based diets have been demonstrated to assist in healthy weight loss. These include the Mediterranean diet (25), the DASH diet (26), and the Healthy U.S. Style Eating Pattern (27). It has been further demonstrated that macronutrient composition of weight loss plans (e.g., low-fat versus low carb, etc.) do not achieve different results in studies lasting longer than one year.

Nutrition should be part of an overall approach to weight loss. Weight loss guidelines, generally issued by the U.S. Preventive Services Task Force, the American Heart Association, the American College of Cardiology (ACC) and The Obesity

Society (TOS), and the Academy of Nutrition and Dietetics (AND) all recommend a multidisciplinary team approach to managing obesity. Included in these approaches are physical activity, counseling, medical nutrition therapy (MNT), as well as a structured approach to behavior change.

8.13 PHARMACOLOGICAL MANAGEMENT OF THE PATIENT WITH OBESITY

The U.S. Food and Drug Administration (FDA) has approved six drugs with acceptable safety profiles for short-term and long-term pharmacological therapy in the area of weight loss (28). Pharmacological treatment for obesity is indicated as an adjunct to lifestyle changes in adults with a BMI at or above 30 kg/m^2 or above 27 kg/m^2 in the presence of at least one weight-related comorbidity. The selection of an obesity drug should be personalized to accommodate consideration for a patient's past medical and social history, including medical and mental health issues and current medications.

The weight loss drugs which have been approved for weight loss and approved patient population are found in Table 8.4.

8.14 SURGERY FOR SEVERE OBESITY

A bariatric surgery is indicated for patients who have a BMI of $\geq$40 kg/m^2 or those with a BMI $\geq$35 kg/m^2 who have comorbid conditions. Mean weight loss at two to three years following a surgical procedure for weight loss ranges between 20% and 34% of initial body weight, depending on the procedure. It is essential to have continued attention to diet, physical activity, and emotional health after bariatric surgery in order to ensure optimal outcomes. Any patient who is considering weight loss surgery should also undergo a comprehensive assessment by a multidisciplinary team of health care providers. This team includes a physician or an advanced practice provider, registered dietitian, and mental health professional (29). Potential bariatric surgical procedures are shown in Figure 8.3.

8.15 ADIPOSITY-BASED CHRONIC DISEASE (ABCD): A NEW DIAGNOSTIC TERM

Mechanick et al. have proposed a new diagnostic term entitled adiposity-based chronic disease (30). These investigators argue that this novel diagnostic term emphasizes dysfunctional adipose tissue that is present in an unfavorable distribution and associated with metabolic disease, including increased risk of CVD and a host of other comorbidities. They further argue that ABCD will allow early intervention in a variety of individuals who have excessive adiposity and foster further opportunities for research, clinical applications, and intensive lifestyle intervention. The intensive lifestyle management advocated for ABCD includes healthy dietary patterns, physical activity, sleep hygiene, stress reduction, and community involvement. Further research is underway to establish parameters and treatments for this interesting, new diagnostic term.

TABLE 8.4

Weight Loss Drugs, DEA Schedule, Weight Loss Effects, and Approved Patient Population

Drug Generic Name	Drug Commercial Name	DEA Schedule	Weight Loss Caused by Drug Compared to Placebo	Approved Patient Population
Drugs approved for short-term weight loss (weight loss effect after a variable period as described in table)				
Phentermine	Adipex, Ionamin, Lomaira	IV	3.6 kg (2–24 weeks) (28)	18 and older. Pregnancy category X
Diethylpropion	Tenuate	IV	3.0 kg (6–52 weeks) (28)	16 and older. Pregnancy category B
Benzphetamine	Didrex	III	3.3 kg (1.6–17 weeks) (28)	12 and older. Pregnancy category X
Phendimetrazine	Bontril, Prelu-2	III	There were no trials to meet the selection criteria (28)	17 and older. Pregnancy category X
Drugs approved for long-term weight loss (weight loss effect after one year of treatment)				
Orlistat	Xenical, Alli	None, over-the-counter drug	3.1% (71)	12 and older. Pregnancy category X
Lorcaserin	Belviq, Belviq SR	IV	3.6% (41)	18 and older. Pregnancy category X
Phentermine-topiramate	Qsymia	IV	6.6% (49)	18 and older. Pregnancy category X
Naltrexone-bupropion	Contrave	None	4.8% (50)	18 and older. Pregnancy category X
Liraglutide	Saxenda	None	5.4% (56)	18 and older. Pregnancy category X

Pasarica M. Pharmacological Management of the Patient with Obesity, in: Rippe JM. *Lifestyle Medicine*, 3rd edition. CRC Press, Boca Raton, 2019. Used with permission.

8.16   FUTURE DIRECTIONS IN OBESITY AND WEIGHT MANAGEMENT

Significant progress is continuing to be made for effective obesity care and prevention. A number of organizations such as the AHA, ACC, and TOS (31) have combined to issue guidance for clinicians who wish to incorporate evidence-based treatment for obesity. In addition, pharmacotherapy is moving toward more targeted

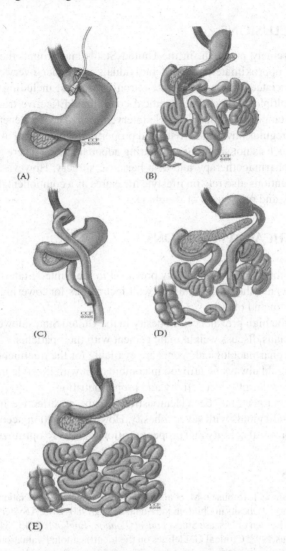

FIGURE 8.3 (a) Laparoscopic adjustable gastric banding (LAGB). (b) Laparoscopic sleeve gastrectomy (LSG). (c) The Roux-en-Y Gastric Bypass (RYGB). (d) Biliopancreatic diversion (BPD). (e) Biliopancreatic diversion with duodenal switch (BPDDS). Kushner R, Neff L. Surgery for Severe Obesity, in: Rippe JM. *Lifestyle Medicine*, 3rd edition. CRC Press, Boca Raton, 2019. Used with permission.

options, which may make it comparable in efficacy to bariatric surgery. Considerable potential exists to utilize precision medicine techniques in the area of obesity, allowing for more tailored options for different obesity phenotypes. The high prevalence of obesity mandates that continued research explore the most effective ways of preventing and treating obesity.

8.17 CONCLUSIONS

Obesity is extremely prevalent in the United States and around the world. In the United States, approximately 70% of individuals are either overweight or obese. Obesity is associated with a number of chronic diseases, including CVD, T2DM, cancer, and multiple other chronic medical conditions. Effective treatment of obesity invariably employs multiple lifestyle interventions to combat energy imbalance. These include regular physical activity and proper nutrition as well as other lifestyle interventions such as not smoking and getting adequate sleep. There are also important roles for pharmacotherapy and also bariatric surgery. However, both of these types of interventions also rely on lifestyle measures as a component of overall treatment of obesity and prevention of weight gain.

8.18 PRACTICAL APPLICATIONS

- Overweight and obesity are very prevalent in the United States.
- All clinicians should be familiar with techniques for lowering the risk of weight gain and obesity.
- Despite the high prevalence of obesity in the United States, fewer than 40% of physicians discuss weight management with their patients.
- Multiple pharmacological agents are available for the treatment of obesity. These should always be utilized in combination with lifestyle interventions such as regular physical activity and proper nutrition.
- Bariatric surgery has been demonstrated to be an effective management tool for individuals with severe obesity. However, attention needs to be paid to both physical activity and proper nutrition in order to optimize outcomes.

REFERENCES

1. Ng M, Fleming T, Robinson M, et al. 2014. Global, Regional, and National Prevalence of Overweight and Obesity in Children and Adults during 1980–2013: A Systematic Analysis for the Global Burden of Disease Study. *Lancet (London, England)*. 2013;384(9945):766–781.
2. Anonymous 1998. Clinical Guidelines on the Identification, Evaluation, and Treatment of Overweight and Obesity in Adults--The Evidence Report. *National Institutes of Health. Obesity Research*. 1998;6(Suppl 2):51S–209S.
3. Allison D, Fontaine K, Manson J, et al. Annual Deaths Attributable to Obesity in the United States. *JAMA*. 1999;282(16):1530–1538.
4. Flegal K, Graubard B, Williamson D, et al. Excess Deaths Associated with Underweight, Overweight, and Obesity. *JAMA*. 2005;293(15):1861–1867.5.
5. Clinical Guidelines on the Identification, Evaluation, and Treatment of Overweight and Obesity in Adults: Executive Summary. Expert Panel on the Identification, Evaluation, and Treatment of Overweight in Adults. *American Journal of Clinical Nutrition*. 1998;68(4):899–917.
6. The Diabetes Prevention Program (DPP) Research Group. The Diabetes Prevention Program (DPP). Description of Lifestyle Intervention. *Diabetes Care*. 2002;25(12):2165–2171.

7. Berger S, Huggins G, McCaffery J, et al. Comparison among Criteria to Define Successful Weight-Loss Maintai ners and Regainers in the Action for Health in Diabetes (Look AHEAD) and Diabetes Prevention Program Trials. *American Journal of Clinical Nutrition.* 2017;106:1337–1346.

8. Kuczmarski R, Flegal K, Campbell S, et al. Increasing Prevalence of Overweight among US Adults. The National Health and Nutrition Examination Surveys, 1960 to 1991. *JAMA.* 1994;272(3):205–211.

9. Flegal K, Kruszon-Moran D, Carroll M, et al. Trends in Obesity among Adults in the United States, 2005 to 2014. *JAMA.* 2016;315(21):2284–2291.

10. Hall K, Sacks G, Chandramohan D, et al. Quantification of the Effect of Energy Imbalance on Bodyweight. *Lancet.* 2011;378(9793):826–837.

11. Leibel R, Rosenbaum M, Hirsch J. Changes in Energy Expenditure Resulting from Altered Body Weight. *New England Journal of Medicine.* 1995;332(10):621–628.

12. Nielsen S, Popkin B. Patterns and Trends in Food Portion Sizes, 1977–1998. *JAMA.* 2003;289(4):450–453.

13. Rankinen T, Zuberi A, Chagnon Y, et al. The Human Obesity Gene Map: The 2005 Update. *Obesity.* 2006;14(4):529–644.

14. Huypens P, Sass S, Wu M, et al. Epigenetic Germline Inheritance of Diet-Induced Obesity and Insulin Resistance. *Nature Genetics.* 2016;48(5):497–499.

15. McAllister E, Dhurandhar N, Keith S, et al. Ten Putative Contributors to the Obesity Epidemic. *Critical Reviews in Food Science and Nutrition.* 2009;49(10):868–913.

16. Flegal K, Troiano R, Pamuk E, et al. The Influence of Smoking Cessation on the Prevalence of Overweight in the United States. *New England Journal of Medicine.* 1995;333(18):1165–1170.

17. Van Cauter, E. Sleep Disturbances and Insulin Resistance. *Diabetic Medicine: A Journal of the British Diabetic Association.* 2011;28(12);1455–1462.

18. Bray G. Identification, Evaluation and Treatment of Overweight and Obesity. In: Rippe JM, Angelopoulos TJ. *Obesity: Prevention and Treatment.* CRC Press (Boca Raton), 2012.

19. Rippe JM, Angelopoulos T. *Obesity: Prevention and Treatment.* CRC Press (Boca Raton), 2012.

20. U.S. Department of Agriculture and U.S. Department of Health and Human Services. *Dietary Guidelines for Americans, 2010* (7th edition). U.S. Government Printing Office (Washington, DC), December 2010.

21. Tremmel M, Gerdtham U, Nilsson P, et al. Economic Burden of Obesity: A Systematic Literature Review. *International Journal of Environmental Research and Public Health.* 2017;14(4). doi:10.3390/ijerph14040435

22. Dor A. Ferguson C, Langwith C. et al. *A Heavy Burden: The Individual Costs of Being Overweight and Obese.* George Washington University School of Public Health and Health Services Department of Health Policy. Washington, DC. 2010.

23. Trogdon J, Finkelstein E, Hylands T, et al. Indirect Costs of Obesity: A Review of the Current Literature. *Obesity Reviews: An Official Journal of the International Association for the Study of Obesity.* 2008;9(5):489–500.

24. Jakicic J, Rogers R, Collins K. *Lifestyle Medicine* (3rd edition). CRC Press (Boca Raton), 2019.

25. Shai I, Schwarzfuchs D, Henkin Y, et al. Weight Loss with a Low-Carbohydrate, Mediterranean, or Low-Fat Diet. *New England Journal of Medicine.* 2008;359:229–241.

26. The DASH Diet Eating Plan. http://dashdiet.org/default.asp. Accessed June 25, 2020.

27. U.S. Department of Health and Human Services and U.S. Department of Agriculture. *2015–2020 Dietary Guidelines for Americans* (8th edition). December 2015. http://hea lth.gov/dietaryguidelines/2015/guidelines/.

28. Pasarica M. *Pharmacological Management of the Patient with Obesity. Lifestyle Medicine* (3rd edition). CRC Press (Boca Raton), 2019.
29. Kushner R, Neff L. *Surgery for Severe Obesity. Lifestyle Medicine* (3rd edition). CRC Press (Boca Raton), 2019.
30. Via M. *Adiposity-Based Chronic Disease: A New Diagnostic Term. Lifestyle Medicine* (3rd edition). CRC Press (Boca Raton), 2019.
31. Guideline for the Management of Overweight and Obesity in Adults. A Report of the American College of Cardiology/American Heart Association Task Force on Practice Guidelines and the Obesity Society. *Circulation.* 2014;129(25 Suppl 2):S102–S138.

9 Pulmonary Medicine

KEY POINTS

- Lung problems and breathing symptoms are extremely common in the United States population.
- Asthma is very common in the U.S. population and a variety of preventative measures as well as effective treatments are available.
- In any given year, 5–20% of persons in the United States are infected with influenza and up to 56,000 people die each year as a result of influenza.
- Indoor air quality can cause a variety of adverse health consequences and should be assessed with a careful history.
- The COVID-19 virus infects many organs, but lung infections are particularly common and often fatal.

9.1   INTRODUCTION

Lung problems are very common in the health care system. Shortness of breath, cough, and wheezing are among the most common symptoms experienced by patients seeking medical care. Thus, it is important for all clinicians to have a general understanding of pulmonary medicine and various respiratory symptoms in order to properly diagnose these individuals. Also, many of these symptoms come from exposures in the environment (e.g., allergies) or from personal habits and actions such as smoking, obesity, or stress. Thus, lifestyle medicine plays a very important role in treating a variety of issues in pulmonary medicine.

With regard to respiratory symptoms, a comprehensive and insightful history is an important starting point which can help clinicians narrow down possible lung issues that underlie symptoms. Further tests, such as pulmonary function tests, spirometry, or pulse oximetry may further elucidate exact causes of underlying symptoms.

9.2   RESPIRATORY SYMPTOMS

- *Dyspnea:* Dyspnea or breathlessness may be experienced in a variety of circumstances or may be experienced by healthy individuals when exercising to the limits of their aerobic capacity or it can represent either primary pulmonary disease or cardiovascular disease (CVD). Dyspnea can also be a manifestation of severe metabolic acidosis. In one large study of 1000 randomly selected adults with dyspnea, approximately 35% of these patients were without known cardiopulmonary pathophysiology, yet dyspnea was associated with increased morbidity and possibly mortality as compared to patients without dyspnea (1).

TABLE 9.1

Descriptors of Dyspnea

1. My breath does not go in all the way
2. My breathing requires effort
3. I feel that I am smothering
4. I feel a hunger for more air
5. My breathing is heavy
6. I cannot take a deep breath
7. I feel out of breath
8. My chest feels tight
9. My breathing requires more work
10. I feel that I am suffocating
11. I feel that my breath stops
12. I am gasping for breath
13. My chest is constricted
14. I feel that my breathing is rapid
15. My breathing is shallow
16. I feel that I am breathing more
17. I cannot get enough air
18. My breath does not go out all the way
19. My breathing requires more concentration

Source: Simon PM, Schwartzstein RM, Weiss JW, et al. 1989. Distinguishable Sensations of Breathlessness Induced in Normal Volunteers. *Am Rev Respir Dis* 140:1021–1027.
Rippe, JM. *Lifestyle Medicine*, 3rd edition. CRC Press, Boca Raton, 2019. Used with permission.

Patients may describe dyspnea in a variety of different ways. These are listed in Table 9.1. Using the description of symptoms, it may be possible to pinpoint the underlying cause of the dyspnea. The management of dyspnea primarily involves treating the underlying pathophysiological process causing the patient's breathlessness. A detailed review of the various causes of dyspnea and the treatment is beyond the scope of this manual, but can be found in multiple other places, including the chapter on respiratory symptoms in the 3rd edition of *Lifestyle Medicine* (1).

- *Cough:* Cough is a sudden expiratory maneuver associated with high intrathoracic pressures intended to clear secretions or foreign material from the airways. The most common causes of cough are outlined in Table 9.2.

Acute cough is one that has been present for less than three weeks (2). The most common cause of acute cough is respiratory infection, which is typically characterized by spittle production and may be accompanied by a raw substernal sensation. Subclinical bronchial spasm may also cause

---

TABLE 9.2

Common Clinical Causes of Cough

Acute Cough
  Respiratory infection, airway inflammation
  Bronchospasm
  Inhalational injury
  Aspiration
Subacute Cough
  Infectious or post-infectious cough (*Bordetella pertussis*)
  Sinus infection/inflammation resulting in post-nasal drip
Chronic Cough with Clear Chest X-ray
  Upper airway cough syndrome (post-nasal drip)
  Bronchospasm
  Gastroesophageal reflux
  Chronic bronchitis
  Bronchiectasis
  Endobronchial neoplasms
  Non-asthmatic eosinophilic bronchitis
Chronic Cough with Abnormal Chest X-ray
  Interstitial lung disease
  Recurrent aspiration
  Endobronchial neoplasm
  Indolent infections (e.g., *Pneumocystis jerovici*, pneumonia, tuberculosis)

Source: Simon PM, Schwartzstein RM, Weiss JW, et al. 1989. Distinguishable Sensations of Breathlessness Induced in Normal Volunteers. *Am Rev Respir Dis* 140:1021–1027.
Rippe, JM. *Lifestyle Medicine*, 3rd edition. CRC Press, Boca Raton, 2019. Used with permission.

---

acute cough. Mild asthma may also present with acute cough. Some exposures to allergens, cold air, or exercising may result in a transient cough. Pulmonary function tests, including spirometry, are often needed to make a specific diagnosis. Hyper-reactive airways without wheezing can present as a chronic cough, which has been termed cough-variant asthma. GERD also is a common cause of chronic cough. Chronic bronchitis which is defined as a productive cough present for more than three months a year for more than two years is another cause of chronic cough. A chest X-ray is often helpful in determining abnormalities that may result in a chronic cough.

• *Hemoptysis:* Hemoptysis is the term that refers to coughing with the expectoration of blood or blood-tinged sputum. It is worth noting that the normal trachealbronchial tree should not bleed even in the presence of a coagulopathy. Thus, hemoptysis even in the setting of anticoagulation should be considered a pathological finding.

The four major sources of blood in the lower respiratory tract are airways, pulmonary parenchyma, pulmonary circulation, and bronchial circulation. Massive hemoptysis is generally defined as production of ≥600 ml of blood in 24 hours. Patients often overestimate the amount of blood they expectorate because of concomitant anxiety, so it is important to encourage a patient to be as explicit as possible in quantifying the amount of blood.

Massive hemoptysis can occur in endobronchial carcinoma, but is more commonly associated with erosions of bronchial vessels in large, intrapulmonary cavities or with bronchiectasis (3). There are ten etiological categories to be considered when evaluating a patient with hemoptysis. These are outlined in Table 9.3.

• *Wheezing:* Wheezing is the sound that emanates from the lower airways (below the larynx) resulting in turbulent airflow (4). The sound is produced by turbulent flow through the narrowed airways and in some cases may reflect a rapid oscillation of airway narrowing. Common causes of wheezing include primary airway reactivity (e.g., asthma) interstitial edema, airway inflammation and mucous hypersecretion, endobronchial obstruction (e.g., neoplasm or foreign body), vocal cord dysfunction, or exercise-induced bronchial obstruction.

• *Snoring and Apnea:* The prevalence of nocturnal respiratory symptoms has increased markedly in the 21st century. The leading cause of the increased frequency and severity of nocturnal respiratory symptoms is likely the increase in obesity in the general population.

Snoring is defined as noisy breathing during sleep and is very common in the general population. Prevalence of snoring varies between studies

---

TABLE 9.3

Etiologic Categories for Hemoptysis

Pulmonary infections

Neoplasms

Collagen-vascular and immunological lung diseases

Cardiovascular diseases (including pulmonary vascular and valvular diseases)

Congenital or acquired vascular disease (arteriovenous malformation)

Structural parenchymal disease (cavitary lesion)

Structural airway disease (bronchiectasis)

Infection (bacterial pneumonia, invasive fungal pneumonia)

Aspiration of foreign bodies

Chest trauma with pulmonary contusion

Source: Simon PM, Schwartzstein RM, Weiss JW, et al. 1989. Distinguishable Sensations of Breathlessness Induced in Normal Volunteers. *Am Rev Respir Dis* 140:1021–1027.

Rippe, JM. *Lifestyle Medicine*, 3rd edition. CRC Press, Boca Raton, 2019. Used with permission.

---

ranging from 10% to 50%. The prevalence of snoring increases with age up to 60 years after which the prevalence decreases (5). Snoring occurs due to vibration of the soft palate and faucial pillars. The likelihood that snoring will occur is dependent on the size of the airway, the tone of the soft tissue structures in the airway, and body positions. The clinical significance of snoring is uncertain. In the absence of observed or measured apneic episodes, snoring is considered to be benign.

Nocturnal apneas are defined as a cessation of airflows during sleep. The term apnea specifically describes a cessation of airflow for ≥10 seconds. Hypopnea is a transient reduction in airflow that lasts ≥10 seconds and is associated with a ≥4% decrease in oxygen saturation. Frequent nocturnal apneas and hypopneas may result in hypoventilation. The diagnostic criteria for clinically significant obstructive sleep apnea is an average of greater than five apneas or hypopneas per hour of sleep. This is typically referred to as "Apnea-Hypopnea Index" (AHI). A sleep study must be performed to accurately measure AHI.

9.3 ASTHMA

- *Clinical features:* Asthma is an inflammatory disease of the airways characterized by intermittent symptoms, including chest congestion, cough, and wheezing. These symptoms are associated with airway responsiveness and variable airway obstruction. In 2016, approximately 20.4 million adults representing 8.3% of the population in the United States had asthma (6,7). Despite advances in therapies, asthma remains a large burden on the health care system accounting for up to 6.2% of physician outpatient visits and emergency visits and over 1.7 million emergency room visits. Unfortunately, asthma resulted in 3615 deaths in the United States in 2015 (8). The prevention and treatment of asthma are highly relevant to all clinicians, particularly to lifestyle medicine clinicians and, of course, pulmonologists.

   The National Asthma Education and Prevention Program (NAEPP) 2007 Guidelines recommend a written asthma action plan for any individual who has asthma based on signs and symptoms (7). This may be particularly helpful for those who have poorly controlled asthma. Action plans also help clarify all of the medications.
- *Treatment:* Environmental control measures, such as avoiding allergens, should be included in all asthma management strategies. This includes seasonal allergens such as grasses and trees. In addition, an important step for controlling allergen-induced asthma is to reduce exposure to indoor and outdoor allergens. Major indoor allergens of particular importance for people with asthma are pet dander, dust mites, mold, mites, and cockroaches. All warm-blooded pets can cause allergic reactions. With regard to outdoor allergens, a variety of tree, grass, and weed pollens and seasonal spores contribute to outdoor allergen loads that affect many asthmatic patients.

TABLE 9.4

Long-Term Control and Quick–Relief Therapies for Asthma

Long-Term Control	Quick Relief
Inhaled corticosteroids	Short-acting beta-2 agonists
Cromolyn	Systemic corticosteroids
Leukotriene modifiers	Ipratropium bromide
Long-acting bronchodilators	
• Long-acting beta-2 agonists	
• Theophylline	
• Tiotropium	
Systemic corticosteroids	
Anti-IgE therapy	
• Omalizumab	
Anti-IL-5 Ab and –IL-5-Receptor Ab	
• Mepolizumab	
• Reslizumab	
• Benralizumab*	
Immunotherapy	

* IL-5 receptor Ab.

Source: Ciccolella DE, D'Alonzo GE. 2019. Asthma in: Rippe, JM. *Lifestyle Medicine*, 3rd edition. CRC Press, Boca Raton, 2019. Used with permission.

- *Pharmacologic therapy:* A variety of pharmacological therapies are available. These are listed in Table 9.4. A description of all of the available pharmacological agents is beyond the scope of this manual. However, the U.S. National Asthma Education and Prevention Program (NAEPP) 2007 Guidelines for Asthma provides detailed descriptions of these therapies.

- *Management of asthma according to severity and control classifications:* A step wise approach has been proposed for pharmacological therapy for asthma. The classification for this approach and when to use various medications may be found in NAEPP Expert Panel Report and is repeated in Table 9.5 (7). In addition, the NAEPP Expert Panel also provided guidance for when to refer patients to an asthma specialist for factors that are associated with increased risk of asthma exacerbation. These are found in Tables 9.6 and 9.7.

- *Other issues in long-term asthma management:* Exercise may bring on asthma attacks. Exercise-induced asthma (EIA) is a transient airway narrowing and airflow obstruction which occurs during or after exercise (9). Nearly 90% of persistent asthmatics have EID. Patients often describe this syndrome as the inability to take a full breath of air during or following exercise (10). Symptoms usually start several minutes after exercise has stopped and usually improve within one hour.

TABLE 9.5

Classification of Asthma Severity ≥12 Years of Age

Components of Severity		Classification of Asthma Severity ≥12 years of age			
		Intermittent	Mild	Moderate	Severe
			Persistent		
Impairment Normal FEV$_1$/FVC: 8–19 yr 85% 20–39 yr 80% 40–59 yr 75% 60–80 yr 70%	Symptoms	≤2 days/week	>2 days/week but not daily	Daily	Throughout the day
	Nighttime awakenings	≤2x/month	3–4x/month	>1x/week but not nightly	Often 7x/week
	Short-acting beta$_2$-agonist use for symptom control (not prevention of EIB)	≤2 days/week	>2 days/week but not daily, and not more than 1x on any day	Daily	Several times per day
	Interference with normal activity	None	Minor limitation	Some limitation	Extremely limited
	Lung function	• Normal FEV, between exacerbations • FEV$_1$ >80% predicted • FEV/FVC normal	• FEV$_1$ >80% predicted • FEV$_1$/FVC normal	• FEV$_1$ >60% but <80% predicted • FEV$_1$/FVC reduced 5%	• FEV$_1$ <60% predicted • FEV$_1$/FVC reduced >5%
Risk	Exacerbations requiring o'al systemic corticosteroids	0–1/year (see note)	≥2/year (see note)		
		Consider severity and interval since last exacerbation Frequency and severity may fluctuate over time for patients in any severity category. Relative annual risk of exacerbations may be related to FEV$_1$			
Recommended Step for Initiating Treatment (See "Stepwise Approach for Managing Asthma" for treatment steps.)		Step 1	Step 2	Step3	Step 4 or Step 5
		In 2–6 weeks, evaluate the level of asthma control that is achieved and adjust therapy accordingly.		and consider short course of oral systemic corticosteroids	

Source: Adapted from National Heart, Lung and Blood Institute. National Asthma Education and Prevention Program: Expert Panel Report 3 (EPR3). Guidelines for the Diagnosis and Management of Asthma. NIH Publication No. 08-4051, Full Report. 2007.

TABLE 9.6
Referral to Asthma Specialist for Consultation or Co-management

1. Patient has had a life-threatening asthma exacerbation
2. Patient has needed more than two bursts of oral corticosteroids in one year or required hospitalization
3. Patient is not meeting the goals of asthma therapy after three to six months of treatment or is unresponsive to therapy
4. Diagnosis unclear
5. Conditions complicating asthma or its diagnosis (e.g., sinusitis, nasal polyps, aspergillosis, severe rhinitis, VCD, GERD, COPD, psychosocial problems)
6. Further diagnostic studies is needed (e.g., allergy skin testing, rhinoscopy, complete pulmonary function studies, provocative challenge, bronchoscopy)
7. Consideration for immunotherapy
8. Patient requires step 4 care or higher or even consider referral for step 3 care
9. Patient education and guidance on complications of therapy, problems with adherence, or allergen avoidance
10. Confirmation of possible occupational or environmental inhalant or ingested substance contributing to asthma

Source: Adapted from National Heart, Lung and Blood Institute. National Asthma Education and Prevention Program: Expert Panel Report 3 (EPR 3). Guidelines for the Diagnosis and Management of Asthma. NIH Publication No. 08-4051, Full Report 2007.

TABLE 9.7
Factors Associated with Increased Risk of Asthma Exacerbations or Mortality

1. Severe airflow obstruction, as detected by spirometry
2. Two or more ED visits or hospitalizations for asthma in the past year; past intubation or ICU admission, especially in past five years
3. Patients feeling in danger or frightened by their asthma
4. Patient characteristics: female, non-white, non-use of ICS therapy, and current smoking
5. Psychosocial factors: depression, increased stress, socioeconomic factors
6. Attitudes and beliefs about taking medications

Source: Adapted from National Heart, Lung and Blood Institute. National Asthma Education and Prevention Program: Expert Panel Report 3 (EPR 3). Guidelines for the Diagnosis and Management of Asthma. NIH Publication No. 08-4051, Full Report 2007.

- *Occupational asthma:* Occupational asthma is also common. It has been estimated that approximately 9–15% of cases of asthma occur in adults of working age. A variety of substances in the workplace have been implicated in the development of asthma, including a variety of animal proteins, flour and grain dust, wood dust, cotton dust, chemical compounds, and even pharmaceuticals.

- *Obesity:* Asthma is more common and more difficult to treat in obese patients because there are a variety of potential contributors to dyspnea and wheeze in obese patients. The diagnosis of asthma in obese individuals should be confirmed by an objective measurement of variable airflow obstruction.
- *Stress:* While asthma is not a psychosomatic illness, there is emerging evidence that stress plays an important role in precipitating asthma attacks and may act as a risk factor.
- *Other causes:* Other causes of asthma include food hypersensitivity, medication-induced asthma, gastroesophageal reflux, and esophageal reflux.
- *Pregnancy and asthma:* Asthma is the most common medical condition in pregnancy occurring in 4–8% of pregnant women (11). The risk of asthma exacerbation during pregnancy is higher in women, especially in the second trimester. The goals of asthma during pregnancy are to prevent acute exacerbation and optimize lung function. If asthma medications are necessary during pregnancy, the benefit of keeping asthma under control must be weighed against the small potential risk of adverse effects from the asthma medication during pregnancy. The majority of asthma medications that are used in practice present little or no risk during pregnancy. The FDA has a five category medication classification system concerning potential of medications to cause harm to the fetus (A-D and X). Most of the asthma medicines are in category B. Inhaled therapies for asthma should be selected over systemic therapy during pregnancy. Obstetricians and primary care physicians should work together to create the safest regimen for a pregnant, asthmatic patient. When questions arise, a local asthma expert, generally an allergist or a pulmonary specialist, should be consulted.

9.4 OCCUPATIONAL AND ENVIRONMENTAL LUNG DISEASES

A variety of occupational and environmental lung diseases have occurred that are of significant concern. For example, work-related asthma (WRA) is responsible for about 15–20% of adult asthma and is associated with high morbidity, disability, and cost (12). Chronic obstructive pulmonary disease (COPD) is a leading cause of morbidity and mortality, especially among non-smokers who have occupational exposure to noxious fumes. Silica, coal, asbestos, and beryllium are important causes of occupational lung disease among workers in the mining, automotive, and construction industries. Hypersensitivity pneumonitis is an immunologically related lung disease caused by a variety of inducing agents. Corticosteroids may be important in therapy as is avoidance of exposure. High-altitude sickness is a group of clinical syndromes which occur in travelers at altitudes above 2500 meters. For all of these reasons, the knowledge of occupational and environmental lung disease is important to every clinician.

- *Work-Related Asthma:* WRA is a chronic inflammatory lung disease characterized by the presence of reversible airway narrowing following exposure to various dust particles, gases, or fumes in the work environment.

Primary prevention of WRA involves education, avoidance of exposure to sensitizing agents, and where this is not possible, a substitution for sensitizing agents with non-sensitizers. Pharmacotherapy represents an adjunct to avoiding sensitizers and irritants and involves similar approaches outlined in the previous section on asthma.

- *Chronic Obstructive Pulmonary Disease:* COPD is an inflammatory lung disease characterized by irreversible airway obstruction (13). Smoking is, by far, the most important risk factor resulting in more than two-thirds of COPD cases (14). COPD affects about 10% of the general population. Its prevalence increases with age and smoking. The diagnosis of COPD should be considered in any patient presenting with a chronic cough, shortness of breath, and sputum production in the context of a smoking history.

    Spirometry is required to make the diagnosis of COPD. A post-bronchial dilator FEV1/FVC <0.70 confirms the presence of persistent airflow limitation and identifies the presence of COPD in patients with appropriate symptoms and predisposing risk factors. Therapy for COPD includes symptom control and improvement of exercise tolerance.

- *Asbestos-related lung disease:* Asbestos-related lung disease is a group of lung diseases caused by exposure to asbestos fibers which are comprised of magnesium silicate minerals (15). These fibers have been widely used in industry because of their high tensile strength, flexibility, and resistance to chemical and thermal degradation. Asbestos fibers are highly carcinogenic and are known to cause lung cancer and malignant mesothelioma. It is estimated that worldwide over 40,000 people die of malignant mesothelioma every year. Individuals exposed to asbestos are mostly asymptomatic with a lengthy period as long 20–30 years between initial exposure and development of the clinically apparent disease. Pleural mesothelioma (PMP) is a dreaded, typically fatal consequence of the asbestos exposure typically occurring in men over the age of 60.

- *Silicosis:* Silicosis is a fibrotic lung disease caused by inhalation of free crystalline silicon dioxide or silica. It is recognized as one of the most important occupational diseases worldwide (16). It most commonly occurs in workplaces where quartz, tridymite, and cristobalite are utilized. This is highest in individuals employed in construction work involving masonry, heavy construction, painting, and steel foundries. In the United States, about 127,000 miners have been exposed to this disease.

- *Berylliosis:* Beryllium is a naturally occurring element which is extracted from ores and processed into metal, oxides, alloys, and composite materials used in the aerospace, automotive, and mining industries (17). It is estimated that about 134,000 workers in government and private industry are at present potentially exposed to beryllium in the United States. The diagnosis of beryllium sensitization is made on the basis of positive blood Beryllium Synthesized Proliferation Tests (BeLPT) in patients with a history of beryllium exposure.

- *Coal Mine Dust Lung Disease (CMDLD):* CMDLD refers to a broad spectrum of lung diseases caused by exposure to coal mine dust (18). Coal is the second largest energy source worldwide and accounts for over 25% of global energy supplies. Consequently, individuals exposed to coal particles are considerable. Within China and India, which are the top consumers of electricity made through coal power, the exposure to coal particles is considerable. In the United States, this disease is largely concentrated in states, including Wyoming, West Virginia, Kentucky, Pennsylvania, and Texas. Diagnosis is made clinically on the basis of a combination of the appropriate exposure history and radiological and pathological findings. Typically chest X-rays show the occurrence of upper lobe predominant small rounded opacities. These may also be found in all lung zones.
- *High-Altitude Illnesses (HAI):* It is estimated that 30 million people each year travel to and from recreational areas with altitudes greater than 2500 meters. For clinicians, it is important to prevent the development of HAI (19). Risk factors for the further development of HAI include preexisting cardiopulmonary disease, heavy exertion at altitude, and low-altitude residence before ascent. Obesity is also a risk factor. Prevention involving gradual ascent into high altitudes which allows for acclimatization is the most effective preventive strategy. It is generally recommended that for altitudes above 3000 meters, daily ascents should not exceed more than 300–500 meters above the previous night with a resting place after every 1000 meters (or every two to three days).
- *Hypersensitivity Pneumonitis (HP):* HP is an immune-mediated inflammatory disease of the lungs that occurs because of the exposure to an inducing agent (20). This often occurs in an occupational or recreational setting and has hence given rise to an extensive list of diseases, including farmers' lung, bird fanciers' lung, and hot tub lung. HP is characterized by lymphocytic inflammation of the lungs due to the accumulation of activated T-lymphocytes in lungs. The cornerstone of HP treatment involves identification of the offending agent and avoidance.

9.5 VENOUS THROMBOEMBOLIC DISEASE (VTE)

VTE disease is a form of deep vein thrombosis (DVT) and pulmonary embolism (PE). It is a common, costly, and morbid condition encountered by clinicians in a variety of medical and surgical fields (21). The true incidence of VTE disease is challenging because of the unknown number of asymptomatic DVT or PE cases. Asymptomatic PE alone is believed to complicate up to 50% of all confirmed cases of DVT. CDC data reports that there are 300,000–600,000 cases of VTE in the United States and 80% of these will occur in the context of at least one or more than one known risk factors. Risk factors for VTE include the following:

- *Immobility:* It has been reported that distal DVT in patients requiring cast immobilization without surgery may be as high as 19%. The risk associated with airline travel is the most intensely scrutinized, although it remains controversial. It has been estimated that DVT in flyers may be twice as that in non-flyers. Immobility not related to airline travel may include prolonged periods of non-flight-related immobility. One study that demonstrated this defined prolonged immobility as sitting for an accumulated 8 hours in a 24-hour period with at least 3 hours unbroken, 10 hours in a 24-hour period with at least 2 hours unbroken, or 12 hours in a 24-hour period with at least one hour of continuous sitting.

- *Obesity:* Obesity is also a risk factor for VTE. It has been theorized that obesity exerts a procoagulant effect. In addition to its impact on the development of the first episode of VTE, obesity has also been observed to increase the risk of recurrence after treatment of the initial event. These data are particularly important for lifestyle medicine clinicians since efforts to reduce BMI through healthier lifestyle choices may have a positive impact on the management of VTE.
- *Smoking:* Smoking has long been demonstrated to be an independent risk factor for the development of atherosclerotic disease. However, its relationship to the development of VTE is less well understood. Some studies have suggested that smoking increases VTE, while others have not.
- *Treatment:* The approach to treatment of VTE is dependent on a variety of diseases and patient factors, which influence choice of therapeutic therapy in patients and duration of anticoagulation therapies. Recent development of direct oral anticoagulants has suggested that they are both safe and effective (21).

The American College of Chest Physicians (ACCP) Anti-Thrombotic Therapy for VTE Disease updated in 2016 is the most widely accepted standard for VTE management. Detailed discussions of these recommendations are beyond the scope of this manual. However, the reader is referred to this ACCP document.

Distal thrombosis of the extremities does not uniformly require anticoagulation. The risk of increased bleeding must be weighed against the efficacy of therapy. One approach to patients with distal DVT includes performing serial duplex ultrasounds of the lower extremities for a period of two weeks off of anticoagulation. An absence of symptoms or clot progression over this surveillance interval suggests that the patient is at low risk for embolization or clot propagation.

9.6 INFLUENZA

Influenza is a contagious acute illness of the respiratory track caused by the influenza virus (22). This is a common disease and is a source of significant illness in the general population and can lead to death, especially in individuals who are at high risk for complications of influenza. Currently, it is estimated that more than 60,000 people die in the United States each year from complications of influenza. The influenza virus evolves through mutation and mixing among humans and other animal species. Thus, current vaccines are imperfect, but useful nonetheless and generally recommended.

There are three basic types of influenza virus: Influenza A, Influenza B, and Influenza C. Influenza A viruses are one of the most virulent and the cause of all the known influenza pandemics. Influenza B tends to cause milder disease than Influenza A and Influenza C causes infections in humans only infrequently and its pattern of infection shows no seasonal variation.

- *Epidemiology:* It is estimated that 5–20% of people in the United States are infected with the influenza virus each year (23). Influenza constitutes an epidemic when there is an outbreak in a particular location. Adults over the age of 65 and children younger than 2 years of age and persons with certain underlying health problems are most likely to suffer serious consequences of the influenza virus infection. Estimates from the CDC suggest that up to 56,000 people in the United States die each year as a result of influenza virus infection and between 145,000 and 700,700 people are hospitalized.
- *Pandemics:* Pandemics often occur outside of the usual influenza season. On average, there have been five pandemics in each century which have been documented in written history. The well-documented influenza pandemic viruses in the past century include 1918 H1N1 "Spanish Flu," H2N2 "Avian Flu" in 1957, and the H3N2 "Hong Kong Flu" in 1958, and the latest pandemic in 2009 "Novel H1N1."
- *Pathophysiology in influenza:* The predominant means of spread of influenza virus from the main infected person to susceptible host is at a distance of 6 feet or less. Large (≥ 5 μm diameters) respiratory droplets are disseminated when the infected person coughs or sneezes.
- *Seasonal influenza:* Influenza virus infection usually presents with an abrupt onset of fever, headache, malaise, myalgia, sore throat, rhinitis, and cough. Up to 25% of infected individuals may present with nausea, vomiting, diarrhea and less, blennorrhea and pharyngitis.
- *Avian influenza:* Sporadic human infection with Influenza A viruses that predominantly affect birds has been noted. Most human cases of Avian influenza are due to either H5N1 or H7N9. These types of infections have not generally resulted in person-to-person transmission. However, in 1997, the first recognized case of severe human illness of H5N1 Avian influenza was reported in Hong Kong. Millions of poultry were slaughtered in order to contain the disease.
- *Prevention* – Vaccination is the best way to prevent influenza virus infection. Some studies have suggested that vaccinating children against influenza may be more effective in preventing the flu in the elderly than vaccinating older adults themselves since children are very effective in spreading influenza and older adults may have a submaximal response to vaccination. More high-potency vaccines are now available for individuals over the age of 65. Currently, the influenza vaccine is recommended yearly for all persons over the age of 6 months.
- *Self-care for persons with influenza:* Most persons with influenza virus infections do not need antiviral drugs or require attention of a medical

professional. Usual activities, including exercise, can be resumed when recovery is adequate and the person who had influenza is ready to take part in these activities. Whether handwashing prevent influenza transmission is unclear as the virus is not known to survive for a long period of time on surfaces. Transmission through the air via respiratory droplets is thought to be the most important means of transmission. However, handwashing has been shown to be helpful in preventing transmission of other respiratory viruses and gastrointestinal illnesses and it is prudent to practice. Covering the mouth when coughing should be practiced routinely no matter what the reason for the cough. The same is true for using a tissue that is discarded in a waste receptacle or by coughing onto one's shoulder if a tissue is not available.

- *Antiviral therapy:* Antiviral medicines active against the influenza virus include the neuraminidase inhibitors (NAIs) and the M2 inhibitors. M2 inhibitors classified as neuraminidase are active only against Influenza A and are less useful due to high levels. DNA inhibitors are active versus both A and B viruses. Antiviral therapy is indicated as early as possible for persons hospitalized with influenza and those with severe progressive illness and those with higher risk of severe illnesses.

9.7   COVID-19

The world is in the midst of the pandemic of the novel coronavirus (SARS-CoV-2). The coronavirus family of viruses is named for the crown like appearance of surface protein called spike proteins. These spike proteins allow the virus to gain entry into the epithelial cells (and other cell types) via receptors on the surface known as angiotensin converting enzyme-ACE II. The virus tricks the cell into swallowing it through the process of endocytosis ACE II which is expressed in multiple organs in the body and has many roles including modulating systemic fluid-salt-balance and blood pressure. ACE II is expressed in the lungs which makes them the primary cite of COVID-19 infection through inhaled respiratory droplets. However, ACE II is also highly enriched in the heart, kidneys and intestines making the COVID-19 infection a problem in multiple organs.

Recent breakthroughs utilizing a messenger RNA platform have allowed vaccines against COVID-19 to be produced by Pfizer and Moderma which are highly effective against the virus. It is hoped that these vaccines will make an enormous difference by lowering the spread of the COVID-19 virus. Because the virus is spread through respiratory droplets, public health measures such as social distancing, mask wearing and regular hand washing have been central in lowering the risk of becoming infected with the COVID-19 virus. As of January 1, 2021 there were over 350,000 people in the United States who have died from COVID-19 infections and over 19 million individuals have been infected. Worldwide there have been over 84 million diagnosed cases of COVID-19 as of January 1, 2021 and over 1.8 million deaths.

9.8   INDOOR AIR QUALITY

Clean environmental air is essential for human health. This is particularly important since as humans we spend up to 90% or more of our time indoors. Indoor air
quality in the United States is regulated by the Federal Government through the
Environmental Protection Agency (EPA) (24,25). One of the most important things
that a clinician can do when meeting the patient for the first time is to take a comprehensive history of environmental exposures both at work and at home. Various issues
related to indoor air quality will be discussed in this section.

- *Secondhand smoke:* Awareness of the adverse consequences of smoking
  is widespread today. Unfortunately, globally smoking remains a highly
  prevalent lifestyle choice around the globe. Secondhand smoke is also a
  leading public health problem. Approximately one non-smoker dies from
  secondhand smoke exposure for every eight smokers who die from smoking. Secondhand smoke is composed of both side stream smoke and smoke
  release from the burning end of the cigarette as well as smoke exhaled by
  the smoker. During cigarette burning, there are over 4000 chemical con-
  centrates which may be toxic. The U.S. Public Health Services National
  Toxicology Program in 2005 unambiguously states that environmental
  tobacco smoke is a known human carcinogen.
- *Radon:* Radon is a gas produced from decay of uranium 238 and radium
  226 which are naturally present in the earth rocks and soil. Radon gas can
  seep into buildings through porous soils. Inhaled radon has been linked
  to an increase in the risk of lung cancer in underground miners. The EPA
  recommends testing for radon in homes and schools below the third floor.
  Its toxic effects have not been reported in high-rise dwellings.
- *Carbon monoxide:* Carbon monoxide is a by-product of the combus-
  tion of carbon fuels and is a colorless, odorless gas. Sources of carbon
  dioxide include gas space heaters, leaking chimneys, furnaces, gas water
  heaters, wood stoves, generators, and other gas-powered equipment,
  as well as automobile exhaust and tobacco smoke. Each year approximately 15,000 emergency department visits and 500 accidental deaths
  in the United States are attributed to accidental inhalation of CO. CO
  levels can be monitored at home with commercially available detectors.
  The Consumer Product Safety Commission (CPSC) recommends that a
  detector be located near the home sleeping areas to alert sleeping members in the event of elevated CO levels. The detector should not be placed
  within 15 feet of heating or cooking appliances or near very humid areas,
  such bathrooms.
- *Indoor mold:* Mold is ubiquitous in the outside environment and plays an
  important role in breaking down organic matter such as trees and leaves.
  The abundance of mold in the outside environment allows for easy
  transmission into the indoor environment. A small subset of mold from
  the indoor environment is known to cause immunoglobulin antibody

responses in humans. The keys to preventing potential harmful effects of mold exposure include both the identification of areas and removal of both mold- and moisture-rich environments. Mold can be successfully removed from hard, non-porous surfaces with simple detergents and water allowing complete drying. Porous areas including ceiling tiles and carpeting should be disposed of as the mold cannot be eliminated with cleaning alone.

- *Animal dander:* Animal dander is most commonly associated with allergies from the dead skins of animals such as cats, dogs, and other furred pets. Epidemiological studies have shown that sensitization to dog and cat allergens is strongly associated with asthma. Reducing exposure to animal dander may be accomplished by using HEPA filters, frequent bathing of the animal, or by removing the animal from the environment altogether.
- *Dust mites:* Dust mites are arthropods from the class of Arachnida that colonize bedding, sofas, carpets, and any other woven materials in the home. Dust mites are the most common allergens worldwide. It is not the mite itself, but its fecal particles that result in strong allergic response in up to 26% of Americans. Thus, mite allergens may worsen existing asthma. A variety of control measures may be implemented to lower the risk of dust mites, including frequent vacuuming and removal of stuffed animals from bedrooms, frequent washing every two weeks of bedding in hot water, and removal of upholstered furniture.
- *Cockroaches:* Cockroaches are a common occurrence in the urban environment and play an important role in poor indoor air quality and the development of asthma in the inner city. Techniques to reduce cockroach antigens involve controlling humidity, improving indoor sanitation, and implementing both chemical and non-chemical extermination.
- *Mice:* Mice and the allergens they release pose a significant health risk for both urban and rural indoor air quality. The most effective way to limit mice impact is to prevent or reduce the chance of exposure. The use of rodent proof construction, improved sanitation, and population control of mice using traps and chemicals may reduce exposure.
- *Electronic cigarettes:* In recent years, there has been a significant gain in the popularity of electronic cigarettes, especially among youth. This is partially due to the perception that they are safer than combustible cigarettes. Based on CDC data in 2016, 3.2% of U.S. adults currently use E-cigarettes. Clinically, E-cigarettes may cause bronchitis symptoms, especially in adolescents. Since a number of individuals have developed severe lung problems from E-cigarettes and there have even been deaths due to E-cigarette use, this is an area of active research. The FDA has delayed rules to regulate E-cigarettes until August 2022, however, the Federal Government and many states have barred flavored E-cigarettes and vaping since flavored cartridges have been associated with increased likelihood of abuse among children and adolescents.

9.9 CONCLUSIONS

Lung problems, including shortness of breath, cough, and wheezing are common symptoms experienced by patients seeking medical care. In addition to various respiratory symptoms, there are very significant lung problems which are common in the U.S. population, including asthma, occupational environmental lung diseases, venous thromboembolic disease, and influenza. Also, indoor air quality can cause considerable health issues, including problems associated with secondhand smoke, carbon monoxide, indoor mold, and animal dander. For all these reasons, clinicians should take a careful history to determine if there are environmental hazards which are causing significant lung problems in patients.

9.10 PRACTICAL APPLICATIONS

- A variety of conditions may cause respiratory symptoms, including dyspnea, wheezing, and cough.
- Snoring and apnea have become increasingly common and are often associated with obesity.
- Asthma is common in the United States, with 8.3% of individuals suffering from this condition.
- For all these reasons, careful pulmonary history should be taken by all clinicians.

REFERENCES

1. Richards J, Schwartzstein R. *Respiratory Symptoms. Lifestyle Medicine* (3rd edition). CRC Press (Boca Raton), 2019.
2. Irwin R, Baumann M, Bolser D, et al. Diagnosis and Management of Cough Executive Summary: ACCP Evidence-Based Practice Guidelines. *Chest.* 2006;129(1 suppl) suppl:1S–23S.
3. Jean-Baptiste E. Clinical Assessment and Management of Massive Hemoptysis. *Critical Care Medicine.* 2000;28:1642–1647.
4. Hollingsworth H. Wheezing and Stridor. *Clinics in Chest Medicine.* 1987;8:231–240.
5. Enright P, Newman A, Wahl P, et al. Prevalence and Correlates of Snoring and Observed Apneas in 5201 Older Adults. *Sleep.* 1996;19:531–538.
6. Centers for Disease Control and Prevention (CDC). Summary Health Statistics Tables for U.S. Adults: National Health Interview Survey(NHIS) Data, 2016. https://www.cdc .gov/nchs/fastats/asthma.htm. www.cdc.gov/nchs/fastats/asthma.htm. Accessed April Accessed July 6, 2020.
7. National Asthma Education and Prevention Program. Expert Panel Report III: Guidelines for the Diagnosis and Management of Asthma; *NIH Publication No. 07-4051,* 2007.
8. National Health Interview Survey. *Summary Health Statistics Tables for US Adults and Children: National Health Interview Survey,* 2015–2018.
9. Storms W. Asthma Associated with Exercise. *Immunology and Allergy Clinics of North America.* 2005;25:31–43.
10. Boulet L, O'Byrne P. Asthma and Exercise-Induced Bronchoconstriction in Athletes. *New England Journal of Medicine.* 2015;372:641–648.

11. Kwon H, Belanger K, Bracken M. Asthma Prevalence among Pregnant and Childbearing-Aged Women in the United States: Estimates from National Health Surveys. *Annals of Epidemiology.* 2003;13:317–324.

12. Tarlo S, Balmes J, Balkissoon R. et al. Diagnosis and Management of Work-Related Asthma: American College of Chest Physicians Consensus Statement. *Chest.* 2008;134 Supplement:1S–41S.

13. Vogelmeier C, Criner GJ, Martinez FJ. et al. Global Strategy for the Diagnosis, Management, and Prevention of Chronic Obstructive Lung Disease 2017 Report. GOLD Executive Summary. *American Journal of Respiratory and Critical Care Medicine.* 2017;195:557–582.

14. Landis S, Muellerova h, Mannino D. et al. Continuing to Confront COPD International Patient Survey: Methods, COPD Prevalence, and Disease Burden in 2012–2013. *International Journal of Chronic Obstructive Pulmonary Disease.* 2014;9:597–611.

15. Suvatne J, Browning R. Asbestos and Lung Cancer. *Disease-a-Month.* 2011;57:55–68.

16. Leung C, Yu S, Chen W. Silicosis. *Lancet.* 2012;379:2008–2018.

17. Balmes J, Abraham J, Dweik R. et al. *An Official American Thoracic Society Statement: Diagnosis* and Management of Beryllium Sensitivity and Chronic Beryllium Disease. *American Journal of Respiratory and Critical Care Medicine.* 2014;190:e34–59.

18. Petsonk E, Rose C, Cohen R. Coal Mine Dust Lung Disease. New Lessons from Old Exposure. *American Journal of Respiratory and Critical Care Medicine.* 2013;187:1178–1185.

19. Schoene R. Illnesses at High Altitude. *Chest.* 2008;134:402–416.

20. Vasakova M, Morell F, Walsh S, et al. Hypersensitivity Pneumonitis: Perspectives in Diagnosis and Management. *American Journal of Respiratory and Critical Care Medicine.* 2017;196:680–689.

21. Belohlavek J, Dytrych V, Linhart A. Pulmonary Embolism II: Management. *Experimental and Clinical Cardiology.* 2013;18(2):139–147.

22. Scully G. *Influenza. Lifestyle Medicine* (3rd edition). CRC Press (Boca Raton), 2019.

23. Lagace-Wiens PR, Rubinstein E, Gumel A. Influenza Epidemiology—Past, Present, and Future. *Critical Care Medicine.* 2010;38(Suppl 4):e1–e9.

24. Sundell J. On the History of Indoor Air Quality and Health. *Indoor Air.* 2004;14(Suppl 7):51–58.

25. Campagna A, Desai D. *Indoor Air Quality. Lifestyle Medicine* (3rd edition). CRC Press (Boca Raton), 2019.

10 Obstetrics and Gynecology

KEY POINTS

- Lifestyle strategies impact in significant ways on a variety of issues related to women's reproductive health.
- Nutrition and lifestyle impact on the likelihood of conception as well as pregnancy outcomes.
- Regular exercise in pregnancy has been recommended by both the American Academy of Pediatrics (AAP) and the American College of Obstetrics and Gynecology (ACOG) as well as the Physical Activity Guidelines for Americans 2018 Scientific Report.
- All clinicians should be familiar with the ways that lifestyle practices and habits impact on women's reproductive health and counsel all women of reproductive age on these interactions.

10.1 INTRODUCTION

Lifestyle measures are very important in all phases of women's reproductive life and also in various health issues, including contraception, prevention screening and treatment of sexually transmitted infections, and reducing the risk of cancers. Lifestyle measures are also very important in the areas of menstrual disorders and menopause. Furthermore, lifestyle measures are also important in the decision of whether or not to breastfeed.

For all of these reasons, individuals who practice obstetrics and gynecology are natural allies in the area of lifestyle medicine. Many of these clinicians have become actively involved in the field of lifestyle medicine.

This chapter will explore some of the issues related to obstetrics and gynecology as they relate to lifestyle medicine. For more details, the interested reader is referred to the excellent section in the 3rd edition of *Lifestyle Medicine* edited by Dr. Amanda McKinney in the area of obstetrics and gynecology (1).

10.2 NUTRITION AND LIFESTYLE TO IMPROVE CONCEPTION AND PREGNANCY OUTCOMES

The live birth rate in the United States is 59.8 live births per 1,000 women aged 15–44 (2). This is the lowest live birth rate ever in the United States. There are a number of factors which may be contributing to low live birth rate, including contraception, delaying childbirth to older ages when the likelihood of becoming pregnant declines, and shift of cultural norms which place more importance on careers and self-fulfillment rather than the rearing of children.

It could also be argued that obesity and diabetes epidemics might also be factors contributing to the declining birth rate. As discussed in multiple chapters in this manual, there has been a steady rise in both obesity and diabetes since 1960. It is well established that maintaining a normal BMI helps retain reproductive capacity.

The likelihood of conceiving during any month of unprotected intercourse is about 20% when a woman is 30 years old and declines to about 5% by age 40, where only 30% of all conceptions actually result in a live birth (3,4). The Centers for Disease Control and Prevention (CDC) has generated data that 71% of adults aged 20 years and above are overweight or obese, which is likely to have affected the capacity for reproduction in various ways (5). Moreover, pregnancy outcomes are also adversely affected by obesity or diabetes.

10.2.1 OVULATORY INFERTILITY

Ovulatory infertility is directly related to polycystic ovarian syndrome (PCOS) (6). From a metabolic standpoint, PCOS represents the constellation of obesity, insulin resistance, and anovulation resulting in infertility, menstrual dysfunction, and hirsutism.

As women become obese, they typically become insulin resistant, which results in increases in circulating insulin that suppresses sex hormone binding globulin (SHBG). This results in free androgens and infrequent ovulation.

It has been estimated that about 30% of overweight and obese women have PCOS versus about 5% in normal-weight women (7).

Dietary behaviors which contribute to obesity and malnutrition are also linked to oxidative disturbances and chronic low-grade inflammation. In one study, consuming 5% of total energy intake from animal protein rather than carbohydrates was associated with a 19% greater risk of ovulatory infertility. There are some data that individuals with PCOS can achieve improved ovarian function with regular exercise which, in turn, improves the chances of conception.

10.2.2 PREGNANCY OUTCOMES

Lifestyle significantly impacts on both maternal and fetal outcomes. One aspect of this is maternal mortality. According to the CDC, the maternal mortality rate in 1915 was 608 deaths per 100,000 live births (8). By 1986, this had fallen to 8.5. Every year since, however, maternal mortality has increased. According to the WHO, the number is now closer to 28 maternal deaths per 1,000 live births. This makes the United States of having the highest maternal mortality rate among all industrialized nations and 60th among all nations. This increase in maternal mortality has partly been due to an increase in women with obesity, diabetes, and pre-pregnancy hypertension, all of which can lead to a variety of complications such as preeclampsia, stroke, and cardiomyopathy.

Preeclampsia is a constellation of signs and symptoms, including hypertension, proteinuria, and edema, and in severe cases, headache, elevated liver enzymes, pulmonary edema, and thrombocytopenia, which can ultimately lead to seizure, stroke, and death for both mother and infant. Within the United States, the incidence of preeclampsia has risen steadily over the past three decades, from 2.4% of pregnancies in 1980 to 3.8% of pregnancies in 2010.

Preeclampsia, like other cardiovascular diseases (CVD), is a result of endothelial dysfunction and inflammation of the blood vessels (9). Preeclampsia and hypertensive disease during pregnancy impact on material health acutely, but also increase the risk of chronic disease in the long term. For example, heart disease is eight times as likely for women who develop diabetes or high blood pressure during pregnancy. In the year after delivery, women with a hypertensive disorder of pregnancy had a 12–25-fold higher risk of hypertension than women with a normotensive pregnancy (10).

For all of these reasons, lifestyle measures discussed in multiple chapters of this book, including regular physical activity and nutrition, are very important for pregnant women. (See also Chapter 12.)

10.2.3 FETAL IMPACT OF MATERNAL LIFESTYLE

Maternal dietary patterns can also impact long-term fetal outcomes. For example, in one study, consumption of a high animal-protein, low-carbohydrate diet in pregnancy was associated with higher adult blood pressure in their offspring.

Fish consumption during pregnancy is also a subject of controversy. There is evidence that long chain fatty acid (DHA) is important for fetal development; however, increased exposure to DHA also leads to increased exposure to mercury, which is neurotoxic (11). Eating a single serving of fish per week during pregnancy results in infants having substantially more mercury in their bodies than they would acquire from as many as six mercury-containing vaccines. Mercury has a 75 day half-life, so for the body to rid itself of 99% of it requires one year. Fish may also have other industrial pollutants. Nonetheless, the current consensus guidelines recommend that women should consume 200 mg per day of DHA during pregnancy. The best way to obtain this is through consumption of algae-based oil, which is nutritionally equivalent to fish oil without contamination.

10.2.4 AUTISM

The incidence of autism spectrum disorders (ASD) has risen dramatically in the last 30 years. In 1981, the incidence was 1 in 10,000. In 2000, it was 1 in 150, and the most current estimate is 1 in 68 (12).

The causes of autism are not completely understood and are hotly debated. An article in the *New England Journal of Medicine* looked at the brains of children with autism who had died of unrelated causes and compared them to brains of unaffected children. It appeared that there were some changes in neuronal circuitry in the brains of children with autism (13). This study implied that abnormalities almost certainly occurred *in utero* during key developmental windows, most likely between 19 and 30 weeks of gestation. The cause of this finding is not known; however, it does appear that maternal inflammation may play a role.

Diseases which have an inflammatory component such as obesity and diabetes may contribute to autism. It has been argued that eating a plant-based diet can create a more favorable component of bacterial species in the gut. This may, in turn, reduce inflammation and oxidative stress. This is an area of active research.

10.3   EXERCISE IN PREGNANCY

Regular aerobic exercise during pregnancy has been repeatedly shown to improve or maintain physical fitness. Although the evidence is limited, there may be some benefits for pregnancy outcomes and no evidence of harm to contraindicate exercise for most pregnant women. The issue of exercise in pregnancy is discussed in more detail in the next section.

Both the CDC (14) and the ACOG (15) encourage regular physical activity during pregnancy since the benefits far outweigh the risks. The Physical Activity Guidelines for Americans 2018 Scientific Report also strongly urges pregnant women to exercise and recommends the level of 150 minutes of moderate intensity physical activity per week.

10.3.1   THE BENEFITS OF EXERCISE

10.3.1.1 Weight Management

As already mentioned, overweight and obesity have continued to increase in the United States. A greater percentage of women are currently entering pregnancy overweight or obese and many are gaining significantly more weight during pregnancy than is recommended. Excessive weight gain is an important predictor of adverse pregnancy outcome. Exercise during pregnancy has been shown to reduce excess weight gain and decrease weight retention postpartum. Many studies have shown that there are multiple benefits of exercise and weight management during pregnancy (16).

Postpartum weight retention is also strongly related to weight gain during pregnancy. In one study of women six months postpartum, women who had excessive weight gain during pregnancy weighed 12% more than they did pre-pregnancy (7.9 kg or 17.4 pounds more) (17). In contrast, women who gained weight at or below the recommended guidelines were only 5.7% heavier at six months postpartum (3.2 kg or 7.1 pounds). Thus, women who exercise during pregnancy are less likely to gain excessive weight during pregnancy and also less likely to retain a significant amount of extra weight in the postpartum time frame.

10.3.2   GLYCEMIC CONTROL

Gestational diabetes mellitus (GDM) is one of the most common pregnancy complications affecting approximately 7% of pregnancies in the United States. GDM (18) is highest among obese and overweight women. Exercise appears to lower the risk of

GDM. In one study, physical activity reduced the risk of GDM by 48% (19). Exercise can also be a component of the treatment for GDM.

10.3.3 REDUCTION OF RISK OF HYPERTENSIVE DISORDERS IN PREGNANCY

Hypertensive disorders occur in approximately 12–22% of pregnancies and are one of the leading causes of maternal mortality in the United States, accounting for 15–20% of maternal deaths (20,21). There are a few small studies that suggest that exercise lowers the risk of hypertension during pregnancy. This is an area of active research.

10.3.4 PSYCHOLOGICAL BENEFITS

Regular exercise during pregnancy may improve maternal mental health. This is important because prenatal depression occurs in approximately 11% of women and postpartum depression in up to 16% (22). Multiple aspects of physical activity have been hypothesized to improve mental health, including self-efficacy, social interaction, and improved body image. Women who engage in regular physical activity report increased vigor, decreased fatigue, less stress and anxiety, and decreased symptoms of negative mood and depression. For all these reasons, a regular exercise regimen seems to be a helpful tool in maintenance of emotional well-being both during pregnancy and postpartum.

10.3.5 OTHER BENEFITS

Women who exercise during pregnancy report that symptoms such as nausea, heart burn, leg cramps, varicose veins, constipation, and insomnia as well as musculo-skeletal discomfort decrease during pregnancy (23). Some studies have suggested that less medical intervention is required during pregnancy in women who exercise routinely during pregnancy.

10.3.6 RISKS OF EXERCISE DURING PREGNANCY

Limited data exists concerning risks of exercise during pregnancy. As already indicated, the guidelines from both the CDC and ACOG as well as PGA 2018 recommend moderate intensity physical activity during pregnancy. There is a small risk of spontaneous abortion, fetal distress, or low birth weight as well as preterm delivery and maternal injury (24). These issues are beyond the scope of this chapter and can be found in the ACOG Guidelines for Exercise during Pregnancy. As already indicated, the multiple potential benefits of exercise during pregnancy far outweigh the potential risks.

10.3.7 CONTRAINDICATIONS TO EXERCISE IN PREGNANCY

When discussing physical activity for a pregnant woman, it is important to discuss any factors that might adversely affect the woman's health and the health of the fetus. It has been argued that a previous history of sedentary lifestyle may be relative or even absolute contraindication to exercise during pregnancy. However, recent guidelines have suggested that when begun carefully, an exercise regimen in pregnancy is safe even for previously inactive women (25).

10.3.8 RECOMMENDATIONS FOR EXERCISE DURING PREGNANCY

The PAGA 2018 (14) and 2008 Physical Activity Guidelines recommend (26) the following four considerations for exercise during pregnancy:

1. Healthy women should get at least 150 minutes per week of moderate intensity physical activity per week during and after pregnancy. This should be broken up into 30 minutes per day, five days per week or similar durations.
2. For previously inactive women without medical contraindication to exercise, it is reasonable to begin moderate intensity exercise regimen.
3. For healthy women who regularly perform vigorous intensity aerobic activity, this can be continued during pregnancy as long as no adverse symptoms occur.
4. Pregnant women should not partake in activities involved in lying directly on one's back or increase the risk of falling or abdominal trauma.

Unfortunately, in the United States, only 16% of pregnant women comply with physical activity recommendations from ACOG and the CDC compared to 26% of non-pregnant women (27). Given the proven benefits of exercise in pregnancy, it is important for clinicians to educate and encourage women to participate in moderate physical activity during the course of their pregnancy.

10.4   BREASTFEEDING

Breastfeeding is a component of lifestyle that promotes health for both the mother and the baby (28). Clinicians and other health care providers play an important role in encouraging, teaching, and helping to manage breastfeeding.

Human breast milk is a physiological form of nutrition for infants and young children. Even though formula feeding is widespread worldwide, a significant body of literature and research strongly supports infant and maternal benefits from breastfeeding. Both ACOG and AAP state that breastfeeding ensures the best possible health outcomes for the child. Both of these organizations recommend exclusive breastfeeding for at least the first six months of life and continue breastfeeding as complementary foods are introduced to the infant's first year of life or longer if mutually desired by the women and her infant. The World Health Organization (WHO) endorses breastfeeding for the first two years of life. Healthy People 2020 guidelines establish a goal of 82% of babies to have been breastfed and a continuation rate of 61% at six months and 34% at one year.

10.4.1   MATERNAL BENEFITS

A lactating mother can expend about 500 kcals/day to produce breast milk; thus, a breastfeeding mother may lose more weight postpartum than a non-breastfeeding mother (29). In addition, data from the Nurses' Health Study also showed that parous women who had breastfed had a reduced risk of developing type 2 diabetes (T2DM). Similar findings were demonstrated in the Women's Health Initiative (WHI). WHI also showed that post-menopausal women with a period of lactation of more than 12 months had a lower prevalence of hypertension, diabetes, and CVD (30). Parous women who had never breastfed were 28% more likely to develop cardiovascular disease than women who had breastfed for 7–12 months.

10.4.2 INFANT BENEFITS

Human breast milk has the appropriate nutrients to supply a growing infant's needs. Extensive studies have shown both significant short- and long-term infant benefits from breastfeeding (31). These include decreased rates of chronic diseases and infectious diseases, improving neural development, and decreasing rates of childhood autoimmune diseases. Among the infant derived benefits from breast feeding are the improvement of the gut flora in the newborn's GI tract and a lower risk of infectious diseases due to immunological factors in breast milk (32). Atopic disease and asthma are also decreased in breastfed babies. A wide range of other diseases may be reduced in infants who are breastfed. In addition, there may be a benefit of neurodevelopment in infants breastfed, although this has been difficult to prove conclusively due to the multiple factors associated with cognitive development.

10.4.3 PRACTICAL MANAGEMENT OF BREASTFEEDING

The WHO has listed "Ten Steps to Successful *Breastfeeding*." These are found in Table 10.1 (33).

TABLE 10.1

Ten Steps to Successful Breastfeeding

1. Have a written breastfeeding policy that is routinely communicated to all health care staff
2. Train all health care staff in skills necessary to implement this policy
3. Inform all pregnant women about the benefits and management of breastfeeding
4. Help mothers initiate breastfeeding within 1 hour of birth
5. Show mothers how to breastfeed and how to maintain lactation, even if they are separated from their infants
6. Give newborn infants no food or drink other than breast milk, unless medically indicated (a hospital must pay fair market price for all formula and infant feeding supplies that it uses and cannot accept free or heavily discounted formula and supplies)
7. Practice rooming-in: allow mothers and infants to remain together—24 hours a day.
8. Encourage breastfeeding on demand
9. Give no artificial teats or pacifiers to breastfeeding infants
10. Foster the establishment of breastfeeding support groups and refer mothers to them on discharge from the hospital or clinic

Source: Adapted from *Evidence for the Ten Steps to Successful Breastfeeding* (Revised), Division of Child Health and Development, World Health Organization, Geneva, Switzerland, 1998.

10.4.4 ASSESSMENT OF INTAKE ADEQUACY

Infants typically lose 5–7% of body weight in the first 5 days of life. This weight is usually regained within two weeks. The AAP recommends a post-discharge hospital visit within 3–5 days of age for all breastfeeding infants. At this time, the infant should be weighed, breastfeeding practices can be assessed, and the mother can be instructed and encouraged.

10.4.5 WEANING

Timing for weaning can be a complex project, depending on multiple factors. The AAP recommends exclusive breastfeeding for six months,

with a gradual introduction of complementary iron-rich foods at six months. Breastfeeding should be continued for a least the first year of life and beyond as desired by both mother and infant.

10.5 CONTRACEPTION

The ability to plan and control reproduction is an essential part of a healthy lifestyle. There are a variety of different approaches to contraception and the risks and benefits associated with each method are important to understand. Despite the many choices available for contraception, unintended pregnancy remains a public health challenge in the United States. Despite decades of study and proposed interventions, a percentage of pregnancies that are mis-timed or unwanted remains 45–50%. Approximately half of the 6.1 million pregnancies in the United States in 2011 were unintended and 42% of these pregnancies ended in elective abortion (34). Interestingly, almost half of these pregnancies occurred among women who reported using some form of reversible contraception at the time of conception. The other half are among women who did not use any contraception even though they did not desire pregnancy. Multiple reasons for contraception failure include failure to adhere to the method, inappropriate use, lack of continuation of the method, inability to access the method regularly, or failure of the method itself.

The available options for contraception are beyond the scope of the current chapter; however, clinicians could individualize the care with each woman, including a discussion of the safety and efficacy of the following potential contraceptive methods (35):

- Combined oral contraceptive pills
- Transdermal contraceptive patch
- Progestin-only method
- Long-acting reversible contraception
- Nexplanon implant
- Intrauterine contraception (IUD)
- Emergency contraception
- Medication or copper IUD: both of these used shortly after unprotected intercourse or possible contraception failure

Women should be educated regarding the use of emergency contraception since it works best if taken as soon as possible after intercourse.

10.5.1 POSTPARTUM CONTRACEPTION

Methods include:

- Nexplanon implant
- IUD
- Sterilization (interrupt the patency of the fallopian tubes or vas deferens in men). These methods are considered permanent and are highly effective methods with a failure rate of less than 1%.

10.6 PREVENTION, SCREENING, AND TREATMENT OF SEXUALLY TRANSMITTED INFECTIONS

More than two million cases of syphilis, gonorrhea, and chlamydia were reported to the CDC in the United States in 2016 (36). This represents the highest number ever. In addition to these infections, many other infections also result in significant morbidity. Adolescents and adults aged 15–24 years are at the highest risk of acquiring STIs (37).

Education is critically important in the prevention of STIs. There are a number of methods for lowering the risk of STI (38):

- Contraceptive counseling
  The best contraceptive method for prevention of STIs continues to be the male condom.
- Vaccines
  One of the most effective means of preventing STIs is exposure immunization. Currently, there are vaccinations available for hepatitis A virus, hepatitis B virus, and human papilloma virus.
- Male circumcision
  By removing the foreskin and thus eliminating a moist environment where infection can proliferate, male circumcision significantly reduces the risk of HVP, HIV, and HSV transmission. Circumcision also reduced a man's risk for penile cancer and genital ulcer disease.

10.6.1 EDUCATION

10.6.1.1 Screening

The first step in screening for STIs is to take a thorough sexual history. This includes the following:

- Partners
- Practices

- Protection from STIs
- Past history of STIs and prevention of pregnancy

10.6.1.2 *Diagnosis and Treatment*

Anyone who has sexual contact is at risk for getting an STI. This includes men and women of all ages, ethnic backgrounds, regions, and economic levels. The best way to prevent getting an STI is not to have sexual contact. The following STIs are relatively common in U.S. population:

- *Chlamydia:* This is the most commonly reported STI in the United States with almost 1.6 million cases reported in 2016. Routine screening of both men and women is recommended for this STI.
- *Gonorrhea:* Gonorrheal infection is the second most common STI with over 800,000 new infections reported in the United States each year. As with chlamydia, most women with active gonorrheal infection are asymptomatic. Because there is increasing resistance to many antibiotics, the only regimen recommended for treatment of gonorrheal infection is dual therapy with 250 mg ceftriaxone intramuscularly plus 1 g of azithromycin orally.
- *Syphilis:* In 2016, there were over 27,000 cases of primary and secondary syphilis reported in the United States. Patients diagnosed with syphilis should be tested for HIV. The treatment for primary, secondary, or early latent syphilis is a single dose of 2.4 million units of intramuscular penicillin G.
- *Hepatitis A virus:* Hepatitis A is a self-limited disease which is primarily transmitted via the fecal oral route, but may also arise from oral anal sexual contact. Rates of hepatitis A have declined by more than 95% since the start of routine vaccination in 1995. It is estimated that 2,800 cases of hepatitis A in the United States in 2015.
- *Hepatitis B virus:* In 2014, there were 2,953 of acute cases of hepatitis B reported in the United States and 850 to 2–2.2 million people in the United States with chronic HBV. It is transmitted by percutaneous sexual and perinatal contact. In the United States, it is most commonly acquired in adolescents or young adulthood by IV drug use, sexual intercourse, or any contact that involves percutaneous or mucosal contact with infectious blood or bodily fluids.
- *Hepatitis C virus:* In 2014, there were 2,194 cases of acute hepatitis C. There are between 2.7 and 3.7 million citizens with chronic HCV infection. HCV affects the liver and is primarily spread through exposure to infected serum through IV drug use, hemodialysis, or blood transfusion.
- *Human immunodeficiency virus:* HIV was first recognized by the CDC in 1981. There were 37,600 new HIV infections in 2014 and 1.2 million persons living with HIV. HIV is transmitted by exposure to blood, vaginal secretions, semen, or breast milk as well as vertical transmission from mother to child. Testing for HIV is recommended once for people aged 13–64 who are at average risk. A number of effective antiviral regimens

have been approved. Because of these regimens, HIV has become a manageable chronic illness.

- *Herpes simplex virus:* Infection with HSV results in genital or labial herpes. One out of six people aged 14–49 has genital herpes. In the United States, 776,000 new cases of herpes are diagnosed each year. There is effective episodic treatment, prophylaxis, and suppression available for HSV. The patient should be treated with oral antiviral at the time of primary infection with a 7–10 day course of acyclovir 400 mg three times per day, valacyclovir 1,000 mg twice per day, or Famciclovir 250 mg three times per day.
- *Human papilloma virus:* HPV can cause cancer of the cervix, vulva, oropharynx, penis, anus, and vagina with an average of over 38,000 of HPV-related cancers diagnosed annually in the United States.

10.7 MENSTRUAL DISORDERS AND MENOPAUSE

A variety of menstrual disorders can be somewhat ameliorated by lifestyle habits and practices (39).

PCOS is a constellation of obesity, insulin resistance, and ovulation, which can result in infertility, menstrual dysfunction, and anovulation. PCOS affects approximately one in eight women in the United States.

A number of conditions besides PCOS can cause abnormal uterine bleeding (AUB). AUB is responsible for one third of all office visits to the gynecologist and approximately 5% of women aged 30–49 will consult a physician each year for treatment; additionally, approximately 30% of all women having had heavy bleeding (40). This can result in significant personal, societal, and economic impact. As already discussed, women with PCOS tend to have insulin resistance, dietary behaviors that may result in obesity, and nutrition as well as oxidative disturbances and chronic low-grade inflammation. One study has linked these issues to consumption of animal protein.

10.7.1 MENOPAUSE

Menopause is defined as literally the end of monthly menstrual cycles. From a medical standpoint, menopause is typically defined as a woman who has had no vaginal bleeding for one year. The age at which menopause occurs varies widely ranging from the late 30s to late 50s. The range of age for most women being 48–55 years.

Perimenopause transition typically lasts for about four years. Estrogen declines during menopause; however, the balance of risks and benefits for hormonal replacement in healthy menopausal women remain uncertain. Vaginal estrogens for local urogenital symptoms appear to be safe.

Other treatment options commonly employed to help reduce vasomotor symptoms of menopause include phytoestrogen such as soy. Current studies utilizing soy have been inconclusive. Some studies evaluating vasomotor symptoms observe a significant placebo effect of up to 30% reduction in hot flashes in the placebo group. Therefore, longer clinical trials are necessary to evaluate the sustainability and affects. Soy may play some role in reducing ovarian cancer. In a large prospective analysis of 46,000 post-menopausal women, those in the highest quintile of soy consumption had a 26.7% reduced risk of endometrial cancer. A 2008 meta-analysis confirmed this and also revealed a 38% lower risk of ovarian cancer in those women consuming the most soy.

10.8 RISK REDUCTION AND SCREENING FOR WOMEN'S CANCERS

Cancer is the second leading cause of death for women in the United States. The World Cancer Research Fund estimates that 20% of all cancers diagnosed in the United States are caused by a combination of excess body weight, physical inactivity, excess alcoholic consumption, and poor nutrition; thus, many of these could be prevented (41). As many as 40–60% of all cancers in women are preventable with lifestyle modifications. Diet and lifestyle impact on the development of breast and endometrial and cervical cancers to a large degree and ovarian cancer to a lesser degree. All of these cancers and the background information on them are discussed in more detail in Chapter 7.

10.9 CONCLUSIONS

Many of the issues in the area of obstetrics and gynecology relate strongly to various lifestyle decisions and practices such as nutrition, weight management, and physical activity. Since many women see their obstetrician or gynecologist as their primary care provider, it is important that individuals in these subspecialties are aware of lifestyle modalities. In addition, all clinicians should be familiar with how lifestyle practices and habits impact on pregnancy, breastfeeding, contraception, sexually transmitted infections, menstrual disorders, and menopause as well as risk factor reduction and screening for women's cancers.

10.10 CLINICAL APPLICATIONS

- Various lifestyle habits and practices such as proper nutrition and exercise significantly impact on women's reproductive health.
- Regular exercise of moderate intensity before and during pregnancy carries multiple benefits for women.
- All clinicians should counsel women of reproductive age and also during menopause concerning the multiple interactions between lifestyle factors and women's obstetric and gynecological health.

REFERENCES

1. Rippe JM. *Lifestyle Medicine* (3rd edition). CRC Press (Boca Raton), 2019.
2. Martin JA, Hamilton BE, Ventura SJ, Osterman MJ, Wilson EC, Mathews TJ. Births: Final Data for 2010. *National Vital Statistics Reports*. 2012;61(1):1–72.

3. Zinaman MJ, Clegg ED, Brown CC, O'Connor J, Selevan SG. Estimates of Human Fertility and Pregnancy Loss. *Fertility and Sterility.* 1996;65:503–509.
4. Ford H, Schust D. Recurrent Pregnancy Loss: Etiology, Diagnosis, and Therapy. *Reviews in Obstetrics and Gynecology.* 2009;2:76–83.
5. http://www.cdc.gov/obesity/data/adult.html. Accessed July 6, 2020.
6. Mehrabian F, Afghani M. Can Sex-Hormone Binding Globulin Considered as a Predictor of Response to Pharmacological Treatment in Women with Polycystic Ovary Syndrome? *International Journal of Preventive Medicine.* 2013;4:1169–1174.
7. Alvarez-Blasco F, Botella-Carretero JI, San Millán JL, et al. Prevalence and Characteristics of the Polycystic Ovary Syndrome in Overweight and Obese Women. *Archives of Internal Medicine.* 2006;166:2081–2086.
8. Say L, Chou D, Gemmill A, et al. Global Causes of Maternal Death: A WHO Systematic Analysis. *Lancet Global Health.* 2014;2:e323–e333.
9. Steegers EA, von Dadelszen P, Duvekot JJ, et al. Pre-Eclampsia. *Lancet.* 2010;376:631–644.
10. Behrens I, Basit S, Melbye M. Risk of Post-Pregnancy Hypertension in Women with a History of Hypertensive Disorders of Pregnancy: Nationwide Cohort Study. *BMJ.* 2017;358:j3078.
11. Zeilmaker M, Hoekstra J, van Eijkeren J, et al. Fish Consumption during Child Bearing Age: A Quantitative Risk-Benefit Analysis on Neurodevelopment. *Food and Chemical Toxicology.* 2013;54:30–34.
12. Developmental Disabilities Monitoring Network Surveillance Year 2010 Principal Investigators; Centers for Disease Control and Prevention (CDC). Prevalence of Autism Spectrum Disorder among Children Aged 8 Years—Autism and Developmental Disabilities Monitoring Network, 11 Sites, United States, 2010. *MMWR Surveillance Summaries.* 2014;63(2):1–21.
13. Stoner R, Chow M. Boyle M, et al. Patches of Disorganization in the Neocortex of Children with Autism. *New England Journal of Medicine.* 2014;370:1209–1219.
14. *2018 Physical Activity Guidelines Advisory Committee Submits Scientific Report.* Office of Disease Prevention and Health Promotion (Washington, DC), 2018.
15. The American College of Obstetrics and Gynecology. https://www.acog.org/patient-r esources/faqs/pregnancy/exercise-during-pregnancy. Accessed July 6, 2020.
16. Clapp J, Little K. Effect of Recreational Exercise on Pregnancy Weight Gain and Subcutaneous Fat Deposition. *Medicine & Science in Sports & Exercise.* 1995;27(2):170–177.
17. Gore SA, Brown DM, Smith DS. The Role of Postpartum Weight Retention in Obesity among Women: A Review of the Evidence. *Annals of Behavioral Medicine.* 2003;26(2):149–159.
18. American Diabetes Association. Gestational Diabetes Mellitus. *Diabetes Care.* 2004;27(Suppl 1):S88–S90.
19. Dempsey JC, Butler CL, Sorensen TK, et al. A Case-Control Study of Maternal Recreational Physical Activity and Risk of Gestational Diabetes Mellitus. *Diabetes Research and Clinical Practice.* 2004;66:203–215.
20. Bung P, Bung C, Artal R, Khodogiuan N, Fallenstein F, Spatling L. Therapeutic Exercise for Insulin-Requiring GDM. Results from a Randomized Prospective Longitudinal Study. *Journal of Perinatal Medicine.* 1993;21:125–137.
21. ACOG. Practice Bulletins Number 33. Diagnosis and Management of Preeclampsia and Eclampsia. *International Journal of Gynecology & Obstetrics.* 2002;77: 67–75.
22. O'Hara M, Swain A. Rates and Risk of Postnatal Depression: A Meta-Analysis. *International Review of Psychiatry.* 1996;8:37–54.

23. Wang S, Zinno P, Fermo L, et al. Complementary and Alternative Medicine for Low Back Pain in Pregnancy: A Cross Sectional Survey. *Journal of Alternative and Complementary Medicine.* 2005;104:65–70.

24. Hjollund N, Jensen T, Bonde J, et al. Spontaneous Abortion and Physical Strain around Implantation: A Follow-Up Study of First Pregnancy Planners. *Epidemiology.* 2000;11(1):18–23.

25. Cavalcante S, Cecatti J, Periera R, et al. Water Aerobics II: Maternal Body Composition and Perinatal Outcomes after a Program for Low Risk Pregnant Women. *Reproductive Health.* 2009;6:1. doi: 10.1186/1742-4755-6-1

26. Physical Activity for Everyone: Healthy, Pregnant or Post-Partum Women, Physical Activity Guidelines for Americans, 2018. https://www.cdc.gov/physicalactivity/basics /pregnancy/index.htm#:~:text=Pregnant%20or%20postpartum%20women%20should ,this%20activity%20throughout%20the%20week. Accessed July 6, 2020.

27. Peterson A, Leet T, Brownson R. Correlates of Physical Activity among Pregnancy Women in the United States. *Medicine & Science in Sports & Exercise.* 2005;37:1748–1753.

28. Head J, Jones S, Richardson M. Breast-Feeding. In: Rippe J, ed., *Lifestyle Medicine* (3rd edition). CRC Press (Boca Raton), 2019.

29. Butte N, Wong W, Hopkinson J. Energy Requirements of Lactating Women Derived from Doubly Labeled Water and Milk Energy Output. *Journal of Nutrition.* 2001;131:53–58 [PubMed: 11208938].

30. Schwarz E, Ray R, Stuebe A, et al. Duration of Lactation and Risk Factors for Maternal Cardiovascular Disease. *Obstetrics & Gynecology.* 2009;113:2601–2610 [PMID: 19384111].\

31. Heinig MJ. Host Defense Benefits of Breastfeeding for the Infant. Effect of Breastfeeding Duration and Exclusivity. *Pediatric Clinics of North America.* 2001;48:105–123.

32. Glass RI, Stoll BJ. The Protective Effect of Human Milk against Diarrhea. A Review of Studies from Bangladesh. *Acta Paediatrica Scandinavica.* 1989;351:131–136.

33. World Health Organization, Division of Child Health and Development. *Evidence for the Ten Steps to Successful Breastfeeding (Revised).* World Health Organization (Geneva, Switzerland), 1998.

34. Facts on Induced Abortion in the United States. The Guttmacher Institute. https://ww w.guttmacher.org/fact-sheet/induced-abortion-united-statesClick here to enter text.. Accessed July 6, 2020.

35. Carlson K, Haider S. Contraception. In: Rippe J, ed., *Lifestyle Medicine* (3rd edition). CRC Press (Boca Raton), 2019.

36. Santelli J, Grilo S, Lindberg L. et al. Abstinence-Only-Until-Marriage Policies and Programs: An Updated Position Paper of the Society for Adolescent Health and Medicine. *Journal of Adolescent Health.* 2017;61(3):400–403. doi: 10.1016/j. jadohealth.2017.06.001.

37. Clark LR, Jackson M, Allen-Taylor L. Adolescent Knowledge about Sexually Transmitted Diseases. *Sexually Transmitted Diseases.* 2002;29(8):436–443.

38. Carlson K. Prevention, Screening and Treatment of Sexually Transmitted Infections. In: Rippe J, ed., *Lifestyle Medicine* (3rd edition). CRC Press (Boca Raton), 2019.

39. McKinney A. Menstrual Disorders and Menopause. In: Rippe J, ed., *Lifestyle Medicine* (3rd edition). CRC Press (Boca Raton), 2019.

40. ACOG. Practice Bulletin #128 "Diagnosis of Abnormal Uterine Bleeding in Reproductive-Aged Women". *Obstetrics & Gynecology.* 2012;120:197–206.

41. McKinney A, Tran Janco J. Risk Reduction and Screening for Women's Cancers. In: Rippe J, ed., *Lifestyle Medicine* (3rd edition). CRC Press (Boca Raton), 2019.

11 Lifestyle Medicine and Brain Health

KEY POINTS

- Brain health has become an area of considerable research with multiple, new understandings.
- Risk factors for decline in brain health and cognition are similar to risk factors for cardiovascular disease.
- Lifestyles modalities such as regular physical activity, healthy nutrition, and stress reduction as well as social interactions can all play significant roles in maintaining cognition and other aspects of optimal brain health.

11.1 INTRODUCTION

A healthy brain is essential for a fulfilling life. Many lifestyle measures play particularly important roles in maintaining brain health. Multiple aspects of brain health will be discussed in this chapter.

Cognitive function is one component of brain health which is essential for maintaining quality of life (QoL) and functional independence, and is a very important component of the aging process. As life expectancy continues to increase in developed countries, the numbers of individuals over the age of 65 will undoubtedly increase dramatically over the next 15–20 years. Currently, it has been estimated that there are 47 million people with dementia worldwide and this is projected to increase to 75 million individuals by 2030 and 131 million individuals by 2050 (1).

There is a particularly strong link between brain health and cardiovascular health. This essential fact is underscored by the Presidential Advisory from the American Heart Association (AHA) and the American Stroke Association (ASA) on "Defining Optimal Brain Health in Adults" (2).

It is clear that positive lifestyle measures play essential roles in maintaining healthy cognition throughout the lifetime. Poor lifestyle factors may compromise brain health and are also associated with poor cardiovascular health. These include uncontrolled hypertension, diabetes mellitus (T2DM), obesity, physical inactivity, smoking, and depression (3). All of these conditions have been shown to be potentially ameliorated to some degree by positive lifestyle measures. Many of these lifestyle measures are included in the seven areas to achieve optimal brain health from the AHA and the ASA. These seven factors will be discussed in some detail in this chapter.

It is also important to stress that many of the manifestations of the spectrum of cognition, ranging from diminished cognition to dementia, occur in individuals in their 50s and 60s and beyond. Playing close attention to risk factors throughout a lifetime is important. This further underscores the importance of lifestyle measures. The recently released Physical Activity Guidelines for Americans 2018 Scientific Report also emphasizes the multiple roles that increased physical activity plays in brain health (4). Benefits of physical activity for brain health are prominent throughout the lifespan and will be emphasized in this chapter.

11.2 COGNITIVE IMPAIRMENT AND DEMENTIA

Sustaining brain health and cognition over a lifetime is critically important to allow individuals to maximize overall functional ability and independence. Maintaining brain health also helps reduce the risk of diversion of economic and health care resources for care and treatment. Poor brain health can ultimately manifest as cognitive impairment or dementia. These underlying disorders include Alzheimer's disease (AD), strokes, and other causes of vascular cognitive impairment, brain trauma, and other neurodegenerative disorders. It has been estimated that in the United States, 2.9 million people are living with dementia. This is the second largest number of individuals with dementia, second only to China, where there is an estimated 5.4 million people with dementia.

Modifiable risk factors for poor cardiovascular health are also relevant to risk factors for dementia and include uncontrolled hypertension, diabetes mellitus, obesity, physical inactivity, smoking, and depression. In addition to dementia, it has been estimated that one in eight adults over the age of 60 have memory loss and that approximately 35% of individuals in this age range report functional difficulties (5). In addition, it is estimated there are 5.1 million individuals in the United States aged 65 and above who have AD. This is predicted to rise to 13.2 million in 2050.

Cognitive impairment and dementia, as well as AD, are among the most expensive conditions to treat with, direct care expenses being greater than for cancer and equal to those of heart disease (6). Direct costs of cognitive impairment are only a portion of the total financial loss. For example, in 2011, more than 15 million Americans spent on average 21.9 hours per week caring for family members with dementia and these costs may actually be more than the direct cost of dementia itself (7). Furthermore, caregivers can experience significant declines in their quality of life. In addition, dementia and cognitive impairment may undercut effective treatment for some concurrent illnesses.

11.3 CARDIOVASCULAR AND STROKE RISK

Cardiovascular disease (CVD) remains the leading cause of mortality in the United States. Risk factors for CVD and stroke are common in the U.S. population. Over 100 million people in the United States (approximately 40% of adults) have hypertension and in over half of these individuals' blood pressure is not controlled (8). Risk factors for both heart disease and brain health also include diabetes mellitus (T2DM) and obesity, both of which have risen significantly in the United States over the past 30 years. Smoking is also a significant risk factor for both heart disease and stroke. Given that these modifiable risk factors are shared for heart disease and stroke and decreased brain function, strategies to ameliorate these risk factors can play a significant role in brain health.

11.4 OPTIMAL BRAIN HEALTH

Most definitions of brain health emphasize the absence of overt or vascular or neurodegenerative injuries such as stroke or AD. Optimal brain health extends this concept to include optimal capacity to function and adapt to the environment (2). This includes cognition as well as lowering the risk of many other insults to the brain such as stroke.

Optimal brain health, including brain function, depends on many of the energy-intensive activities in the brain. This, in turn, depends on vascular supply to the brain. There is very little energy reserve within the brain. Thus, normal brain function is highly dependent on delivery of oxygen and glucose, which are, in turn, delivered by cerebral blood flow. All of these depend on both cardiovascular and cerebral vascular health.

There are multiple parallels between cardiovascular and cerebrovascular health and brain health. Aging has profound effects on multiple physiologic systems, including the structure and function of the cerebral vascular system. Furthermore, age-related alterations in various organs such as the liver, kidneys, lung, and immune systems can also have secondary deleterious effects on the brain. Conversely, brain dysfunction may lead to adverse effects on the CV system. Therefore, the health of the brain is inextricably related to both cardiovascular and cerebrovascular health.

According to the Presidential Advisory from the AHA and ASA, optimal brain health is defined as "optimal capacity to function adaptively in the environment." This encompasses multiple competencies, including the ability to pay attention, perceive, recognize sensory input, to learn and remember, to solve problems and make decisions, to have mobility, and to regulate emotional states. All of these domains are ultimately attributable to functions of the brain. Furthermore, bodily functions such as sleep, continence, and appetite are also affected by the brain.

Thus, brain health impacts on an enormous number of other health-related parameters, which, in turn, are clearly associated with various lifestyle habits and practices. For example, according to the Physical Activity Guidelines for Americans 2018 Scientific Report (PAGA 2018), the level of physical activity profoundly affects the level of cognition (4). Furthermore, physical activity improves various biomarkers of brain health, including neurotropic factors, task-evoked brain activity, volume, and connectivity. Furthermore, physical activity lowers the risk of impaired cognitive function.

11.5 BRAIN HEALTH ACROSS THE LIFESPAN

Many brain disorders tend to become manifest later in life, but, in fact, just like risk factors for cardiovascular disease, they are established throughout the life course. For example, the risk of stroke, which becomes more prevalent in the fifth and sixth decades of life, depends not only on blood pressure at the time of these strokes, but also accumulated levels of blood pressure throughout life. This makes interventions focused on modifiable risk factors and protective factors important to modify even in young adulthood and perhaps even as far back as childhood.

An intriguing body of information exists about the role of physical activity throughout the lifespan with the development of what researchers have called "cognitive reserve." These investigators have argued that the primary effect of physical activity and exercise on the human brain is to build cognitive reserve (9). Cognitive reserve is hypothesized as the capacity of the mature brain to sustain function and resist the effects of disease or injury sufficient to cause decline in cognition or clinical dementia. It has been suggested that individuals who experience these declines have less cognitive reserve than individuals who do not and that physical activity helps to build and maintain this cognitive reserve. Cognitive reserve is further classified as either active reserve or passive reserve. The former refers to the efficiency and adaptability of neuro-circuits to respond to cognitive challenge, as exemplified by compensation and use of other parts of the brain. The concept of passive reserve refers to structural anatomic processes such as density of brain tissue, white matter integrity, and vascularity.

There is also a very strong association between brain health and the concept of QoL. This concept relates to the way that individuals perceive and react to their health status for non-medical aspects of their life. The relationship of various components of lifestyle, including stress reduction and physical reaction, is strong. This is particularly true in older adults (i.e., over the age of 50, and primarily over the age of 65). There is also strong evidence that individuals aged 18–65 who participate in regular physical activity improve health-related QoL compared to no physical activity.

11.6   RISK FACTORS

There is considerable interest and research in the area of how to achieve healthy brain aging and reduce the risk of stroke and cognitive decline. For example, T2DM has been associated with cognitive impairment and dementia presumably through potential mechanisms, including vascular and neuronal damage as well as diminished cerebral blood flow. Smoking is also highly correlated with risk of cognitive decline and dementia. Obesity, dyslipidemia, and high blood pressure also contribute to decreased vascular brain health. Adherence to healthy dietary patterns such as the Mediterranean (10) or DASH Diet (11) has been associated with reduced cognitive decline. Some evidence has suggested that obesity and hypertension are associated with cognitive decline, although the exact mechanisms remain uncertain.

Multiple studies have shown that levels of physical activity are strongly related to cognitive health outcomes (2,4). There is strong evidence that acute responses to vigorous physical activity yield transient benefits for various domains of cognition such as memory, processing speed, and executive control. These findings are particularly true in children and older adults. There is also evidence for chronic effects of moderate and vigorous physical activity, particularly in individuals over the age of 50, related to improved cognition. There is further evidence that physical activity can improve diminished cognition related to such diseases as attention-deficit hyper-activity disorder, schizophrenia, multiple sclerosis, Parkinson's disease, and stroke (4). The most dramatic improvements in cognitive function associated with physical activity have been shown to involve executive function. Multiple studies supporting the relationship between physical activity and improved cognition have been sum-marized in the PAGA 2018 Scientific Report.

11.7 METRICS FOR DEFINING OPTIMAL BRAIN HEALTH

In the Presidential Advisory from the AHA and ASA, the core concept for defin-ing risk factors for declining brain health utilizes the AHA's "Life's Simple 7" (12). The reason for utilizing this framework is that these parameters are common in their impact on both brain health and cardiovascular health. Furthermore, these are factors that, to a large extent, can be measured and can be modified through life-style decisions. The following seven factors are listed as components of both optimal brain health and Life's Simple 7:

1. *Manage Blood Pressure*

    High blood pressure is a major risk factor for heart disease and stroke. When your blood pressure stays within healthy range, you reduce the strain on your heart, arteries, and kidneys, which keeps you healthier longer.

2. *Control Cholesterol*

    High cholesterol contributes to plaque, which can clog arteries and lead to heart disease and stroke. When you control your cholesterol, you are giv-ing your arteries their best chance to remain clear of blockages.

3. *Reduce Blood Sugar*

    Most of the food we eat is turned into glucose (or blood sugar) that our bodies use for energy. Over time, high levels of blood sugar can damage your heart, kidneys, eyes, and nerves.

4. *Get Active*

    Living an active life is one of the most rewarding gifts you can give yourself and those you love. Simply put, daily physical activity increases your length and quality of life.

5. *Eat Better*

    A healthy diet is one of your best weapons for fighting cardiovascular disease. When you eat a heart-healthy diet, you improve your chances of feeling good and staying healthy—for life!

6. *Lose Weight*

    When you shed extra fat and unnecessary pounds, you reduce the burden on your heart, lungs, blood vessels, and skeleton. You give yourself the gift of active living, you lower your blood pressure, and you help yourself feel better, too.

7. *Stop Smoking*

    Cigarette smokers have a higher risk of developing cardiovascular dis-ease. If you smoke, quitting is the best thing you can do for your health.

(https://www.heart.org/en/healthy-living/healthy-lifestyle/my-life-check--lifes-simple-7)

There are other factors that impact on brain health. These include education and literacy that may be mediated by higher socioeconomic conditions, which, in turn, influence healthy aging and lifestyle choices. In addition to educational level, the quality of education in early life also is known to contribute to cognitive outcomes later in life (13,14). Other factors have been studied, including air pollution, but results have not been consistent and therefore are typically not considered as a metric for optimal brain health.

11.8 MAINTENANCE OF BRAIN HEALTH

There are multiple longitudinal observational studies that show that lifestyle-related factors such as blood pressure control, T2DM, dyslipidemia, weight management, and smoking appear to influence the trajectory of optimal brain health. In the PREDIMED Study, individuals who were randomized into the Mediterranean Diet had modestly better cognition after four years compared to the control diet group (15). In the FINGER Study (16), individuals randomized to exercise, cognitive training, and coaching for vascular risk reduction, as well as adherence to the Mediterranean Diet, had a better cognitive performance at two years with particular emphasis on improvement in executive function. It should be noted that some studies have had neutral results with regard to maintenance of cognition. It has been speculated that a number of these studies only employed lifestyle measures for a period toward the end of life. This suggests that prevention of risk factors in the first place appears to be a more effective strategy for improving brain health, when compared to later in life interventions.

11.9 PHYSICAL ACTIVITY, ANXIETY AND DEPRESSION, AND STRESS REDUCTION

Anxiety, depression, and stress are all endemic in the modern, fast-paced world. Lifestyle interventions have been demonstrated to play an effective role in ameliorating all three of these conditions.

- *Anxiety:* Within mental health disorders, anxiety is the most common. The overall prevalence of anxiety disorders in the population has been reported as over 30%. Regular physical activity has been demonstrated in multiple studies to lower both state anxiety and trait anxiety (17). State anxiety has been shown to be reduced immediately following a single session of exercise, while trait anxiety appears to require training periods of at least ten weeks. The studies which have explored anxiety typically utilize 30 minutes of moderate intensity physical activity per session.
- *Depression* (18): Depression is also quite common, with a lifetime risk of significant depression of 10% in the U.S. population. Even in the absence of significant depressive disorders, the symptoms of depression can negatively

influence health and quality of life. Physical activity has been repeatedly shown to decrease symptoms of depression. Typical levels of physical activity employed in research in this area have involved at least 30 minutes of moderate intensity physical activity performed on a regular basis.

- *Stress* (19): Stress is quite common in the modern society. Some estimates have suggested that more than 30% of individuals have enough stress in their daily lives to hinder their performance at home or at work. Multiple lifestyle medicine modalities have been demonstrated to be effective for stress reduction, including regular physical activity, mindfulness meditation, and others. These issues are dealt with in more detail in Chapter 4.

11.10 SLEEP

Sleep is an underestimated component of brain health. Sleep is an important determinant of health and well-being across the lifespan, and multiple lifestyle factors play important roles in sleep. Sleep is essential for biological function and also important for neural development, learning, memory, and emotional regulation of cardiovascular and metabolic health (20).

Three meta-analyses and three systematic reviews have all reported positive effects of greater amounts of physical activity on one or more aspects of sleep, including total sleep time, sleep efficiency, sleep quality, daytime sleepiness, insomnia, and obstructive sleep apnea (OSA). These results from physical activity have been demonstrated across the lifespan, including beyond middle age and older men and women.

Improvements in sleep also carry significant public health impact. Approximately 10% of adults suffer from clinically diagnosed insomnia and 26% of adults between the ages of 30 and 70 years suffer from OSA. The prevalence of OSA appears to be rising since the major risk factor for this condition is obesity. Weight loss is a highly effective treatment for OSA. In addition to specific disorders, 25% of the population reports getting inadequate sleep on at least 15 out of every 30 days and 25–48% of the population reports sleep problems of some kind.

Sleep problems are also associated with multiple health issues, including CVD risk factors, obesity, stroke, and all-cause mortality. In addition, sleep issues impact significantly on motor vehicle accidents. The National Highway Traffic Safety Administration estimates that 2.5% of fatal vehicle accidents and 2% of non-fatal accidents involve drowsiness while driving. Other estimates suggest that the estimate may be as high as 15–33%. Issues related to risk factors for both heart disease and improved brain health have the potential for improving multiple aspects of sleep.

11.11 FUTURE DIRECTIONS

The Presidential Advisory from the AHA and ASA also anticipates that there will be future research to expand components of optimal brain health. For example, there is a limited, but increasing body of knowledge related to childhood exposures that later affect cognition. Intrauterine and early life exposures may also play important roles in neurocognitive development, as may stress in early life. These factors are subject to ongoing research and will undoubtedly be included in future considerations of defining and enhancing optimal brain health. Optimal brain health is also an important component of successful aging for not only CVD risk but also other components of this emerging concept. (See also Chapter 16 for further discussion of the components for successful aging.)

11.12 CONCLUSIONS

Optimal brain health is a key component of all stages of the lifespan. Optimal brain health predicts quality of life, functional independence, and risk of institutionalization in the older population. Advances in understanding of risk factors for optimal brain health have concluded that many of the same risk factors for declining cognition are shared between brain health and risk of cardiovascular disease. As the population continues to age, issues related to maintenance of healthy cognition and also decreasing the risk of dementia, including Alzheimer's disease, will become increasingly important. Lifestyle factors play an important role in virtually every aspect of optimizing brain health.

11.13 PRACTICAL APPLICATIONS

- Risk factors for heart disease and declines in brain health are similar. Thus, both of these considerations should be part of every patient encounter.
- Lifestyle measures such as increased physical activity, healthy nutrition, and stress reduction are all key components of maintaining a high level of cognition.
- Clinicians should discuss brain health with patients on every encounter.
- Lifestyle measures also are important for reducing the risk of dementia, including Alzheimer's disease.
- Risk factors for decreased brain health are similar to those of CVD risk and are summarized by the American Heart Association's "Life's Simple 7" framework.

REFERENCES

1. Winblad B, Amouyel P, Andrieu S, et al. Defeating Alzheimer's Disease and Other Dementias: A Priority for European Science and Society. *Lancet Neurology.* 2016;15:455–532.
2. Gorelick P, Furie K, Iadecola C, et al. Defining Optimal Brain Health in Adults: A Presidential Advisory from the American Heart Association/American Stroke Association. *Stroke.* 2017;48(10):e284–e303.
3. Gorelick P, Scuteri A, Black S, et al. on behalf of the American Heart Association Stroke Council, Council on Epidemiology and Prevention, Council on Cardiovascular Nursing, Council on Cardiovascular Radiology and Intervention, and Council

on Cardiovascular Surgery and Anesthesia. Vascular Contributions to Cognitive Impairment and Dementia: A Statement for Healthcare Professionals from the American Heart Association/American Stroke Association. *Stroke.* 2011;42:2672–2713.

4. Physical Activity Guidelines Advisory Committee. *2018 Physical Activity Guidelines Advisory Committee Scientific Report.* U.S. Department of Health and Human Services (Washington DC), 2018.

5. Centers for Disease Control and Prevention (CDC). Self-Reported Increased Confusion or Memory Loss and Associated Functional Difficulties among Adults Aged ≥60 Years −21 States, 2011. *Morbidity and Mortality Weekly Report.* 2013;62:347–350.

6. Hurd M, Martorell P, Delavande A, et al. Monetary Costs of Dementia in the United States. *New England Journal of Medicine.* 2013;368:1326–1334.

7. Alzheimer's Association. 2013 Alzheimer's Disease Facts and Figures. *Alzheimers Dement.* 2013;9:208–245.

8. Merai R, Siegel C, Rakotz M, et al. CDC Grand Rounds: A Public Health Approach to Detect and Control Hypertension. *Morbidity and Mortality, Weekly Report* 2016;65:1261–1264.

9. Kayes M, Hatfield B. The Influence of Physical Activity on Brain Aging and Cognition: The Role of Cognitive Reserve, Thresholds for Decline, Genetic Influence, and the Investment Hypothesis. In: Rippe JM, ed., *Lifestyle Medicine* (3rd edition). CRC Press (Boca Raton), 2019.

10. Shai I, Schwarzfuchs D, Henkin Y, et al. Weight Loss with a Low-Carbohydrate, Mediterranean, or Low-Fat Diet. *New England Journal of Medicine.* 359:229–241.

11. The DASH Diet Eating Plan. http://dashdiet.org/default.asp. Accessed June 25, 2020.

12. American Heart Association. Life's Simple 7®, 2010. https://www.heart.org/en/profe ssional/workplace-health/lifes-simple-7. Accessed July 6, 2020.

13. Alley D, Suthers K, Crimmins E. Education and Cognitive Decline in Older Americans: Results from the AHEAD Sample. *Research on Aging.* 2007;29:73–94.

14. Cagney KA, Lauderdale DS. Education, Wealth, and Cognitive Function in Later Life. *Journals of Gerontology, Series B: Psychological Sciences and Social Sciences.* 2002;57:P163–P172.

15. Estruch R, Ros E, Salas-Salvadó J, et al. Primary Prevention of Cardiovascular Disease with a Mediterranean Diet. *New England Journal of Medicine.* 2013;368:1279–1290.

16. Ngandu T, Lehtisalo J, Solomon A, et al. A 2 Year Multi-Domain Intervention of Diet, Exercise, Cognitive Training, and Vascular Risk Monitoring versus Control to Prevent Cognitive Decline in At-Risk Elderly People (FINGER): A Randomised Controlled Trial. *Lancet.* 2015;385:2255–2263.

17. Gaudlitz K, von Lindengerger B, Strohle A. Physical Activity and Anxiety. In: Rippe JM, ed., *Lifestyle Medicine* (3rd edition). CRC Press (Boca Raton), 2019.

18. Fair K, Rethorst C. Physical Activity and Depression. In: Rippe JM. *Lifestyle Medicine* (3rd edition). CRC Press (Boca Raton), 2019.

19. Loiselle E, Mehta D, Proszynski J. Behavioral Approaches to Manage Stress. In: Rippe JM, ed., *Lifestyle Medicine* (3rd edition). CRC Press (Boca Raton), 2019.

20. Physical Activity Guidelines Advisory Committee. *2018 Physical Activity Guidelines Advisory Committee Scientific Report.* U.S. Department of Health and Human Services. Brain Health (Washington, DC). 2018;F3-1–F3-49.

12 Women's Heath

KEY POINTS

- Physical activity, healthy nutrition, weight management, and avoiding tobacco products all profoundly impact on lowering the risk of various chronic diseases in women.
- Despite the abundance of evidence, less than half of physicians currently counsel women patients on the importance of lifestyle measures such as physical activity and maintenance of a healthy body weight during routine visits.
- Only 20% of physicians recognize that heart disease is the leading cause of death in women.

12.1 INTRODUCTION

A number of lifestyle factors play critically important roles in enhancing women's health. For example, both coronary heart disease (CHD) and type 2 diabetes (T2DM) are significantly impacted by lifestyle factors. In addition, various cancers are impacted by lifestyle factors such as physical activity and nutrition. Weight management and obesity are other areas of interaction between lifestyle factors and both weight gain and adiposity. An increasing array of factors such as brain health and cognition, as well as bone health and osteoporosis, also have strong interactions with various lifestyle factors (1).

Physical activity, nutrition, and weight management are also very important both during pregnancy and in the postnatal period. However, these factors will not be considered in this chapter. They have already been considered in Chapter 10.

This chapter will focus on lifestyle factors such as physical activity, nutrition, obesity, and weight management, as well as cigarette smoking—there is abundant evidence that these factors play a significant role in both prevention and treatment of chronic conditions.

12.2 PHYSICAL ACTIVITY

Regular physical activity conveys multiple benefits for women throughout the lifespan (2). These benefits range from reducing the likelihood of dying from multiple causes to reducing specific risk factors for coronary heart disease (CHD) obesity, diabetes (T2DM), and certain cancers. Cognition and affect and other aspects of brain health can also be improved in women by regular physical activity throughout the lifespan.

Multiple organizations, including the American Heart Association (AHA) (3), Physical Activity Guidelines for Americans 2008 (PAGA 2008) (4) and 2018 (PAGA 2018) (5), and the American College of Sports Medicine (ACSM) (6), have all issued guidelines and recommendations for regular exercise. These guidelines involve 30 minutes of moderate intensity physical activity on most days or perhaps intense physical activity of at least 25 minutes two to three days per week. The PAGA 2018 recommends 150 minutes of moderate intensity physical activity per week and two strength training sessions per week. Unfortunately, only approximately 28% of women exercise enough to meet these basic guidelines and 41% engage in no physical activity at all (3).

Aerobic activity has been the focus of most research on health benefits for women. Resistance exercise, however, may also confer healthy benefits, particularly in the area of bone density and musculoskeletal function (7). Yet only 17.5% of women engage in strength training at least twice a week, which is recommended by the current guidelines.

Multiple risk factors which are related to lifestyle decisions also significantly impact on the likelihood of developing chronic diseases, including coronary heart disease (CHD) and type 2 diabetes (T2DM). For example, the Nurses' Health Study demonstrated that 84% of all CHD and 91% of T2DM could be eliminated if women followed five simple practices: regular physical activity (30 minutes on most days), maintain a healthy weight (BMI <25 kg/m^2), follow sound nutritional practices (e.g., more fruits and vegetables, whole grains, and several fish meals per week), do not smoke cigarettes, and consume only moderate amounts of alcohol (one alcoholic beverage per day) (8). In this section, we will focus attention on the benefits of physical activity.

12.2.1 ALL-CAUSE MORTALITY

Multiple studies have shown inverse relations between physical activity and all-cause mortality. PAGA 2008 Scientific Report estimated a 30% decrease in all-cause mortality when comparing the least to most active individuals. Further decreases were noted in the PAGA 2018 Scientific Report.

Even individuals who engage in physical activity for only 30 minutes per week achieve a 20% decrease in all-cause mortality. Individuals who exercise 1.5 hours per week have a further 30% reduction in all-cause mortality.

Recent studies using accelerometers showed a 60–70% reduction in risk factors for heart disease in women when comparing the lowest to highest levels of physical activity (9). A meta-analysis of 22 cohort studies involving 643,000 women and 335,000 men who performed 2.5 hours per week of moderate intensity physical activity experienced a 19% reduction in all-cause mortality compared to less active individuals (10). Those who performed 30 minutes of moderate activity on a daily basis reduced their mortality by 24%. These findings were duplicated in the National Institutes of Health (NIH) AARP Diet and Health study which involved 253,000 women. In this study, those who engaged in moderate intensity physical activity of 3 hours or greater per week experienced a 27% decrease in mortality compared to those with no physical activity (11). It should be noted that a number of studies have also shown that time spent in sedentary living represents an independent risk factor for all-cause mortality (12). Those who were involved in sedentary occupations yet managed to maintain recommended levels of physical activity were able to substantially ameliorate this risk.

12.2.2 CORONARY HEART DISEASE

Physical activity plays a substantial role in reducing the risk of CHD in women (12). This is important since CHD is the leading cause of death in women.

Since women tend to get serious manifestations of heart disease such as myocardial infarction (MI) and sudden cardiac death at a later age than men, women who develop CHD have a significantly worse prognosis than men. Unfortunately, in a national survey of physician awareness of CHD prevention in women, fewer than one in five physicians knew that more women than men die each year of CHD (1). Multiple studies have shown that 30 minutes per day of moderate intensity physical activity substantially lowers the risk of CHD in women. This includes Women's Health Initiative Observational Study where brisk walking for two hours per week, or approximately 30 minutes five times per week resulted in a 30% reduction in cardiovascular events over a 3.2 year follow-up (13). Multiple other studies have shown similar reductions in CHD based on moderate intensity aerobic activity.

In addition to aerobic physical activity, women who engage in resistance training more than 30 minutes per week are 23% less likely to develop CHD over an eight-year period. Yet, unfortunately, only 17.5% of women engage in strength training at this level (14).

12.2.3 PHYSICAL ACTIVITY, TYPE 2 DIABETES, AND PREDIABETES

A number of studies have demonstrated that regular physical activity lowers the risk of T2DM in women. In the Women's Health Study, participants who reported walking 2–3 hours per week were 34% less likely to develop T2DM over a 7-year period compared to those who reported not walking. Multiple other studies have yielded similar responses (15).

A number of effects of regular physical activity undoubtedly contribute to reducing the progression to T2DM. These include lowering body weight, increasing insulin sensitivity, improving glycemic control, lowering blood pressure, improving lipid profile, enhancing endothelial function, and yielding more effective inflammatory defense systems (16). In addition, regular physical activity in prediabetes lowers the risk of developing diabetes. This was demonstrated in both the Diabetes Prevention Program (DPP) (16) and the Finnish Diabetes Study (17). More details about the relationship between physical activity and diabetes in both men and women may be found in Chapter 6.

12.2.4 WEIGHT CONTROL

Regular physical activity is an important component of weight loss programs and very significant in lowering the risk of weight gain in healthy women. Numerous studies have documented that both caloric restriction and physical activity play important roles in long-term maintenance of weight loss (18). More details concerning the link between physical activity and reducing the risk of weight gain and obesity may be found in Chapter 8.

12.2.5 CANCER

Physical activity has been shown to significantly reduce the risk of multiple cancers in women. As a result of this, the American Cancer Society and PAGA 2018 Scientific Report both recommend 30 minutes of moderate to vigorous physical intensity activity five or more times per week. Both the World Cancer Research Fund and the American Institute of Cancer Research (WCRF/AICR) noted that regular physical activity yields significant reductions in the prevalence and risk of 13 different cancers including breast, endometrial, and colon cancers in women (19).

12.2.6 BREAST HEALTH

In addition to lowering the risk of breast cancer, physical activity improves other aspects of breast health and creates positive body image (20). Regular exercise can lower body weight, which, in turn, reduces the risk of breast cancer due to overweight and obesity.

12.2.7 BRAIN HEALTH/COGNITIVE FUNCTION

Physical activity has been associated with multiple aspects of improved cognitive function and brain health throughout the lifespan in women (21–23). In 2009, a meta-analysis of 16 prospective studies reported individuals at the highest level of physical activity experience a 28% reduction in the risk of dementia and 46% reduction in the risk of Alzheimer's disease compared to individuals in the lowest activity category (24). Regular physical activity is particularly associated with improvements in executive function as well as improved affect, including a lower risk of both depression and anxiety (25).

12.2.8 PREGNANCY AND POSTPARTUM

Physical activity yields multiple benefits during pregnancy and postpartum. For this reason, both the American College of Obstetrics and Gynecology (ACOG) and the PAGA 2018 Scientific Report recommend regular physical activity for women who are pregnant. This is discussed in more detail in Chapter 10.

12.2.9 MENOPAUSE

Regular physical activity may be an important component of both physical and psychological well-being during menopause. Individuals in menopause who participate in regular physical activity report more energy and a better sense of well-being. In addition, as already discussed, aerobic exercise is well known for yielding multiple benefits, including lowering the risk of cardiovascular disease (CVD), T2DM, weight gain, and obesity (26).

12.2.10 BONE HEALTH/OSTEOPOROSIS

Regular weight-bearing exercise is important for ongoing bone health. A number of randomized controlled trials (RCTs) have assessed the relationship between physical activity and bone mineral density (BMD) in women. In 2011, a meta-analysis of 43 such trials in post-menopausal women showed slower bone loss of 3.2% in the vertebral column and 1% in the hip (27). Both of these are highly significant. The mechanism for reduction in risk of osteoporosis appears to be related to increasing bone strength and also lowers the risk of falls.

12.2.11 PHYSICAL ACTIVITY AND BODY COMPOSITION

Physical activity also carries multiple benefits for improving body composition. Studies have shown that regular physical activity improves lean muscle and reduces adiposity (28). Muscular strength with regular activity also enhances physical independence and the ability to perform activities of daily living and enjoy recreational pursuits. Regular activity such as resistance strength training also helps prevent age-related loss of muscle and reduces the risk of muscle frailty.

12.3 NUTRITION

Recent studies have focused more on the whole diet and dietary patterns rather than on single nutrient or food. The dietary patterns that have been recommended by a variety of organizations include increased whole grains, unsaturated omega-3 fatty acids, nuts, legumes, fish, poultry, and an abundance of fruits and vegetables with a minimal intake of refined grains, sugar-sweetened beverages, and red meat.

These dietary patterns have been shown to lower the risk of CVD and other conditions such as T2DM. Food patterns that fit into these recommendations include the Mediterranean Diet (29), the U.S. Healthy Foods Diet (30), and the DASH diet (31). The Lyon Diet Heart Study showed that the Mediterranean style diet resulted in a 72% lower risk of recurrent MI for cardiac death with a mean follow-up for 3.8 years compared to a control diet (32). A study of the DASH diet showed that it resulted in significantly lower blood pressure in individuals with hypertension.

The Nurses' Health Study compared a "prudent" diet recommended by the American Heart Association versus a typical "Western" dietary pattern on the development of CVD and T2DM (33). The prudent pattern featured higher intakes of fruits, vegetables, legumes, fish, poultry, and whole grains, whereas the Western pattern had higher intakes of red and processed meats, sweets and desserts, French fries, and refined grains. The Western diet pattern was associated with a higher risk of CHD by 46% and T2DM by 49% over 14–16 years of observation. There is a high level of consistency among diets for overall health and cardiovascular health.

These guidelines are summarized in the recommendations from the AHA Dietary Guidelines 2006 (34).

12.3.1 FRUITS AND VEGETABLES

Health authorities uniformly recommend five or more servings of fruits and vegetables on a daily basis. Most U.S. adults do not meet this guideline. For example, only 36% of women eat at least two servings of fruit daily and only 32% eat at least three servings of vegetables (men are even less likely to eat fruit and vegetables. The likelihood for fruit and vegetable consumption in men is 29% and 22%, respectively). A meta-analysis from 13 prospective cohort studies on 278,000 participants with a mean follow-up of 11 years found that people who regularly eat the required amount of fruits and vegetables were substantially at lower risk of developing CHD by about 17% (35). Similar data are available for stroke with a 26% reduction for individuals who ate the recommended servings of fruits and vegetables.

It has also been suggested that fructiferous and green leafy vegetables as well as citrus fruit and juices are particularly protective against CVD and ischemic stroke. Fruits and vegetables, particularly those that are deeply colored (e.g., spinach, carrots, peaches, and berries), contain numerous compounds, including folate, potassium, flavonoids, phytoestrogens, and antioxidants. Vitamin C, E, carotenoids, fiber, and many other phytochemicals may contribute to their protective effect.

12.3.2 CARBOHYDRATES

Multiple expert organizations have recommended that within the area of carbohydrates, individuals should choose whole grain, high-fiber foods. These foods are typically classed as "low glycemic index" and have been shown to lower the risk of both CHD and stroke, particularly among overweight and obese women (36). Prospective cohort studies show a significant inverse association between intake of whole grains and fiber and the risk of CVD. A pooled analysis from ten cohort studies in the United States and Europe which followed 245,000 women and 91,000 men for six to ten years showed that for each 10 g/day increment of dietary fiber, there was a 14% decrease in risk of coronary events and a 27% decrease in the risk of coronary mortality. Prospective studies have also shown that whole grains or cereal fiber protect again T2DM. A recent meta-analysis of data from nine large prospective cohort studies with follow-up of 6–16 years showed that the risk of diabetes was reduced by 33%, which is related to a higher intake of cereal fiber but not fruit and vegetable fiber (37). Whole grains improve insulin sensitivity and glucose metabolism as well as blood pressure, LDL cholesterol, and endothelial function.

12.3.3 DIETARY FATS

The American Heart Association recommends to "limit intake of saturated fat to less than 7% mg, trans fat to less than 1% of energy and cholesterol to less than 300 mg/day." Dietary intervention trials indicate that replacing saturated fat with polyunsaturated fat is likely to be more effective than reducing total fat intake for CHD risk reduction (37). Polyunsaturated fat exerts a beneficial influence on blood lipids, insulin sensitivity, and inhibition of thrombosis and also increases the threshold for ventricular fibrillation.

In a 20-year follow-up from the Nurses' Health Study, polyunsaturated fat intake lowered the risk of CHD by 25% after adjustment for dietary and other factors. Substituting unsaturated for saturated fat also increases insulin sensitivity in some small intervention trials in individuals with T2DM.

While several studies suggest a decrease for CHD in women, caution should be observed since there was no significant inverse association between polyunsaturated fat and T2DM except in lean men. In the large Women's Health Initiative Dietary Modification Trial, total fat consumption comparing 20% of calories from fat along with increased fruit and vegetable intake to greater than five servings per day, and grain intake to greater than six servings per day when compared to the "usual diet" did not lower the risk of CHD or stroke after eight years of follow-up (38).

Trans fat is an industrially produced fat generated by partial hydration of vegetable oils and has typically represented 2–3% of total calorie consumption in the United States. The major sources of trans fat are deep-fried fast foods, French fries, some bakery products, and some packaged snack foods. A number of dietary trials have shown that trans fats have significantly unfavorable effects on blood lipids, including lowering HDL-C and raising LDL-C (39). The current recommendation is to not exceed 1% of calories from trans fat.

12.3.4 FISH

The American Heart Association recommends that individuals "consume fish, especially oily fish, at least twice per week." The results of most observational trials indicate that healthy women and men who eat fish which contains polyunsaturated omega-3 fatty acids EPA and DHA experience significant reductions in CVD. In some studies, daily fish oil supplements have also been shown to lower the risk of CHD (40). Based on this evidence, the AHA has recommended that CHD patients consume a gram a day of EPA or DHA. Since this translates into more than one fish meal per day, fish oil supplements may be a more realistic way to comply with this recommendation.

12.3.5 SALT

The AHA and other authorities recommend restricting sodium intake to less than 2,300 mg (this translates to one teaspoon of salt per day) (41). Some organizations have recommended that the optimal may be no more than 1,500 mg per day particularly in individuals at high risk for hypertension. The average consumption for men and women combined in the United States is 3,400 mg per day and for women is 3,000 mg per day, about 80% of which is found in canned and processed foods and restaurant meals (42). There are some data to suggest that these levels of consumption may be more beneficial in terms of reduction of CHD than the more restrictive recommendations from the American Heart Association. Thus, this is an area where there is considerable scientific debate.

12.3.6 ALCOHOL

The American Heart Association recommends: "if you consume alcohol, do so in moderation" (43). It is well known that heavy alcohol use increases the risk of cardiovascular mortality, while moderate daily consumption of alcohol provides protection against CHD, ischemic stroke, and T2DM in both men and women. Some studies have shown that moderate alcohol consumption reduces coronary risk factors by 30–50% among moderate drinkers compared to non-drinkers (44). The protective effect of alcohol does not depend on the type of alcoholic beverage consumed.

The recommendations are for men to not consume more than two alcoholic drinks per day or women one alcoholic drink per day. It has been postulated that the antioxidant value of bioflavonoids in red wine increases its potential to reduce CVD risk. However, epidemiological data do not support this contention.

Experimental and observational data suggest that 50% of the CHD risk reduction attributed to alcohol is explained by increases in HDL-C. Some studies have also shown alcohol reduces platelet activation and aggregation and improves insulin sensitivity. It should be noted, however, that the anti-clotting effects of alcohol may translate into an increased risk of hemorrhagic stroke.

Even at moderate levels, alcoholic consumption has also been linked in some studies to increased risk of breast cancer and higher risk for colorectal and esophageal cancers. Finally, women are more susceptible to alcoholic liver disease and ethanol-induced cardiomyopathy than are men, likely due to differences in alcoholic metabolism and absorption (45). The final recommendation is that women (or men) who do not drink, do not begin to do so in an effort to prevent CHD ischemic stroke or type 2 diabetes.

12.3.7 SUGAR-SWEETENED BEVERAGES

Sugar-sweetened beverages are the largest single source of calories in the U.S. diet contributing to 7% of total energy intake (46, 47). The AHA recommends that individuals "minimize intake of beverages and food with added sugars." In the Nurses' Health Study, regular consumers of sugar-sweetened soft drinks were significantly more likely to develop type 2 diabetes than individuals who did not consume sugar-sweetened beverages. This pattern held true even when controlling for potential increases in weight. There is some controversy related to the findings of sugar-sweetened beverages with some investigators maintaining that sugar-sweetened beverage consumption is a marker for an unhealthy lifestyle rather than direct negative consequences of the sugar-sweetened beverage per se.

12.3.8 VITAMIN SUPPLEMENTS

Randomized trials in both primary and secondary prevention settings indicate that antioxidant vitamin supplements are ineffective in reducing the risk of CVD and type 2 diabetes and should not be taken for these purposes (46). Whether a daily multi-vitamin is useful for primary prevention is being tested in the ongoing Physicians' Health Study in middle-aged and older men.

12.4 OBESITY AND WEIGHT MANAGEMENT

Overweight and obesity are very prevalent in both men and women in the United States and in many other countries around the world. Between 1980 and 2004, the prevalence of obesity among U.S. adults doubled. In 2006, it was estimated that 35% of women were obese and 62% of U.S. women were overweight or obese (48). Excess weight is a major risk factor for a variety of metabolic diseases, including CVD and T2DM.

It used to be thought that adipocytes were largely a reservoir for excess fat; however, it is now clear that they are metabolically very active. In particular, obesity has been demonstrated to increase inflammation, insulin resistance, and elevations of thrombotic markers such as fibrinogen and plasminogen activator inhibitor-1. Among inflammatory markers increased with excess adipose tissue are interleukin-6 (IL-6), tumor necrosis factor-alpha (TNF-α), and c-reactive protein.

12.4.1 CORONARY HEART DISEASE

CHD risk increases as people gain weight and are overweight or obese. In fact, risk of CHD starts to increase rapidly after a BMI of >22 kg/m^2. In the Nurses' Health Study, even in the healthy weight range, there was an increased risk of CHD (49). Relative risks continue to increase with increasing degrees of overweight; relative risk is over six times as high for people who are obese with a BMI >31 compared to individuals with a BMI of 22 (50). Many long-term cohort studies have shown a strong relationship between excess weight and CHD.

In addition, weight gain is also associated with an increased risk of CHD. Compared with women who are stable weight, women who gain 5–7.9 kg were 25% more likely to develop CHD compared to those who were stable weight, and those who gained more than 20 kg were 2.65 times as likely to develop CHD. In other words, CHD risks increased by 3.1% for every kilogram gained.

Regional distribution of fat also impacts on cardiovascular risk. Adipose tissue in the waist, abdomen, and upper body is more metabolically active than the hip, thigh, or buttocks (51). Abdominal fat accumulation is an important predictor for dyslipidemia, hypertension, T2DM, and CHD. This is because abdominal fat cells appear to be more metabolically active than those in the buttocks or thighs.

12.4.2 STROKE

Despite the fact that increased weight increases blood pressure, lipids, and blood glucose, the relationship between weight gain, obesity, and stroke is not as clear as it is for CHD.

A 14-year follow-up of 235,000 middle-aged Korean male civil service workers showed that for each one unit increase in BMI, there was a significant 6% increase in ischemic stroke risk and a 2% increase in hemorrhagic stroke risk.

12.4.3 Type 2 Diabetes

Obesity leads to insulin resistance and compensatory hyperinsulinemia, which has been implicated in T2DM. Abdominal obesity is particularly worrisome. The dramatic increase in obesity in U.S. adults has been accompanied by a 61% increase in diabetes over the past 20 years (52). Of the five lifestyle variables, obesity, physical inactivity, poor diet, current smoking, and alcohol abstinence, which were examined in the Nurses' Health Study, excess body weight was, by far, the most predictive in the onset of type 2 diabetes (53). The risk of developing diabetes over 16 years in follow-up was 40-fold higher in women with a BMI of >35 and 20-fold higher in women with a BMI of >30–34.9 compared to women with a BMI ≤23. Even BMI in women in the high normal range (23.0–23.9) was associated with a threefold increase in diabetes compared to women with a BMI of <23 (54). Other studies have found similar results.

In addition, weight gain during adulthood was also significantly associated with the risk of diabetes (55). In NHANES data, individuals who gained between 5.0 and 7.9 kg over the preceding decade experienced the doubling of risk of diabetes over a nine-year period compared to weight-stable counterparts (56) Those who gained ≥20 kg had a fourfold increase.

Intentional weight loss either through calorie restriction or combined with physical activity improves glucose levels and insulin action among individuals with type 2 diabetes and lowers diabetes risk among overweight individuals. Weight loss in the Diabetes Prevention Program (DPP) study and the Finnish Diabetes Study showed that weight loss and increased physical activity significantly lower the risk of prediabetes turning into diabetes.

12.5 CIGARETTE SMOKING

An enormous body of scientific literature shows that cigarette smoking leads to adverse health consequences. Cigarette smoking is the leading preventable cause of death in the United States (57). Even though cigarette smoking has decreased in both men and women in the past two decades, unfortunately, 15.5% of adults still smoke a pack per day of cigarettes (58). Unfortunately, one in five high school students is a cigarette smoker (59). Cigarette smoking significantly increases the risk of coronary heart disease, stroke, and T2DM. The adverse consequences of cigarette smoking are well known and handled in detail in multiple other documents and will not be described in detail in this chapter.

12.6 PROMOTING HEALTHY LIFESTYLES: THE ROLE OF HEALTH CARE WORKERS

Cardiometabolic diseases with significant a lifestyle component are major causes of morbidity and mortality among U.S. women and men. While there has been some increased level of physical activity and better control of cholesterol and blood pressure, unfortunately, the prevalence of both obesity and T2DM have sharply increased.

It is now estimated that 80–85% of all diseases in the United States and in other developed countries have a lifestyle component. For this reason, it is imperative that clinicians counsel every patient on the important role of regular physical activity, healthy nutrition, weight management, and avoiding tobacco products.

Unfortunately, only one in three adults who saw a physician in the past year were counseled about physical activity and less than half of obese individuals who went to their physicians for a routine checkup received advice about weight loss. In addition to counseling individual patients, clinicians should also work to encourage government, community, and workplace policies that promote healthy weight, increase in physical activity, and disease prevention.

12.7 CONCLUSIONS

The role of positive lifestyle measures is critically important for multiple aspects of women's health. Enormous data exist in support that physical activity can lower the risk of coronary artery disease, T2DM, and cancer in women. Regular physical activity is also important for weight control, breast health, brain health, and bone health. Healthy nutrition, including increased consumption of fruits and vegetables, healthy carbohydrates (whole grains and fiber), polyunsaturated fats, and no more than moderate consumption of alcohol are also associated with positive health benefits. Both obesity and weight gain significantly increase the risk of heart disease and T2DM. For all of these reasons, it is imperative that clinicians focus on multiple lifestyle interventions to preserve the health of all women that they see.

12.8 CLINICAL APPLICATIONS

- Clinicians should counsel every female patient during every visit about the powerful health-promoting benefits of a number of lifestyle measures.
- Increased physical activity lowers the risk of multiple diseases, including coronary heart disease, T2DM, and cancer in women.
- Regular physical activity also improves brain health and cognition.
- Healthy nutrition, including more fruits and vegetables, whole grains and fiber, healthy fats (polyunsaturated), fish, and no more than moderate consumption of alcohol are all important lifestyle-related, health-promoting nutritional factors and should be stressed in every clinical visit.
- Both adult weight gain and obesity are associated with an increased risk of heart disease and T2DM in women and should be addressed at every clinical visit.

REFERENCES

1. Bassuk S, Manson JE. Lifestyle and Risk of Cardiovascular Disease and Type 2 Diabetes in Women: A Review of the Epidemiologic Evidence. *American Journal of Lifestyle Medicine*. 2008;2:191–213.

2. Rippe J. *Lifestyle Medicine Physical Activity and Health in Rippe J: Increasing Physical Activity: A Practical Guide.* CRC Press (Boca Raton) 2020.

3. The American College of Obstetricians and Gynecologists. https://www.acog.org/Abou t-ACOG/ACOG-Departments/Deliveries-Before-39-Weeks/ACOG-Clinical-Guidelin es?IsMobileSet=false. Accessed July 6, 2020.

4. U.S. Department of Health and Human Services. 2008 Physical Activity Guidelines for Americans, 2008. https://health.gov/paguidelines/2008/. Accessed July 6, 2020.

5. Physical Activity Guidelines Advisory Committee. *2018 Physical Activity Guidelines Advisory Committee. 2018 Physical Activity Guidelines Advisory Committee Scientific Report. Women Who Are Pregnant or Postpartum.* U.S. Department of Health and Human Services (Washington, DC), 2018.

6. American College of Sports Medicine. *2018 Guidelines for Exercise Testing and Prescription* (10th edition). Wolters Kluwer (Philadelphia), 2018.

7. Gregg W, Cauley J, Seeley D, et al. Physical Activity and Osteoporotic Fracture Risk in Older Women. Study of Osteoporotic Fractures Research Group. *Annals of Internal Medicine.* 1998;129:81–88.

8. Liu S, Stampfer M, Hu F, et al. Whole-Grain Consumption and Risk of Coronary Heart Disease: Results from the Nurses' Health Study. *American Journal of Clinical Nutrition.* 1999;70:412–419.

9. Lee I, Shiroma E, Evenson K, et al. Accelerometer-Measured Physical Activity and Sedentary Behavior in Relation to All-Cause Mortality: The Women's Health Study. *Circulation.* 2018;137:203–205.

10. Woodcock J, Franco O, Orsini N, et al. Non-vigorous Physical Activity and All-Cause Mortality: Systematic Review and Meta-Analysis of Cohort Studies. *International Journal of Epidemiology.* 2011;40:121–138.

11. Hamer M, Chida Y. Walking and Primary Prevention: A Meta-Analysis of Prospective Cohort Studies. *British Journal of Sports Medicine.* 2008;42:238–243.

12. Patel A, Bernstein L, Deka A, et al. Leisure Time Spent Sitting in a Relation to Total Mortality in a Prospective Cohort of US Adults. *American Journal of Epidemiology.* 2018;172:419–429.

13. Manson J, Greenland P, LaCroix A, et al. Walking Compared with Vigorous Exercise for the Prevention of Cardiovascular Events in Women. *New England Journal of Medicine.* 2002;347:716–725.

14. Tanasescu M, Leitzmann M, Rimm EB, et al. Exercise Type and Intensity in Relation to Coronary Heart Disease in Men. *JAMA.* 2002;288:1994–2000.

15. Weinstein A, Sesso H, Lee I, et al. Relationship of Physical Activity vs. Body Mass Index with Type 2 Diabetes in Women. *JAMA.* 2004;292:1188–1194.

16. Knowler W, Barrett-Connor E, Fowler S, et al. Diabetes Prevention Program Research Group. Reduction in Incidence of Type 2 Diabetes with Lifestyle Intervention or Metformin. *New England Journal of Medicine.* 2002;346:393–403.

17. Tuomilehto J, Lindstrom J, Eriksson J, et al. Prevention of Type 2 Diabetes Mellitus by Changes in Lifestyle among Subjects with Impaired Glucose Tolerance. *New England Journal of Medicine.* 2001;344:1343–1350.

18. Centers for Disease Control and Prevention. Adult Obesity Facts, 2018. https://www .cdc.gov/obesity/data/index.html. Accessed September 2, 2020.

19. World Cancer Research Fund and the American Institute for Cancer Research. *Food, Nutrition, Physical Activity and the Prevention of Cancer: A Global Perspective.* American Institute for Cancer Research (Washington, DC), 2007.

20. Dupree B. Breast Health: Lifestyle Modification. In: Rippe JM. *Lifestyle Medicine* (2nd edition). CRC Press (Boca Raton), 2013.

21. Kramer A, Erickson K, Colcombe S. Exercise, Cognition, and the Aging Brain. *Journal of Applied Physiology*. 2006;101:1237–1242.
22. Weuve J, Kang JH, Manson JE, et al. Physical Activity, Including Walking, and Cognitive Function in Older Women. *JAMA*. 2004;292:1454–1461.
23. Yaffe K, Barnes D, Nevitt M, et al. A Prospective Study of Physical Activity and Cognitive Decline in Elderly Women: Women Who Walk. *Archives of Internal Medicine*. 2001;161:1703–1708.
24. Hamer M, Chida Y. Physical Activity and Risk of Neurodegenerative Disease: A Systematic Review of Prospective Evidence. *Psychological Medicine*. 2009;39:3–11.
25. Colcombe S, Kramer A. Fitness Effects on the Cognitive Function of Older Adults: A Meta-Analytic Study. *Psychological Science* 2003;14:125–130.
26. Gass M. Menopause. In: Rippe JM. *Lifestyle Medicine* (2nd edition). CRC Press (Boca Raton), 2013.
27. Howe T, Shea B, Dawson LJ et al. Exercise for Preventing and Treating Osteoporosis in Postmenopausal Women. *Cochrane Database of Systematic Reviews*. CD000333. 2011.
28. Peeke PM. Women's Body Composition and Lifestyle. In: Rippe, JM. *Lifestyle Medicine* (2nd edition). CRC Press (Boca Raton), 2013.
29. Shai I, Schwarz Fuchs D, Henkin Y, et al. Weight Loss with a Low-Carbohydrate, Mediterranean, or Low-Fat Diet. *New England Journal of Medicine*. 2008;359:229–241.
30. *2015–2020 Dietary Guidelines for Americans*. U.S. Department of Health and Human Services and U.S. Department of Agriculture (8th edition), 2015. Epub December 2015. Available at http://health.Gov/dietaryguidelines/2015/guidelines/. Accessed July 6, 2020.
31. Obarzanek E, Sacks F, Vollmer W, et al. Effects on Blood Lipids of a Blood Pressure-Lowering Diet: The Dietary Approaches to Stop Hypertension (DASH) Trial. *American Journal of Clinical Nutrition*. 2001;74:80–89.
32. de Lorgeril M, Salen P, Martin J, et al. Mediterranean Diet, Traditional Risk Factors, and the Rate of Cardiovascular Complications after Myocardial Infarction: Final Report of the Lyon Diet Heart Study. *Circulation*. 1999;99:779–785.
33. Fung T, Willett W, Stampfer M, et al. Dietary Patterns and the Risk of Coronary Heart Disease in Women. *Archives of Internal Medicine*. 2001;161:1857–1862.
34. Gidding S, Lichtenstein A, Faith M, et al. Implementing American Heart Association Pediatric and Adult Nutrition Guidelines: A Scientific Statement from the American Heart Association Nutrition Committee of the Council on Nutrition, Physical Activity and Metabolism, Council on Cardiovascular Disease in the Young, Council on Arteriosclerosis, Thrombosis and Vascular Biology, Council on Cardiovascular Nursing, Council on Epidemiology and Prevention, and Council for High Blood Pressure Research. *Circulation*. 2009;119:1161–1175.
35. He F, Nowson C, Lucas M, MacGregor G. Increased Consumption of Fruit and Vegetables is Related to a Reduced Risk of Coronary Heart Disease: Meta-Analysis of Cohort Studies. *Journal of Human Hypertension*. 2007;21:717–728.
36. Liu S, Willett W, Stampfer M, et al. A Prospective Study of Dietary Glycemic Load, Carbohydrate Intake, and Risk of Coronary Heart Disease in US Women. *American Journal of Clinical Nutrition*. 2000;71:1455–1461.
37. Meyer K, Kushi L, Jacobs D Jr, Slavin J, Sellers TA, Folsom AR. Carbohydrates, Dietary Fiber, and Incident Type 2 Diabetes in Older Women. *American Journal of Clinical Nutrition*. 2000;71:921–930.
38. Salmeron J, Hu FB, Manson JE, et al. Dietary Fat Intake and Risk of Type 2 Diabetes in Women. *American Journal of Clinical Nutrition*. 2001;73:1019–1026.

39. Mozaffarian D, Katan MB, Ascherio A, Stampfer MJ, Willett WC. Trans Fatty Acids and Cardiovascular Disease. *New England Journal of Medicine*. 2006;354:1601–1613.

40. He J, Ogden L, Vupputuri S, et al. Dietary Sodium Intake and Subsequent Risk of Cardiovascular Disease in Overweight Adults. *JAMA*. 1999;282:2027–2034.

41. Briefel R, Johnson C. Secular Trends in Dietary Intake in the United States. *Annual Review of Nutrition*. 2004;24:401–431.

42. Dickinson B, Havas S. Reducing the Population Burden of Cardiovascular Disease by Reducing Sodium Intake: A Report of the Council on Science and Public Health. *Archives of Internal Medicine*. 2007;167:1460–1468.

43. Di Castelnuovo A, Rotondo S, Iacoviello L, et al. Meta-Analysis of Wine and Beer Consumption in Relation to Vascular Risk. *Circulation*. 2002;105:2836–2844.

44. Stampfer M, Colditz G, Willett W, et al. A Prospective Study of Moderate Alcohol Consumption and the Risk of Coronary Disease and Stroke in Women. *New England Journal of Medicine*. 1988;319:267–273.

45. Urbano-Marquez A, Estruch R, Fernandez-Sola J, Nicolas JM, Pare JC, Rubin E. The Greater Risk of Alcoholic Cardiomyopathy and Myopathy in Women Compared with Men. *JAMA*. 1995;274:149–154.

46. Kris-Etherton P, Lichtenstein A, Howard B, et al. Antioxidant Vitamin Supplements and Cardiovascular Disease. *Circulation*. 2004;110:637–641.

47. Schulze MB, Manson JE, Ludwig DS, et al. Sugar-Sweetened Beverages, Weight Gain, and Incidence of Type 2 Diabetes in Young and Middle-Aged Women. *JAMA*. 2004;292(8):927–934.

48. Ogden C, Carroll M, Curtin L, et al. Prevalence of Overweight and Obesity in the United States, 1999–2004. *JAMA*. 2006;295:1549–1555.

49. Ashton W, Nanchahal K, Wood D. Body Mass Index and Metabolic Risk Factors for Coronary Heart Disease in Women. *European Heart Journal*. 2001;22:46–55.

50. Willett WC, Manson JE, Stampfer MJ, et al. Weight, Weight Change, and Coronary Heart Disease in Women: Risk within the 'Normal' Weight Range. *JAMA*. 1995;273:461–465.

51. Despres J, Lemieux I. Abdominal Obesity and Metabolic Syndrome. *Nature*. 2006;444:881–887.

52. Mokdad A, Ford E, Bowman B, et al. Prevalence of Obesity, Diabetes, and Obesity-Related Health Risk Factors, 2001. *JAMA*. 2003;289:76–79.

53. Hu F, Manson J, Stampfer M, et al. Diet, Lifestyle, and the Risk of Type 2 Diabetes Mellitus in Women. *New England Journal of Medicine*. 2001;345:790–797.

54. Field A, Coakley E, Must A, et al. Impact of Overweight on the Risk of Developing Common Chronic Diseases during a 10-Year Period. *Archives of Internal Medicine*. 2001;161:1581–1586.

55. Colditz G, Willett W, Rotnizky A, et al. Weight Gain as a Risk Factor for Clinical Diabetes Mellitus in Women. *Annals of Internal Medicine*. 1995;122:481–486.

56. Ford E, Williamson D, Liu S. Weight Change and Diabetes Incidence: Findings from a National Cohort of US Adults. *American Journal of Epidemiology*. 1997;146:214–222.

57. Hennekens C. Risk Factors for Coronary Heart Disease in Women. *Cardiology Clinics*. 1998;16:1–8.

58. Centers for Disease Control and Prevention. Smoking and Tobacco Use. Data and Statistics, 2020. https://www.cdc.gov/tobacco/data_statistics/index.htm. Accessed: September 14, 2020.

59. Centers for Disease Control and Prevention. Tobacco Use among Adults—United States, 2005. *Morbidity and Mortality Weekly Report*. 2006;55:1145–1148.

13 Immunology and Infectious Disease

KEY POINTS

- Lifestyle modalities, in general, and exercise, in particular, play a significant role in improving and enhancing the immune system and lowering the risk of infectious disease.
- Regular physical activity lowers both inflammation and the risk of upper respiratory tract infections (URTIs).
- Excessive exercise (uncommon, although found in some marathon runners and some other long-distance athletes) may actually reduce the immune response and result in an increase in URTIs. However, individuals exercising at this level are very unusual.
- Regular exercise also can improve symptoms and multiple physiological factors in people who are living with HIV.

13.1 INTRODUCTION

Various lifestyle measures have been demonstrated to have a positive impact on the immune system and the likelihood of acquiring infectious diseases. Perhaps most prominent in this area is the relationship between exercise, inflammation, and respiratory infection (1). There is also some research suggesting that regular exercise possibly impacts on overall immune function. Moreover, there is good evidence that exercise may play a role in reducing the likelihood and extent of HIV infection. Exercise is particularly important as individuals grow older and their immune system becomes less efficient.

13.2 EXERCISE, INFLAMMATION AND RESPIRATORY INFECTION

The field of how exercise impacts on the immune system is a relatively new area of scientific endeavor. Most of the papers in this area have been published within the past 25 years. The areas of particular interest to lifestyle medicine clinicians are the chronic anti-inflammatory influence of exercise training and the reduction in risk of URTIs from regular, moderate exercise training.

Acute inflammation is a normal physiological function. Markers for inflammation include cytokines, interleukin—IL-6, IL-8, IL-10, and IL-1—as well as receptor antagonists (IL-1ra), granulocyte colony-stimulating factor (GCSF), tumor necrosis factor (TNF-α), and macrophage migratory inhibitory factor (MIF). C-reactive protein (CRP) may be elevated following heavy exertion, but the increase is delayed in comparison to most of the above-referenced cytokines. These inflammatory markers may be elevated after prolonged exercise, such as a marathon race, but regular exercise decreases these inflammatory markers when they are measured at rest. In contrast, inflammatory markers are typically elevated in overweight or unfit adults. For example, CRP levels in long-distance runners in the resting state typically are below 0.5 mg/L in comparison to 3-4 mg/L in obese, post-menopausal women (2).

A persistent increase in inflammatory markers is defined as chronic or systemic inflammation. Systemic inflammation has been linked to multiple disorders, including atherosclerosis and cardiovascular disease (CVD), metabolic syndrome, diabetes mellitus (T2DM), sarcopenia, arthritis, osteoporosis, chronic obstructive pulmonary disease (COPD), dementia, depression, and various types of cancer (3,4).

Recent literature has suggested that inflammation plays a deleterious and widespread role in the human body. The inverse association between physical activity and inflammation may be somewhat related to its activity on fat mass, but even studies that control for fat mass demonstrate lower levels of inflammation for physically active individuals (5).

The mechanism for why regular physical activity or exercise training may exert anti-inflammatory results is still not completely understood. It may be mediated in part through muscle-derived peptides. It should be noted, however, that the recommended exercise regimen of 30 minutes moderate intensity physical activity on most, if not all, days has small influences on visceral fat (5). It has been suggested that moderate physical activity training must be increased to higher levels (e.g., 60 minutes/day) and combined with weight loss and improved dietary quality to achieve reduction in systemic inflammation (6).

The impact of regular, moderate intensity physical activity has been studied in a variety of settings with regard to URTIs (7). There are more than 200 different viruses which cause the common cold. Either rhino viruses or corona viruses are responsible for 25–60% of the URTIs (7). It has been reported by the National Institute of Allergies and Infectious Disease that people in the United States suffer one billion URTIs each year with an incidence of two to four per year for the average adult and six to ten for the average child.

Regular physical activity improves immune function and lowers URTI risk (8). However, sustained and intense exertion may have the opposite effect. It should be noted that marathon race competitors and heavy exercise training regimens may increase URTI risk, but relatively few individuals exercise to this level (9).

A number of studies have shown that moderate physical activity lowers the risk of URTI. In one epidemiological study of 547 adults, a 23% reduction in the URTI risk was found in those engaging in regular versus irregular participation in physical activity. Randomized controlled studies of smaller groups of individuals showed that individuals who exercise regularly reduce URTI symptoms (5.1 versus 10.8 days) during a 15-week period compared to sedentary controls (8).

Changes which occur in the immune system during moderate exercise include recirculation of immunoglobulins, neutrophils, and natural killer (NK) cells. These are cells that play a critical role in immune defenses. These data suggest that moderate exercise favorably influences overall immune surveillance against pathogens.

Regular physical activity should be combined with other lifestyle changes to more effectively reduce URTI risk. These strategies may include stress management, regular sleep, avoidance of poor nutritional habits, and proper hygiene (10). Nonetheless, lifestyle strategies such as regular physical activity in combination with other positive lifestyle approaches appear to have great benefits for lowering the burden of URTI. In addition, as already indicated, reducing inflammation can result in lowering the risk of CVD, T2DM, various kinds of cancer, and dementia. While many questions remain, this is an area of continuing and important scientific research.

13.3   CHRONIC EXERCISE AND IMMUNITY

Regular exercise influences a number of aspects of host defense and indices of immune function (11). This may result in decreased inflammation, improved wound healing, and improved efficacy of vaccines. Research has shown that regular exercisers have a lower number of circulating leukocytes at rest, which may contribute to anti-inflammatory effects such as lowered IL-6 and CRP (12).

Monocytes have both innate and adaptive immune functions. They can respond to infection or tissue damage by traveling to the lymph nodes or migrating to the site of the insult where they can differentiate into tissue-specific macrophages. Chronic, low-grade activation of the monocytes/macrophage lineage is thought to contribute to inflammation, obesity, insulin resistance, and perhaps the development of atherosclerosis (13). There is strong evidence that regular exercise can reduce monocyte/macrophage-induced inflammation, although data in this area are not conclusive and further research is ongoing.

NK cells are cytotoxic lymphocytes and a major constituent of the innate immune system (14). There is an ongoing debate about whether or not exercise training has an impact on NK cells. Neutrophils are polymorphonuclear cells and are the most abundant leukocyte subtype. Neutrophils are the first responders of the innate immune system and migrate to the site of infection or injury within minutes. In individuals who exercise regularly, resting neutrophil number is similar to sedentary individuals. Regular exercise training can impact on neutrophil number, which may, in turn, decrease inflammation (15). T and B cells are primary circulating cells of the adaptive immune system. These cells are involved in some cell-mediated immunity and are primarily responsible for producing antigen-specific antibodies (humoral immunity). Currently, a lack of consensus exists on the effects of regular exercise on lymphocyte proliferative response (16).

Excessive training can result in a wide range of negative clinical signs and symptoms. Resting immunity is not different between athletes and healthy sedentary individuals. Intensive training, however, has been demonstrated to potentially negatively affect several immune measures such as changes in NK cell activity and B cell function after intensive training regimens. Athletes who train hard are frequently reported to have an increased incidence of upper respiratory tract symptoms (URS). Once again, the data in this area are mixed, and it is an area of ongoing research (17).

There is increasing evidence that inflammation plays a variety of roles in chronic disease processes. Exercise is known to provide substantial benefits for the prevention and management of chronic diseases. There is growing evidence that one of the major components of these benefits is that exercise has anti-inflammatory effects. Still in dispute is whether or not there is an intensity threshold for the anti-inflammatory effects of exercise and whether or not it is separate from decreases in body fat.

Aging and chronic conditions are also known to slow the rate of wound healing. In one small study of 28 older adults, a significantly improved healing rate was demonstrated in individuals who exercised versus those who were sedentary. In this study, 55% of the individuals who exercised regularly showed complete healing of an experimental wound on day 4 compared to 0% in the non-exercise group (18). Further research is ongoing in this area. It will offer a substantial benefit if this turns out to be proven in subsequent studies.

Exercise training has been demonstrated to potentially improve immune competence in older adults who have been given the influenza vaccine (19). In several cross-sectional studies in which physically active older adults were compared to sedentary controls, the exercising adults were shown to have a greater immune response. Numerous longitudinal studies have further supported this idea (20,21). In one study of 144 sedentary older adults who were randomized either to a ten-month aerobic training program ($N = 74$) or to a flexibility and balance program ($N = 70$), those in the exercise group demonstrated a significant increase in seroprotection determined by hemagglutination inhibition (HI). This suggests that they were experiencing an enhanced vaccine response. It should be noted, however, that there was no significant difference in URTI between the two groups, although the exercising group exhibited reduced overall illness severity and less sleep disturbance.

13.4   HIV AND EXERCISE

Living with HIV has become more the management of a chronic condition in recent years than the battle of opportunistic infection of the immune system as it was in the first two decades of the epidemic (22). For this reason, lifestyle measures are particularly important in the area of HIV. In particular, healthy lifestyle choices such as healthy diet and regular exercise have now become very important in this population. Exercise alone has been demonstrated to have a positive impact on health across all populations of HIV regardless of disease or health status and carries both psychological and physiological benefits.

Significant improvements in health and quality of life for people living with HIV/AIDS have now been demonstrated in a number of studies (23). The widespread use of antiretroviral therapy (ART) has changed the way HIV is handled (24). People living with HIV/AIDS (PLWHA) have multiple psychological stressors at all stages of the illness. Immediately upon diagnosis, these individuals must face life-changing issues such as managing the illness, affording appropriate health care, and the daily struggles that accompany living with the stigmatization of HIV. Some techniques for managing psychological stressors include mindful meditation and motivational interviewing.

Individuals living with HIV also experience a wide variety of both physical and psychological symptoms. Physical symptoms with ART include diarrhea, loss of appetite, nausea, muscle weakness, peripheral neuropathy, fever, dry skin, and persistent cough (25). Thus, the management of these symptoms become a daily task for PLWHA and ultimately leads to a chronic state of deconditioning leading to functional aerobic impairment. As in other populations with individuals with chronic diseases, there is a growing body of evidence that health benefits can be obtained by incorporating short-term aerobic and resistance exercise into an individual's recovery and/or treatment plan with HIV.

A number of studies have shown that cardiorespiratory fitness improves with regular exercise in people with HIV. There may also be potential benefits for blood lipids, including increases in HDL cholesterol following regular moderate intensity aerobic exercise. Body composition may also improve with regular moderate physical activity. Central fat accumulation is a common side effect of various ART regimens, and this may be somewhat ameliorated by regular physical activity.

Psychological benefits may also be yielded by regular physical activity, including reduction in anxiety and depression, particularly following individuals learning of seropositive status (26). Several studies after the advent of HIV have also shown improvement in anxiety and depression.

The recommended amount of physical activity for individuals with HIV have been documented by both the Physical Activity Guidelines for Americans (PAGA) 2018 Scientific Report (27) and the American College of Sports Medicine (ACSM) Exercise Management for Persons with Chronic Disease and Disability (4th edition) (28). Both of these guidelines recommended a total of 150 minutes of moderate intensity physical activity on a weekly basis as well as two days per week of resistance training. It is strongly recommended by ACSM that anyone with HIV or AIDS must receive medical clearance from their primary health care provider prior to beginning an exercise program.

13.5 COVID-19

The world is in a midst of a pandemic of COVID-19 infections, Over 1.8 million individuals worldwide have died from this novel coronavirus and there have been over 84 million infections with this virus as of January 1, 2021. Individuals who are obese or who have hypertension are up to three times as likely to die from coronavirus as are individuals who are within the healthy weight range and do not have hypertension. These factors underscore the importance of daily habits and actions. More information concerning the COVID-19 virus is found in the chapter on Pulmonary Medicine

13.6 EXERCISE, AGING, AND IMMUNITY

Regular, moderate intensity physical activity may improve antibody and some immune responses and reduce the state of chronic inflammation in older adults. The mechanisms for these beneficial effects on the immune system are not completely understood. It has been suggested that these benefits occur by adipose tissue modulation stimulation of the parasympathetic nervous system and perhaps alteration of the gut microbiome.

It has been recognized that normal aging is associated with a state of chronic low-grade inflammation characterized by elevated levels of circulating IL-6, CRP, TNF-α, all of which may be involved in the pathogenesis of numerous age-related diseases (29).

Regular physical activity may attenuate age-induced low-grade inflammation in the aging population. Several large population cohorts such as the third National Health and Nutrition Examination Survey (NHANES III), the Cardiovascular Health Study (CHS), and the Health ABC study all support this inverse relationship (21). All have reported negative correlations between physical activity and levels of circulating anti-inflammatory markers. There is further information that this inverse relationship occurs in a dose-dependent manner with the lowest levels of inflammatory markers observed in elderly persons who report the highest level of physical activity.

Regular physical activity may lower the amount of adipose tissue in elderly individuals. In addition, there may be a relationship between improving gut microbiomes and regular physical activity. In addition, both T cell and B cell immunity may be improved in the elderly by regular physical activity. For example, one cross-sectional examination of antibody response to influenza vaccine in older, highly fit men and women compared to less fit older adults demonstrated that the highly physically active individuals had greater antibody response to both H1N1 strains of the influenza vaccine than their less active counterparts (30). In addition, the highly physical subjects had greater production of more potent IgG2 after recall vaccination of a tetanus toxoid booster, which suggests an exercise effect on antibody isotype switching. Once again, individuals who exercise vigorously had higher antibody responses.

For all of these reasons, it is highly recommended that individuals over the age of 65 must engage in regular physical activity. The effects on the immune system, including anti-inflammatory effects, may underlie much of the reduction of risk of chronic disease for physically active older adults.

13.7   CONCLUSIONS

The beneficial effects of regular physical activity on the immune system and the reduction of risk of infectious diseases make an important case for why lifestyle medicine clinicians should be recommending regular physical activity for all adults, particularly for individuals over the age of 65. While there are still a number of issues to be resolved for why regular physical activity improves the immune response and lowers infectious disease, there is, however, enough evidence to suggest that these benefits are substantial and that they may contribute to one of the reasons why regular physical activity lowers the risk of a variety of chronic diseases in the general adult population, particularly in those above 65 years of age. This is particularly important since low-grade inflammation is a common component of the aging process.

13.8   PRACTICAL APPLICATIONS

- Regular physical activity carries many benefits for all adults, particularly for individuals over the age of 65.

- Regular exercise enhances both cellular and humoral immunities.
- Regular exercise helps combat the age-associated increase in low-grade inflammation.
- Clinicians should counsel all individuals on regular physical activity, and immunological and infectious disease benefits add another component to why this is so important.

REFERENCES

1. Dudgeon W, Nieman D, Kelley E. *Exercise, Inflammation and Respiratory Infection. Lifestyle Medicine* (3rd edition). CRC Press (Boca Raton), 2019.
2. Nieman D, Henson D, Smith L, et al. Cytokine Changes after a Marathon Race. *Journal of Applied Physiology.* 2001;91:109–114.
3. Khansari N, Shakiba Y, Mahmoudi M. Chronic Inflammation and Oxidative Stress as a Major Cause of Age-Related Diseases and Cancer. *Recent Patents on Inflammation & Allergy Drug Discovery.* 2009;3:73–80.
4. Devaraj S, Valleggi S, Siegel D, Jialal I. Role of C-Reactive Protein in Contributing to Increased Cardiovascular Risk in Metabolic Syndrome. *Current Atherosclerosis Reports.* 2010;12:110–118.
5. Beavers K, Brinkley T, Nicklas B. Effect of Exercise Training on Chronic Inflammation. *Clinica Chimica Acta.* 2010;411:785–793.
6. Pedersen BK. The Diseasome of Physical Inactivity—And the Role of Myokines in Muscle—Fat Cross Talk. *Journal of Physiology* 2009;587(Pt 23):5559–5568.
7. National Institute of Allergy and Infectious Diseases. The Common Cold, 2009. http://www.niai d.nih.gov/topics/commoncold. Accessed July 7, 2020.
8. Matthews C, Ockene I, Freedson P, et al. Moderate to Vigorous Physical Activity and Risk of Upper-Respiratory Tract Infection. *Medicine & Science in Sports & Exercise* 2002;34:1242–1248.
9. Nieman D. Is Infection Risk Linked to Exercise Workload? *Medicine & Science in Sports & Exercise* 2000;32(suppl 7):S406–S411.
10. Fondell E, Christensen S, Bälter O, et al. Adherence to the Nordic Nutrition Recommendations as a Measure of a Healthy Diet and Upper Respiratory Tract Infection. *Public Health Nutrition.* 2011;14:860–869.
11. Markofski M, Coen P, Flynn M. *Chronic Exercise and Immunity. Lifestyle Medicine* (3rd edition). CRC Press (Boca Raton), 2019.
12. Johannsen N, Swift D, Johnson W. et al. Effect of Different Doses of Aerobic Exercise on Total White Blood Cell (WBC) and WBC Subfraction Number in Postmenopausal Women: Results from DREW. *PLoS One.* 2012;7(2): e31319.
13. Rogacev K, Ulrich C, Blomer L. et al. Monocyte Heterogeneity in Obesity and Subclinical Atherosclerosis. *European Heart Journal.* 2010;31(3):369–76.
14. Moro-Garcia M, Fernandez-Garcia B, Echeverria A. et al. Frequent Participation in High Volume Exercise throughout Life is Associated with a More Differentiated Adaptive Immune Response. *Brain, Behavior, and Immunity.* 2014;39:61–74.
15. Smith J, Telford R, Mason I. et al. Exercise, Training and Neutrophil Microbicidal Activity. *International Journal of Sports Medicine.* 1990;11(3):179–87.
16. Rall L, Rubenoff R, Cannon J. et al. Effects of Progressive Resistance Training on Immune Response in Aging and Chronic Inflammation. *Medicine & Science in Sports & Exercise.* 1996;28(11):1356–65.
17. Heath G, Ford E, Craven T. et al. Exercise and the Incidence of Upper Respiratory Tract Infections. *Medicine & Science in Sports & Exercise.* 1991;23(2):152–7.

18. O'Brien J, et al. Evaluating the Effectiveness of a Self-Management Exercise Intervention on Wound Healing, Functional Ability and Health-Related Quality of Life Outcomes in Adults with Venous Leg Ulcers: A Randomised Controlled Trial. *International Wound Journal*. 2017;14(1):130–137.

19. Goodwin K, Viboud C, Simonsen L. Antibody Response to Influenza Vaccination in the Elderly: A Quantitative Review. *Vaccine*. 2006;24(8):1159–69.

20. Woods J, Lowder T, Keylock K. Can Exercise Training Improve Immune Function in the Aged? *Annals of the New York Academy of Sciences*. 2002;959:117–27.

21. Nicklas B, Brinkley T. Exercise Training as a Treatment for Chronic Inflammation in the Elderly. *Exercise and Sport Sciences Reviews*. 2009;37(4):165–70.

22. Samaras K. Prevalence and Pathogenesis of Diabetes Mellitus in HIV-1 Infection Treated with Combined Antiretroviral Therapy. *Journal of Acquired Immune Deficiency Syndromes*. 2009;50(5):499–505.

23. Thompson M, Aberg j, Hoy J. et al. Antiretroviral Treatment of Adult HIV Infection: 2012 Recommendations of the International Antiviral Society-USA Panel. *JAMA*. 2012;308(4):387–402.

24. Anuurad E, Semrad A, Berglund L. Human Immunodeficiency Virus and Highly Active Antiretroviral Therapy-Associated Metabolic Disorders and Risk Factors for Cardiovascular Disease. *Metabolic Syndrome and Related Disorders*. 2009;7(5):401–10.

25. Portillo C, Holzemer W, Chou F. HIV Symptoms. *Annual Review of Nursing Research*. 2007;25:259–91.

26. Robinson F, Mathews H, Witek-Janusek L. Stress and HIV Disease Progression: Psychoneuroimmunological Framework. *Journal of the Association of Nurses in AIDS Care*. 1999;10(1):21–31.

27. Physical Activity Guidelines Advisory Committee. *2018 Physical Activity Guidelines Advisory Committee Scientific Report*. U.S. Department of Health and Human Services (Washington, DC), 2018.

28. Moore G, Durstine J, Painter P. *American College of Sports Medicine: ACSM's Exercise Management for Persons with Chronic Diseases and Disabilities* (4th edition). Human Kinetics (Champaign, IL), 2016.

29. Beavers K, Hus F-D, Isom S. et al. Long-Term Physical Activity and Inflammatory Biomarkers in Older Adults. *Medicine & Science in Sports & Exercise*. 2010;42(12):2189–96.

30. Vu T, Farsih S, Jenkins M. et al. A Meta-Analysis of Effectiveness of Influenza Vaccine in Persons Aged 65 Years and Over Living in the Community. *Vaccine*. 2002;20(13–14):1831–6.

14 Pediatrics

KEY POINTS

- Healthy behaviors are important to establish among children.
- Habits established in childhood often carry into adulthood.
- Issues related to physical activity, healthy nutrition, weight management, avoidance of tobacco products, and sleep, all are very important to discuss with children and their parents.

14.1 INTRODUCTION

It is well known that many chronic diseases which become manifested in adults have their roots in childhood (1). Thus, it is very important to explore how lifestyle issues can play a role in the health and well-being of children as well as reduce their risk of chronic disease in later life.

Numerous studies have shown that regular physical activity, proper nutrition, and weight management can have beneficial effects of reducing multiple risk factors for cardiovascular disease (CVD), diabetes, hypertension, and dyslipidemia (2). There is also emerging literature to show that such lifestyle modalities as physical activity can improve academic performance and feelings of well-being. These benefits apply to both children and adults.

Physical inactivity is a global health problem and has its roots in childhood. The current physical activity guidelines from multiple sources in the United States and around the world call for children and youth to participate in at least 60 minutes of moderate or vigorous physical activity on a daily basis (3,4).

Studies have shown that ideal cardiovascular health is only about 12–18% heritable, which means that approximately 80–85% of ideal cardiovascular health is related to maintaining a healthy lifestyle through healthy diet and physical activity (5,6). Disturbingly, an increasing proportion of children is exhibiting sufficiently poor lifestyle behaviors such that conditions previously only seen in adulthood are now presenting in childhood requiring efforts not only to prevent but to treat. Most estimates indicate that fewer than 5% of individuals reach the age of 50 having maintained ideal cardiovascular health (7,8). Several studies have shown that dietary factors are associated with a substantial portion of deaths from heart disease, stroke, and type 2 diabetes (9). This means that clinicians' jobs can only be accomplished by promoting a healthy lifestyle all the way from fetuses, to infants, to school-age children and adolescents. All of these factors will be discussed in this chapter.

14.2   LIFESTYLE BEHAVIORS

As discussed in Chapter 4, there are numerous models of behavior change. Lifestyle behaviors including diet, physical activity, sedentary behavior, and sleep are all key components of lifestyle medicine from childhood through the rest of the lifespan and are central to preventing the progression of multiple, non-communicable diseases, including obesity, heart disease, cancer, and diabetes. Fostering healthy lifestyle behaviors early in life has been strongly supported by evidence showing that multiple lifestyle-related habits and actions, including sedentary lifestyle, poor nutrition, and obesity, are often established in childhood.

One theoretical model that is widely used is the social ecological model (10). This model posits that multiple levels of influence act on behavior, including personal decisions and community, regional, and public policies. With regard to changing behavior in childhood, a key concept is continual reinforcement. Thus, it is particularly important to reinforce positive behaviors such as physical activity and healthy eating habits. Thus, lifestyle medicine practitioners should help parents and children establish such behaviors as self-monitoring, goal setting, stimulus control, behavior reversal, and regular feedback. These strategies are time consuming, which will be expedited if the physician shares these responsibilities with other members of their clinical staff such as nurses and, if available, nutritionists.

14.3   LIFE COURSE APPROACH TO PREVENTION OF CHRONIC DISEASE

Increased research has now demonstrated that intrauterine exposure to maternal issues such as nutritional deficiency, obesity, diabetes, and smoking are associated with an increased risk of chronic disease among offspring (11). If children are exposed to problems while in the uterus, they are more likely to demonstrate early signs of chronic disease and potentially set into motion a vicious cycle. Numerous fetal exposures have been identified which can carry adverse effects through childhood and throughout the life cycle. A summary of some of these intrauterine exposures is found in Table 14.1.

14.4   PHYSICAL ACTIVITY

Physical activity is one of the key habits and practices that should be encouraged in all children. Regular physical activity has been shown in multiple studies to reduce various risk factors for CVD, including improving lipids, blood pressure, and blood glucose (12). Regular physical activity also can play a very important role in body composition, aerobic fitness, muscular strength, motor skills, and bone health. The Physical Activity Guidelines for Americans (PAGA) 2018 Scientific Report and the American College of Sports Medicine (ACSM) recommend that youth participate in at least 60 minutes of moderate or vigorous physical activity on a daily basis. Unfortunately, 80% of adolescents do not achieve these recommended levels (3,4). According to the 2016 U.S. Report Card on Physical Activity in Children and Youth,

TABLE 14.1
Early Life Exposures and Associated Outcomes

Exposures and Associated Outcomes

Fetal undernutrition   Total calories
         Atherogenic lipid profile
         Disturbed blood coagulation
         Obesity
         Breast cancer
         Insulin resistance
         Obstructive airway disease
         Microalbuminuria
       Folic acid
         Neural tube defects
       Iron
         Obesity
         Hypertension
         Impaired kidney development
       Calcium
         Hypertension
       Vitamin D
         Increased adiposity

Fetal overnutrition   Maternal diabetes
         Obesity
         Glucose intolerance, type 2 diabetes
         Increased blood pressure
         Endothelial dysfunction
         Atherogenic lipid profile
         Metabolic syndrome
       Maternal obesity
         Increased birthweight, obesity, adiposity
         Increased blood pressure
         Metabolic syndrome
       Suboptimal macronutrient profile
         Obesity, increased adiposity
         Increased blood pressure
       Methyl donors
         Increased weight
         Metabolic syndrome

Other intrauterine exposures Physical activity (protective)
         Reduced fat mass at birth
       Smoking
         Obesity, increased adiposity
         Increased blood pressure
         Asthma
         Attention-deficit hyperactivity disorder
       Endocrine disrupting chemicals

(Continued)

TABLE 14.1 (CONTINUED)
Early Life Exposures and Associated Outcomes
Exposures and Associated Outcomes

	Obesity
	Metabolic syndrome
	Asthma, respiratory tract infections
Postnatal exposures	Breastfeeding (protective)
	Reduced obesity, adiposity
	Fewer infections
	Lower blood pressure
	Less type 2 diabetes
	Improved cognitive development
	Shared environment
	Child diet follows maternal diet
	Parental support increases child activity

Source: Sauder K, Dabelia D. Life Course Approach to Prevention of Chronic
Disease, in: Rippe JM. *Lifestyle Medicine*, 3rd edition. CRC Press,
Boca Raton, 2019. Used with permission.

the overall grade for physical activity performance levels is D- (13). Sedentary
behaviors are also very prevalent and also received a D-, and school programs are
not doing much better with the rating of a D+.

- *Physical activity and cardiometabolic health:* An inactive lifestyle is associated with development of CVD, type 2 diabetes (T2DM), and many other
metabolic diseases (14–17). Meta-analyses have routinely shown that physical activity results in lowering of plasma triglycerides and also plasma insulin levels. There is also some suggestion that regular physical activity in
children raises HDL cholesterol. All of these findings represent a strong
rationale for recommending a physically active lifestyle for children as well
as trying to lower their risk of sedentary lifestyle.
- *Physical activity and cardiovascular fitness:* There is a strong relationship
between regular physical activity and cardiovascular fitness in children
aged 3–17 (18–20). Multiple different methods can be used to improve cardiovascular fitness. One that has proved to be very effective is school interventions both during and after school.
- *Physical activity and muscular fitness:* Regular physical activity programs
have also been shown to improve muscular fitness (3,21). This is important
for pursuing activities in daily living and also pursuing aerobic activities
with less risk of injury. The PAGA 2008 and 2018 guidelines both recommend three sessions of muscle-strengthening exercises per week. Just like
aerobic conditioning, muscular fitness achieved in childhood and adolescence is likely to carry over into the adult years.

- *Body weight and adiposity:* The prevalence of childhood obesity has increased significantly since the 1980s. Regular physical activity can play an important role in both lowering the risk of weight gain and reducing chronic disease factors in both overweight and obese children (22). Children who are obese are more susceptible to comorbid conditions such as T2DM, dyslipidemia, and the metabolic syndrome. Children who are obese also have reduced quality of life. Treating childhood obesity is challenging (see also Chapter 8) since many of the pharmaceutical options available to adults are less available or not applicable to children and many practicing clinicians report a lack of training in childhood obesity. Criteria for childhood obesity are as follows:
  - Overweight (BMI >85th to 94th percentile for age or sex)
  - Obese (BMI >95th percentile for age or sex)
  - Severely obese (BMI >120 percentile)
- *Bone health:* Multiple studies of physical activity interventions which include high-impact exercise such as hopping, skipping, jumping, and tumbling have been demonstrated to yield increased bone mass and bone density (3,23). For this reason, the PAGA 2018 Scientific Report recommended these types of exercises for all youth.
- *Sedentary behavior:* Children and adolescents in the United States spend a substantial amount of time engaged in sedentary behaviors (24,25). These include television viewing and other forms of screen time such as cell phone, tablets, and other devices. It has been estimated that U.S. children and adolescents spend six to eight hours per day in sedentary behavior, and the majority spend more than two hours a day watching television or are engaged in other types of screen time. A number of studies have shown that sedentary behavior results in adverse health consequences.
- *Cognitive function and academic achievement:* Numerous studies have shown that increased physical activity positively affects cognitive function in children (26). Single bouts of physical activity have been shown to improve short-term cognitive functioning. Other studies have shown that increased physical activity results in improved academic achievement and engagement in school (27). Other studies have also demonstrated that physical activity results in improvement in self-perception and enhanced self-esteem.
- *Family, school, community, and government strategies:* There are some data to suggest that families, schools, communities, and governments can play very important roles in encouraging children to become more physically active. The 2014 Report on Physical Activity in Youth, for example, demonstrated that 84.6% of children aged 12 years or younger live near at least one park or playground (28). Many other aspects of the built environment can impact on the likelihood that children will increase physical activity. Schools are often not open to children after school hours. Health care workers and physicians should encourage family members to see if there are ways that the school facilities can be utilized at longer hours.

14.5   CARDIOVASCULAR RISK AND DIET IN CHILDREN

More than one-third of U.S. children between the ages 2 and 19 are overweight and 17% are obese (see next section) (29). Pediatric obesity is associated with a broad range of health problems, including dyslipidemia and hypertension and other CVD risk factors. Pediatric CVD risk factors tend to track into adulthood as do eating behaviors. Therefore, it is important to establish healthy nutritional patterns from the earliest time in childhood.

A CVD-protective diet emphasizes unprocessed fruits and vegetables and whole grains with energy, fat, carbohydrates, and protein in proportions based on age, which are recommended in the 2015–2020 Dietary Guidelines. One good nutritional pattern is outlined in the CHILD diet (Cardiovascular Health-Integrated Lifestyle Diet), which was developed to help improve lipids in children. There are two such diets, the CHILD One and CHILD Two. CHILD Two is more aggressive in terms of lipid management. A comparison of the CHILD One and CHILD Two diet is found in Table 14.2.

Other dietary patterns which have been recommended for adults would also be highly appropriate for children. These include the DASH diet and the Mediterranean Diet. These have the advantage of conveying health benefits for the entire family. A description of the Mediterranean and DASH diets is found in Chapter 2.

14.6   CHILDHOOD OBESITY

Childhood obesity has significantly increased in the last three decades. The prevalence of obesity in 2–19-year-olds in the United States is 18.5% and continues to

---

TABLE 14.2

Comparing the Nutritional Intervention Approaches in the Cardiovascular Health-Integrated Lifestyle Diet-1 and Diet-2 for LDL-Cholesterol and Non-HDL-Cholesterol Lowering in Children >2 Years of Age

Nutrient target for LDL-lowering	CHILD-1	CHILD-2
Total dietary fat	25–30% of calories	25–30% of calories
Saturated fat	<10% of daily calories	<7% of daily calories
Trans fat	Avoided	Avoided
Monounsaturated Fat	Up to 10–15% of calories	Up to 10–15% of calories
Polyunsaturated Fat	Up to 10% of calories	Up to 10% of calories
Cholesterol	300 mg or less	200 mg or less
Dietary Fiber	Child's age+ 5 g up to 14 g/1000 calories	Child's age+ 5 g up to 14 g/1000 calories
Simple Carbohydrates	Reduction of SSB	Reduction of SSB

Source: Hildebrandt J, Couch S. Cardiovascular Risk and Diet in Children, in: Rippe JM. *Lifestyle Medicine*, 3rd edition. CRC Press, Boca Raton, 2019. Used with permission.

rise across all age groups and disproportionately affects black, Hispanic, and other minority groups (30). Comorbid conditions such as type 2 diabetes (T2DM) are projected to increase dramatically as generations of children carry obesity into adulthood.

Clinicians should screen all children in primary care at least annually for excess weight gain using age- and sex-specific percentile (for children ≥ 2 years old), or weight-to-length percentile (<2 years old). Clinicians should also screen for other lifestyle factors that may contribute to obesity. Motivational interviewing and behavioral change techniques should be utilized to identify lifestyle factors, which will help identify factors to select and implement to achieve attainable lifestyle goals for overweight or obese children. In 2007, an Expert Committee from the American Academy of Pediatrics recommended treatment to achieve permanent healthy lifestyle:

- Patient/family early identification to help prioritize behaviors reflective of their values and preferences and paired goal setting
- Motivational interviewing
- Implementation of self-monitored and planned reinforcements
- Optimization of multidisciplinary expertise to physical and psychosocial needs of the family
- Excellent communication with a primary care provider

Nutritional interventions include balanced, hypocaloric eating, physical activity, and sedentary behavior interventions.

Sleep is also a relatively new target for pediatric obesity interventions. This will be handled in a subsequent section in this chapter. For individuals with severe obesity (BMI >35) which affects approximately 8.5% of 12–19 year olds, an option may be available for bariatric surgery. This should be handled with a team that is skilled in this type of significant intervention.

14.7 IDENTIFICATION AND MANAGEMENT OF CHILDREN WITH DYSLIPIDEMIA

It is well known that CVD has its roots in childhood. Lipid abnormalities start the process of atherosclerosis. Therefore, it is critically important to identify and treat children with dyslipidemia (31).

Optimal, borderline, and high lipid classifications are found in Table 14.3. Cholesterol screening recommendations are found in Table 14.4. As noted in this table, it is recommended that all children and adolescents between the ages of 9 and 11 years and again between 17 and 21 years be screened at least once each time for dyslipidemia. Lifestyle interventions are relevant to any child with dyslipidemia and should involve utilization of the CHILD One or CHILD Two diet and weight loss, if necessary, as well as increased physical activity and decreased sedentary time.

TABLE 14.3

Cholesterol Level Classification for Children and Adolescents (in md/dL)

Lipid Category	Optimal	Borderline-High	High	Low
TC	<170	170–199	>200	
LDL-C	<110	110–129	>130	
Non-HDL-C	<120	123–144	>145	
TG				
0–9 yr	<75	75–99	>100	
10–19 yr	<90	90–129	>130	
HDL-C	>45	40–45		<40
Cholesterol Level Classification for Young Adults (20–24 years, in mg/dL)[7]				
TC	<190	190–224	>225	
LDL-C	<120	120–159	>160	
Non-HDL-C	<50	150–189	>190	
TG	<115	115–149	>150	
HDL-C	>45	40–45		<40

Source: Brothers J, Daniels S. Identification and Management of Children with Dyslipidemia, in: Rippe JM. *Lifestyle Medicine*, 3rd edition. CRC Press, Boca Raton, 2019. Used with permission.

TC, total cholesterol; LDL-c, low density lipoprotein cholesterol; non-HDL-c, non- high density lipoprotein cholesterol; TG, triglycerides; HDL-c, high density lipoprotein cholesterol.

14.8 DIAGNOSIS AND MANAGEMENT OF CHILDREN WITH HYPERTENSION

Approximately 3–4% of children have hypertension (32). Hypertension in youth is an accepted risk factor for hypertension in adulthood. In adulthood, hypertension is a major cause of heart failure, CVD, and stroke. Hypertension in children is defined by an in office systolic or diastolic blood pressure >95th percentile for age persistent over three to four occasions. In 2017, the American Academy of Pediatrics listed recommended actions for evaluating and treating hypertension in children (33). These are found in Table 14.5.

14.9 PREVENTION OF OSTEOPOROSIS IN CHILDREN AND ADOLESCENTS

Osteoporosis is a disorder of compromised bone strength (34). Research has shown that osteoporosis actually often begins in childhood. Bone accrual occurs dramatically during the first two decades of life and, to a lesser extent, during the third decade of life until bone mass is achieved. The development of peak bone mass is important for lifelong bone health.

TABLE 14.4
Cholesterol Screening Recommendations by Age 7

Age	Screening Recommendation	Labs to Obtain
<2 years	No screening	
2–8 years	No routine screening	
	Screening if:	FLPx2*
	• + family history of early heart disease	
	• Parent has TC >240 mg/dL	
	• Family history is unknown	
	• High risk condition (see Table 5)	
9–11 years	Universal Screening	
	If non-HDL-c>145 or HDL-c<40	Non-FLP
	Then obtain	FLPx2*
	If LDL-c>130 or	FLP
	non-HDL-c>145 or	
	HDL-c<40 or	
	TG > 100 (age< 10 yr) or > 130 (age >10 yr)	
	Then obtain	Repeat FLP*
12–16 years	No routine screening	
	Screening if:	FLPx2*
	New knowledge of CVD risk, same as 2–8 yr	
17–21 years	Universal Screening	
	Ages 17–19:	
	If non-HDL-c>145 or HDL-c<40	Non-FLP
	Then obtain	FLPx2*
	If LDL-c>130 or non-HDL-c>145 or	FLP
	HDL-c<40 or	
	TG > 100 (age< 10 yr) or > 130 (age >10 yr)	
	Then obtain	Repeat FLP*
	Ages 17–21:	
	If non-HDL-c>190 or HDL-c<40	Non-FLP
	Then obtain	FLPx2*
	If LDL-c>160 or non-HDL-c>190 or	FLP
	HDL-c<40 or TG>150	
	Then obtain	Repeat FLP*

Source: Brothers J, Daniels S. Identification and Management of Children with Dyslipidemia, in: Rippe JM. *Lifestyle Medicine*, 3rd edition. CRC Press, Boca Raton, 2019. Used with permission.

FLP, fasting lipid profile; non-FLP, non-fasting lipid profile; LDL-c, low-density lipo-protein cholesterol; HDL-c, high-density lipoprotein cholesterol; non-HDL-c, non-high-density lipoprotein cholesterol (total cholesterol – high-density lipoprotein cholesterol); TG, triglycerides.

* 2nd lipid profile should be obtained two weeks to three months after the first lipid profile obtained.

TABLE 14.5
Clinical Applications and Recommended Actions

Key action statement	Evidence quality and reported strength of recommendation
1. BP should be measured annually in children and adolescents ≥3 years of age.	C, Moderate
2. BP should be checked in all children ≥3 years of age at every health care encounter if they have obesity, are taking medications known to increase BP, or have renal disease, a history of aortic arch obstruction/coarctation, or diabetes.	C, Moderate
3. Trained health care professionals in the office setting should make a diagnosis of HTN if a child or adolescent has auscultatory-confirmed BP readings ≥95th percentile at three different visits.	C, Moderate
4. Organizations with EHRs used in an office setting should consider including flags for abnormal BP values, both when the values are being entered and when they are being viewed.	C, Weak
5. Oscillometric devices may be used for BP screening in children and adolescents. When doing so, providers should use a device that has been validated in the pediatric age group. If elevated BP is suspected on the basis of oscillometric readings, confirmatory measurements should be obtained by auscultation.	B, Strong
6. ABPM should be performed for confirmation of HTN in children with office BP measurements in the elevated BP category for a year or more or with Stage 1 HTN over three clinic visits.	C, Moderate
7. Routine performance of ABPM should be strongly considered in children with high-risk conditions (see Table 8) to assess HTN severity and determine whether abnormal circadian BP patterns are present which may indicate increased risk for target-organ damage.	B, Moderate
8. ABPM should be performed using a standardized approach (see Table 9) with monitors that have been validated in a pediatric population, and studies should be interpreted using pediatric normative data.	C, Moderate
9. Children with suspected WCH should undergo ABPM. Diagnosis is based on the presence of mean systolic and diastolic BP <95th percentile and systolic and diastolic BP load <25%.	B, Strong
10. Home BP monitoring should not be used to diagnose HTN, masked HTN, or WCH but may be a useful adjunct to office and ambulatory BP measurement after HTN has been diagnosed.	C, Moderate
11. Children >6 years of age do not require an extensive evaluation for secondary causes of HTN if they have a positive family history of HTN, are overweight or obese, and/or do not have history or physical examination findings (Table 12) suggestive of a secondary cause of HTN.	C, Moderate
12. Children who have undergone coarctation repair should undergo ABPM for the detection of HTN (including masked HTN).	B, Strong

(Continued)

TABLE 14.5 (CONTINUED)
Clinical Applications and Recommended Actions

Key action statement	Evidence quality and reported strength of recommendation
13. In children and adolescents being evaluated for high BP, the provider should obtain a perinatal history, appropriate nutritional history, physical activity history, psychosocial history, and family history, and should perform a physical examination to identify findings suggestive of secondary causes of HTN.	B, Strong
14. Clinicians should NOT perform electrocardiography in hypertensive children being evaluated for LVH.	B, Strong
15-1. It is recommended that echocardiography be performed to assess cardiac target-organ damage (LV mass, geometry, and function) at the time of consideration of pharmacologic treatment for HTN.	C, Moderate
15-2. LVH should be defined as LV mass>51 g/m (boys and girls) for children greater than eight years of age and defined by LV mass>115 g/BSA for boys and LV mass >95 g/BSA for girls.	
15-3. Repeat echocardiography may be performed to monitor improvement or progression of target-organ damage at 6- to 12-month intervals. Indications to repeat echocardiography include persistent HTN despite treatment, concentric LV hypertrophy, or reduced LV ejection fraction.	
15-4. In patients without LV target-organ injury at initial echocardiographic assessment, repeat echocardiography at yearly intervals may be considered in those with Stage 2 HTN, secondary HTN, or chronic Stage 1 HTN incompletely treated (noncompliance or drug resistance) to assess for the development of worsening LV target-organ injury.	
16. Doppler renal ultrasonography may be used as a noninvasive screening study for evaluation of possible renal artery stenosis in normal-weight children and adolescents ≥8 years of age who are suspected of having renovascular HTN and who will cooperate with the procedure.	C, Moderate
17. In children and adolescents suspected of having renal artery stenosis, either CTA or MRA may be performed as noninvasive imaging studies. Nuclear renography is less useful in pediatrics and should generally be avoided.	D, Weak
18. Routine testing for microalbuminuria is not recommended for children with primary HTN.	C, Moderate
19. In children with diagnosed HTN, the treatment goal with non-pharmacologic and pharmacologic therapy should be a reduction in SBP and DBP to <90th percentile and <130/80 mm Hg in adolescents.	C, Moderate
20. At the time of diagnosis of elevated BP or HTN in a child or adolescent, clinicians should provide advice on the DASH diet and recommend moderate to vigorous physical activity at least three to five days per week (30–60 minutes per session) to help reduce BP.	C, Weak

(*Continued*)

TABLE 14.5 (CONTINUED)
Clinical Applications and Recommended Actions

Key action statement	Evidence quality and reported strength of recommendation
21. In hypertensive children who have failed at least six months of lifestyle modifications—particularly those who have LV hypertrophy on echocardiography, symptomatic HTN, or Stage 2 HTN without a clearly modifiable factor (e.g., obesity)—clinicians should initiate pharmacologic treatment with an ACE inhibitor, ARB, long-acting calcium channel blocker, or thiazide diuretic.	B, Moderate
22. ABPM may be used to assess treatment effectiveness in children with HTN, especially when clinic and/or home BP measurements indicate insufficient BP response to treatment.	B, Moderate
23-1. Children and adolescents with CKD should be evaluated for HTN at each medical encounter.	B, Strong
23-2. Children or adolescents with both CKD and HTN should be treated to lower BP to MAP <50th percentile by ABPM.	
23-3. Regardless of apparent control of BP with office measures, children with CKD and a history of HTN should have BP assessed by ABPM at least yearly to screen for masked HTN.	
24. Children with CKD and HTN should be evaluated for proteinuria.	B, Strong
25. Children with CKD, HTN, and proteinuria should be treated with an ACE inhibitor or ARB.	B, Strong
26. Children and adolescents with T1 DM or T2DM should be evaluated for HTN at each medical encounter and treated if BP >95th percentile or >130/80 mm Hg in adolescents >13 years of age.	C, Moderate
27. In children and adolescents with acute severe HTN and life-threatening symptoms, immediate treatment with short-acting antihypertensive medication should be initiated and BP should be reduced by no more than 25% of the planned reduction over the first eight hours.	EO/D, Weak
28. Children and adolescents with HTN may participate in competitive sports once hypertensive target-organ effects and risk have been assessed.	C, Moderate
29. Children and adolescents with HTN should receive treatment to lower BP below Stage 2 thresholds before participation in competitive sports.	C, Moderate
30. Adolescents with elevated BP or HTN (whether or not they are receiving antihypertensive treatment) should typically have their care transitioned to an appropriate adult care provider by 22 years of age (recognizing that there may be individual cases in which this upper age limit is exceeded, particularly in the case of youth with special health care needs). There should be a transfer of information regarding HTN etiology and past manifestations/complications of the patient's HTN.	X, Strong

Source: Flynn JT et al. Clinical Practice Guidelines for Screening and Management of High Blood Pressure in Children and Adolescents. *Pediatrics*, 2017, 140(3) e20171904.

Baker-Smith C, Gidding S. Diagnosis, Management and Treatment of Systemic Hypertension in Youth, Updates from the 2017 American Academy of Pediatrics Clinical Practice Guideline, in: Rippe JM. *Lifestyle Medicine*, 3rd edition. CRC Press, Boca Raton, 2019. Used with permission.

Whole-body bone mass increases over 20-fold in the first two decades of life. Bone mass is acquired particularly during childhood, but with a peak increase at the onset of puberty. Approximately 39% of peak bone mass is achieved around the four years surrounding peak high velocity. This provides an ideal opportunity to maximize peak bone mass development.

High levels of physical activity are associated with greater bone mass, density, and strength. Adequate nutrient intake is also critically important for children and adolescents who achieve their genetic potential for bone mass, density, and strength. Fruit, vegetables, and dairy food consumption are positively associated with bone mass and density.

Calcium intake is the most studied nutrient in relation to bone accrual, but vitamin D status is also important. Some research studies have shown that protein intake is also important for bone mass in children and adolescents, which implies that dairy products have a major impact on bone density. Phosphorous and magnesium are also important in bone mass accumulation and may also constitute beneficial components of dairy products.

Fruits and vegetables are rich sources of potassium, magnesium, vitamin C, vitamin K, and flavonoids and are also important for bone mass. Carbonated beverage intake, on the other hand, has been associated with reduced bone density in some studies, possibly because of its displacement of dairy products. Tobacco use also exerts deleterious effects on bone health.

Sleep also plays a role in bone health. Recent research studies have suggested that sleep duration is particularly important (see next section.) Of all the modifiable lifestyle factors, physical activity is one of the most important. An enormous body of evidence demonstrates that high levels of physical activity are associated with greater bone mass density and cross-sectional dimensions (e.g., cortical diameter and thickness). Physical activity results in local loads (strains) that can possibly affect bone modeling and remodeling.

14.10 SLEEP

Recent attention has been focused on the issue of sleep and health in children and adolescents (35). The national chronic sleep patterns are becoming an important issue in all groups of children. The National Sleep Foundation reported that children and adolescents are sleeping far less than the amount recommended leading to a chronic problem of sleep deprivation. Poor sleep patterns in childhood tend to persist into adulthood and often develop into chronic sleep problems. In addition, short sleep duration has been shown to influence a variety of important hormones, including leptin, ghrelin, insulin, cortisol, and growth hormone.

A variety of metabolic conditions are associated with short sleep durations, most prominently childhood obesity. In the Heartfelt Study of almost 400 adolescents, the odds of obesity increased by 80% for each hour of sleep lost (36).

The relationship between sleep and diet behaviors is also important. In one study, adolescents were found to have diets with higher glycemic index after five nights of sleep restriction (6.5 hours in bed/night) compared to healthy sleep (10 hours in bed/night). Sleep timing is also associated with dietary habits. Adolescents who go to bed after midnight have been shown to consume larger quantities of sugary or caffeinated beverages. In addition, adolescents who have a late bedtime tend to skip breakfast and consume most of their meals late in the day.

The relationship between physical activity levels and sleep has been inconsistent. It is not clear that physical activity improves or worsens sleep in children and adolescents. However, sleep efficiency has been improved by moderate to vigorous physical activity.

For all these reasons, it is important for clinicians to inquire about sleep, particularly if a sleep disorder is suspected. Input from both the child and their parents may be helpful. Questions should focus on typical bedtimes, wake times, and any bedtime routine or preparation. Some clinical applications for addressing sleep issues in children are found in Table 14.6.

TABLE 14.6
Clinical Applications for Addressing Sleep Issues in Children

Presenting Problem	Possible Diagnoses	Recommended Treatment
All Ages		
Snoring, pauses in breathing, gasping for air during sleep	Obstructive Sleep Apnea	Polysomnography; referral to pediatric sleep clinic
Irregular sleep/wake times	Poor sleep habits in the absence of a discrete sleep disorder	Scheduled, consistent, bed/wake times
Poor sleep habits (e.g., use of electronics at bedtime and/or to fall asleep)	Poor sleep habits in the absence of a discrete sleep disorder	Sleep hygiene recommendations
Younger Children		
Difficulty falling asleep independently (need for parent presence to fall asleep or return to sleep after night wakings)	Insomnia	Behavioral treatments for independent sleep; referral to pediatric behavioral sleep medicine specialist
Bedtime resistance	Insomnia	Bedtime routine; positive reinforcement; referral to pediatric behavioral sleep medicine specialist
Older Children/Adolescents	Insomnia	
Difficulty falling asleep	Insomnia	Cognitive-behavioral therapy for insomnia (CBT-I); referral to pediatric behavioral sleep medicine specialist
Frequent night wakings	Insomnia	CBT-I; referral to pediatric behavioral sleep medicine specialist

Source: Kaar J, Simon S. Sleep and Obesity Prevention in Children and Adolescents, in: Rippe JM. *Lifestyle Medicine*, 3rd edition. CRC Press, Boca Raton, 2019. Used with permission.

14.11 CONCLUSIONS

It is well known that the roots of many chronic diseases that become manifest in adults originate in childhood. Such positive lifestyle measures as regular physical activity, healthy nutrition, weight management, and healthy amounts of sleep as well as avoidance of tobacco products are all important to assess as lifestyle issues in children. These are particularly important since habits which begin in childhood often carry into adulthood and carry adverse health consequences. Therefore, these lifestyle issues should be discussed at every clinical visit with children and their parents.

14.12 PRACTICAL APPLICATIONS

- Clinicians should focus on positive lifestyle habits in children, including regular physical activity, healthful nutrition, weight management, avoidance of tobacco products, and adequate amounts of sleep.
- Tools and guidelines are available from various organizations such as the American Academy of Pediatrics to guide in these discussions.
- Behaviors established in childhood are often carried into later years, so it is particularly important to establish positive lifestyle behaviors in children.

REFERENCES

1. Miller J, Boles R, Daniel S. *Pediatric Lifestyle Medicine. Lifestyle Medicine* (3rd edition). CRC Press (Boca Raton), 2019.
2. Eriksson J, Forsen T, Tuomilehto J. et al. Early Growth and Coronary Heart Disease in Later Life: Longitudinal Study. *BMJ.* 2001;322(7292):949–953.
3. Physical Activity Guidelines Advisory Committee. *2018 Physical Activity Guidelines Advisory Committee Scientific Report.* U.S. Department of Health and Human Services (Washington, DC), 2018.
4. U.S. Department of Health and Human Services. *Physical Activity Guidelines for Americans* (2nd edition). U.S. Department of Health and Human Services (Washington, DC), *2018 Physical Activity Guidelines for Americans* (2nd edition). Chapter 3: Active Children and Adolescents, 2008, pp. 46–55.
5. Lloyd-Jones D, Hong Y, Labarthe D. et al. Defining and Setting National Goals for Cardiovascular Health Promotion and Disease Reduction: The American Heart Association's Strategic Impact Goal through 2020 and Beyond. *Circulation.* 2010;121(4): 586–613.
6. Allen N. Abstract 17245: The Heritability of Ideal Cardiovascular Health: The Framingham Heart Study. *Circulation.* 2018;122, Issue suppl 21.
7. Bambs C, et al. Low Prevalence of "Ideal Cardiovascular Health" in a Community Based Population the Heart Strategies Concentrating on Risk Evaluation (Heart SCORE) Study. *Circulation.* 2011;123(8):850–857.
8. Lloyd-Jones D, Hong Y, Labarthe D, et al. Defining and Setting National Goals for Cardiovascular Health Promotion and Disease Reduction: The American Heart Association's Strategic Impact Goal through 2020 and Beyond. *Circulation.* 2010;121:586–613.
9. Micha R, et al. Association between Dietary Factors and Mortality from Heart Disease, Stroke, and Type 2 Diabetes in the United States. *JAMA: The Journal of the American Medical Association.* 2017;317(9):912–924.

10. Bronfenbrenner U. *The Ecology of Human Development*. Harvard University Press (Cambridge, MA), 1979.
11. Sauder K, Dabelea D. *Lifecourse Approach to Prevention of Chronic Disease. Lifestyle Medicine* (3rd edition). CRC Press (Boca Raton), 2019.
12. Rippe J. Physical Activity a Practical Guide. CRC Press (Boca Raton), 2020.
13. National Physical Activity Plan Alliance. *The 2016 United States Report Card on Physical Activity for Children and Youth*. National Physical Activity Plan Alliance (Washington, DC), 2016. https://www.physicalactivityplan.org/reportcard/2016FINAL _USReportCard.pdf. Accessed on July 7, 2020.
14. Chinapaw M, Proper K, Brug J, et al. Relationship between Young Peoples' Sedentary Behaviour and Biomedical Health Indicators: A Systematic Review of Prospective Studies. *Obesity Reviews*. 2011;12(7):e621–e632.
15. Tremblay M, LeBlanc A, Kho M, et al. Systematic Review of Sedentary Behaviour and Health Indicators in School-Aged Children and Youth. *International Journal of Behavioral Nutrition and Physical Activity*. 2011;8:98. doi:10.1186/1479-5868-8-98.
16. Carson V, Hunter S, Kuzik N, et al. Systematic Review of Sedentary Behaviour and Health Indicators in School-Aged Children and Youth: An Update. *Applied Physiology, Nutrition, and Metabolism*. 2016;41(6 suppl 3):S240–S265.
17. Cliff D, Hesketh K, Vella S, et al. Objectively Measured Sedentary Behaviour and Health and Development in Children and Adolescents: Systematic Review and Meta-Analysis. *Obesity Reviews*. 2016;17(4):330–344.
18. Beets M, Beighle A, Erwin H, et al. After-School Program Impact on Physical Activity and Fitness: A Meta-Analysis. *American Journal of Preventive Medicine*. 2009;36(6):527–537.
19. Larouche R, Saunders T, Faulkner G, et al. Associations between Active School Transport and Physical Activity, Body Composition, and Cardiovascular Fitness: A Systematic Review of 68 Studies. *Journal of Physical Activity and Health*. 2014;11(1):206–227.
20. Sun C, Pezic A, Tikellis G, et al. Effects of School-Based Interventions for Direct Delivery of Physical Activity on Fitness and Cardiometabolic Markers in Children and Adolescents: A Systematic Review of Randomized Controlled Trials. *Obesity Reviews*. 2013;14(1):818–838.
21. *2008 Physical Activity Guidelines for Americans Advisory Committee Report*. U.S. Department of Health and Human Services (Washington DC), 2008.
22. Kelley G, Kelley K, Pate R. Effects of Exercise on BMI Z-Score in Overweight and Obese Children and Adolescents: A Systematic Review with Meta-Analysis. *BMC Pediatrics*. 2014;14:225. doi:10.1186/1471-2431-14-225.
23. Hind K, Burrows M. Weight-Bearing Exercise and Bone Mineral Accrual in Children and Adolescents: A Review of Controlled Trials. *Bone*. 2007;40:14–27.
24. LeBlanc A, Spence J, Carson V, et al. Systematic Review of Sedentary Behaviour and Health Indicators in the Early Years (Aged 0–4 Years). *Applied Physiology, Nutrition, and Metabolism*. 2012;37(4):753–772.
25. Wu L, Sun S, He Y, et al. The Effect of Interventions Targeting Screen Time Reduction: A Systematic Review and Meta-Analysis. *Medicine (Baltimore)*. 2016;95(27):e4029.
26. Donnelly J, Hillman C, Castelli D, et al. Physical Activity, Fitness, Cognitive Function, and Academic Achievement in Children: A Systematic Review. *Medicine & Science in Sports & Exercise*. 2016;48:1197–1222.
27. Owen K, Parker P, Van Zanden B, et al. Physical Activity and School Engagement in Youth: A Systematic Review and Meta-Analysis. *Educational Psychologist*. 2016;51:129–145.

28. American Academy of Pediatrics Council on Communications and Media. Policy Statement - Children, Adolescents, Obesity and the Media. *Pediatrics.* 2011;128:201–208.

29. Hildebrandt J, Couch S. *Cardiovascular Risk and Diet in Children. Lifestyle Medicine* (3rd edition). CRC Press (Boca Raton), 2019.

30. Moore J, Haemer M. *Childhood Obesity. Lifestyle Medicine* (3rd edition). CRC Press (Boca Raton), 2019.

31. Brothers J, Daniels S. *Identification and Management of Children with Dyslipidemia. Lifestyle Medicine* (3rd edition). CRC Press (Boca Raton), 2019.

32. Baker-Smith C, Gidding S. *Diagnosis, Management, and Treatment of Systemic Hypertension in Youth, Updates from the 2017 American Academy of Pediatrics Clinical Practice Guideline. Lifestyle Medicine* (3rd edition). CRC Press (Boca Raton), 2019.

33. Flynn J, Kaelber D, Baker-Smith C, et al. Clinical Practice Guideline for Screening and Management of High Blood Pressure in Children and Adolescents. *Pediatrics.* 2017;140(3):E20171904.

34. Kalkwarf H. *Prevention of Osteoporosis in Children and Adolescents. Lifestyle Medicine* (3rd edition). CRC Press (Boca Raton), 2019.

35. Kaar J, Simon S. *Sleep and Obesity Prevention in Children and Adolescents. Lifestyle Medicine* (3rd edition). CRC Press (Boca Raton), 2019.

36. Gupta N, Mueller W, Chan W, et al. Is Obesity Associated with Poor Sleep Quality in Adolescents? *American Journal of Human Biology.* 2002;14(6):762–768.

15 The Practice of Lifestyle Medicine

KEY POINTS

- The field of lifestyle medicine has now been defined by various organizations and gives practitioners a framework for thinking about this branch of medicine.
- Lifestyle medicine is strongly related to and is a component of allopathic medicine since both are based on high levels of evidence.
- Core competencies in lifestyle medicine have been developed and published.
- Clinical processes in lifestyle medicine have also been developed for those who wish to develop a practice based on lifestyle medicine.
- As the field of lifestyle medicine has matured, high-intensity therapeutic lifestyle change has also emerged for those who wish to have advanced training and specialization in lifestyle medicine.

15.1 INTRODUCTION

There is no longer any serious doubt that daily habits and actions profoundly impact on short- and long-term health and quality of life (1). The scientific and medical literature that supports this concept is now overwhelming. Thousands of studies provide the evidence that regular physical activity, maintenance of a healthy body weight, not smoking cigarettes, as well as following sound nutrition, stress reduction, and other health-promoting practices all profoundly impact on health. Conversely, an inactive lifestyle, obesity, high levels of stress, and cigarette smoking or exposure to cigarette smoke and other pollutants all adversely impact on health.

All of these issues are central to the emerging field of lifestyle medicine. In the past decade, a consensus has arisen that study of these habits and practices will coalesce under the umbrella of "lifestyle medicine." Simultaneously, many health care workers are either devoting their entire careers to lifestyle medicine or utilizing lifestyle medicine principles and practices as a component of their practice.

So, what is lifestyle medicine? I am proud to have named the field of lifestyle medicine in the academic literature with the 1st edition of my major textbook of that same name, which was published in 1999 (2). In that book I defined lifestyle medicine as "the integration of lifestyle practices into the modern practice of medicine both to help to lower the risk for chronic disease and/or if disease is already present, serve as an adjunct in therapy."

Lifestyle medicine brings together sound scientific evidence in diverse health-related fields to assist the clinician in the process of not only treating disease, but also

203

promoting good health. Even though this definition was put forth over two decades ago, it has largely stood the test of time. Other organizations have also offered definitions of lifestyle medicine, but those are very similar to the initial definition that was offered in the 1st edition of my *Lifestyle Medicine* textbook. The 3rd edition of *Lifestyle Medicine* was published in 2019 and addressed the continuing evolution of the field.

In this chapter, we will explore issues related to the practice of lifestyle medicine. The intent is to provide an overall summary for the current state of lifestyle medicine and offer guidance to individuals who are contemplating utilizing lifestyle medicine either as the focal point of their practice or as a component of their overall medical practice.

15.2   DEFINING LIFESTYLE MEDICINE

While many investigators have utilized the phrase "lifestyle medicine," it appears to have been first used by the epidemiologist Ernst Wynder, when he was discussing smoking and lung cancer risk in 1988 (3). Wynder utilized this phrase at a symposium in 1988. Hans Diehl heard Wynder use the term and sought to copyright it in the United States by 1988. However, his request was denied because authorities deemed the individual words to have widespread common use and the combination was not distinct. Following the publication of the 1st edition of my textbook, *Lifestyle Medicine*, in 1999, which was the first text to define the field in academic medicine, Garry Egger, Andrew Binns, and Stephan Rossner published *Introduction of Lifestyle Medicine* in 2007 (4). References to the phrase "lifestyle medicine" in PubMed numbered 208 in January of 2018.

The American College of Lifestyle Medicine, which is a professional organization dealing with health care practitioners who wish to focus on lifestyle medicine, defined the term as "dealing primarily with the application of evidence based, non-drug therapy for the treatment of chronic, non-communicable diseases" (5). Other important milestones in the development of lifestyle medicine came from the founding of the Coronary Health Improvement Project (CHIP), which was developed by Hans Diehl and initially focused on the treatment as well as risk reduction of coronary heart disease (CHD) with nutrition, exercise, and other lifestyle modifications (6). Dean Ornish also published a randomized controlled trial utilizing various techniques in lifestyle medicine to show their effect on the reversibility of CHD (7).

As the field of lifestyle medicine has expanded, the use of the term and development of concepts have broadened to include both social and political effects. This allowed the field to expand beyond the direct responsibility of individuals and into the realm of public health. Other aspects of lifestyle medicine have included components of self-care and self-management as well as concepts related to an overall approach to a healthy environment. Various definitions of lifestyle medicine were brought together by the American College of Lifestyle Medicine in 2012 and published as a document entitled "The Lifestyle Medicine Standards," which is available online (8).

It should also be noted that a number of professional organizations have also become active in the area of lifestyle medicine. For example, the American Heart Association changed the name of one of its Councils from the "Council on Nutrition, Physical Activity and Metabolism" to the "Council on Lifestyle and Cardiometabolic Health" in 2013 (9). Furthermore, both the American Academy of Family Practice and the American College of Preventive Medicine have established educational tracks in the area of lifestyle medicine.

Importantly, a new health care organization, American College of Lifestyle Medicine (ACLM), was formed in 2005. This organization is devoted to providing a professional home for individuals who wish to emphasize lifestyle medicine in their medical practice. ACLM has doubled its membership each year for the past five years, making it the most rapidly growing medical organization in the United States. ACLM has also spawned initiatives to develop curricula and encourage education of medical students as well as physicians and other health care professionals. Lifestyle medicine has also become an international movement with the development of the Lifestyle Medicine Global Alliance (10).

In addition, a peer-reviewed academic journal *American Journal of Lifestyle Medicine*, was launched in 2007, and which now has over 13,000 subscribers and over 100,000 downloads of full text articles on an annual basis (11).

It should also be noted that a number of organizations have participated in developing criteria for the practice of lifestyle medicine. In 2010, representatives from the American Academy of Pediatrics, the American College of Sports Medicine, the Academy of Nutrition and Dietetics, the Academy of Family Practice, and the American College of Preventive Medicine worked together to establish the first Summary of Competencies for Physicians that clinicians should possess to understand the practice of lifestyle medicine. These criteria were published in the *Journal of the American Medical Association* (8).

15.3   DIMENSIONS OF THE DEFINITION

As the field of lifestyle medicine continues to evolve, it will be important to incorporate a number of different concepts into this broad area of medicine. These will include such concepts as primary, secondary, and tertiary prevention, but lifestyle medicine is much broader than this. Lifestyle medicine principles and practices are already recognized as central components of the treatment of most chronic diseases.

When the concepts of lifestyle medicine are brought together, it necessitates different models of clinicians working with a wide variety of health care professionals, including nutritionists, coaches, exercise physiologists, nurses, and many others. Lifestyle medicine, to be successful, will need to also work in allopathic medicine and will also involve concepts that relate to behavior change (see Chapter 4 for more details).

It is also essential that clinicians practice healthy lifestyle practices in their own lives to not only improve their own health, but to also underscore its value to their patients. Perhaps most importantly, clinicians will need to adopt a "partnership mentality" recognizing that the ultimate arbiter of positive lifestyle practices and habits will be the patients themselves. This is different from the "expert" model which is predominant in allopathic medicine.

It is essential that lifestyle medicine is based on the highest level of evidence. It is very difficult to conduct studies with multiple aspects of lifestyle medicine under consideration at the same time. However, there is an enormous amount of evidence in the specific components of lifestyle medicine such as physical activity, nutrition, and weight management. This large body of evidence needs to continue to be emphasized not only to patients but also to other clinicians.

Finally, lifestyle medicine clinicians have an important opportunity to work with the public to create environments that encourage lifestyle medicine modalities such as physical activity and proper nutrition. All of these will be essential in order to bring the enormous benefits of lifestyle medicine to the widest possible patient population.

15.4   CATEGORIES OF MEDICINE

It is important to place lifestyle medicine within the context of other medical constructs. This can help avoid confusion concerning what else lifestyle medicine is and is not (12).

- *Allopathic medicine:* This has been the domain of standard medical practice for over 120 years. Allopathic medicine applies the knowledge of normal physiology and pathophysiology as well as the application of evidence-based surgical and pharmacologic treatment. The cornerstone of allopathic medicine has been evidence-based medicine (EBM). Within this, the randomized controlled trial (RCT) has become the primary tool for understanding how to treat disease. While non-drug therapies have been included in allopathic medicine, they are not typically emphasized.
- *Lifestyle medicine:* Lifestyle medicine is based on the recognition that lifestyle plays a critical role in many chronic disease conditions. Lifestyle medicine brings together, under one umbrella, thousands of studies in disciplines such as physical activity, nutrition, weight management, and smoking cessation. In a sense, lifestyle medicine is very similar to allopathic medicine with its reliance on EBM. However, the focus in lifestyle medicine is on daily lifestyle habits and actions and their impact on health. With this emphasis, lifestyle medicine clearly fits within the framework of allopathic medicine with regard to the emphasis on EBM.
- *Complementary or alternative medicine:* Neither complementary nor alternative medicine is typically considered a part of conventional allopathic medicine. There are many components of complementary medicine for which there is very little evidence. For example, aroma therapy, which utilizes the scents from various oils, flowers, herbs, and so forth, in complementary medicine is thought to promote health and well-being. This type of therapy is not widely accepted in allopathic medicine. Some practices that could be included in complementary medicine may overlap with lifestyle medicine, such as practicing mindfulness.

In contrast, alternative medicine is often used in place of conventional allopathic medicine. For example, an alternative therapy might be use of a special diet to treat cancer in place of undergoing surgery, radiation, or chemotherapy. Other components of alternative medicine may include aspects of medicine as practiced in other cultures such as Chinese medicine or Ayurveda medicine. While some alternative medicine therapies may be acceptable in allopathic medicine, many are not.

- *Mind/body medicine:* This form of medicine focuses on the interaction among brain/mind/body and behavior and the powerful ways that mind/body interact with each other. Just as in alternative or complementary medicine, there may be some overlap with lifestyle medicine and also some overlap with allopathic medicine, although much less current evidence is available in mind/body medicine compared with allopathic or lifestyle medicine.
- *Integrative medicine:* This form of medicine combines allopathic medicine and alternative medicine. This has gained more adherence within normal medicine using benefits from combining some elements of alternative medicine with regular allopathic medicine.
- *Preventive medicine:* This form of medicine focuses on medical care and therapies designed to prevent health problems. Portions of preventive medicine are similar to those in lifestyle medicine, although lifestyle medicine is a much broader, more inclusive term. A section on preventive medicine is one of many sections included in the 3rd edition of the textbook that I edited: *Lifestyle Medicine* (1).

15.5 THE UNIQUE ROLE OF LIFESTYLE MEDICINE WITHIN ALLOPATHIC MEDICINE

A distinct and important advantage of lifestyle medicine compared to other categories such as complementary, alternative, or integrative medicine is that lifestyle medicine is, at its core, EBM, but applies to decisions that people make in their daily lives. Because of the enormous body of evidence that supports lifestyle medicine, it fits within allopathic medicine and extends its boundaries in very significant ways. For example, it is now estimated that over 80% of all chronic illnesses have a significant lifestyle component. Thus, lifestyle medicine offers an important way that allopathic medicine can be extended to deal with the realities of the enormous evidence base that exists in the area of the health consequences of daily habits and actions such as physical activity, healthy nutrition, and weight management.

15.6 HEALTH PROVIDER CORE COMPETENCIES IN LIFESTYLE MEDICINE

As lifestyle medicine has continued to grow, it has become increasingly important to develop a core body of competencies which define lifestyle medicine and educate individuals who wish to incorporate lifestyle medicine and its principles as either part of their medical practice or as the cornerstone of their practice.

With the goal of establishing a core group of practices to define lifestyle medicine, in 2009, a group of health care professionals representing a variety of organizations met to develop a national consensus for what constitutes the core principles of lifestyle medicine. Participants included representatives from the American Academy of Family Physicians, the American Medical Association, the American College of Physicians, the American Osteopathic Association, the American Academy of Pediatrics, the American College of Sports Medicine, and the American College of Lifestyle Medicine. These individuals established a consensus definition of lifestyle medicine which is as follows:

> The evidenced based practice of helping individuals and families adopt and sustain healthy behaviors that affect health and quality of life.

The Consensus Panel also established a list of core competencies which are provided in Table 15.1.

This list of competencies has subsequently been expanded and refined to include the following key competencies:

- Lifestyle medicine basics
- Healthy behavior change
- Effective clinical processes
- Providers' personal health and community advocacies
- Healthy nutrition
- Physical activity
- Mental and emotional well-being
- Sleep health
- Tobacco cessation
- Managing risky alcohol use
- Weight management

For individuals who want to explore more details concerning this, please refer to Chapter 83 in the 3rd edition of *Lifestyle Medicine* textbook by Liana Lianov who has been a leader in developing these competencies.

15.7　LIFESTYLE MEDICINE CLINICAL PROCESSES

The next important step in the development of the field of lifestyle medicine has come from various individuals taking the core competencies and turning them into clinical processes (13).

These processes include a standard set of procedures and approaches that form the core of how to practice lifestyle medicine. These include a lifestyle medicine history that focuses on risk factors that predispose individuals to developing preventive lifestyle-related disease (e.g., physical activity levels, nutrition, stress, and sleep),

TABLE 15.1

Lifestyle Medicine Core Competencies Identified by National Consensus Panel

Competency Domain	Core Competencies
Leadership	Promote healthy behaviors as foundational to medical care, disease prevention, and health promotion
	Seek to practice healthy behaviors and create school, work, and home environments that support healthy behaviors
Knowledge	Demonstrate knowledge of the evidence that specific lifestyle changes can have a positive effect on patients' health outcomes
	Describe ways that physician engagement with patients and families can have a positive effect on patients' health behaviors
Assessment skills	Assess the social, psychological, and biological predispositions of patients' behaviors and the resulting health outcomes
	Assess patient and family readiness, willingness, and ability to make health behavior changes
	Perform a history and physical examination specific to lifestyle-related health status, including lifestyle "vital signs" such as tobacco use, alcohol consumption, diet, physical activity, body mass index, stress level, sleep, and emotional well-being. Based on this assessment, obtain and interpret appropriate tests to screen, diagnose, and monitor lifestyle-related diseases
Management skills	Use nationally recognized practice guidelines (such as those for hypertension and smoking cessation) to assist patients in self-managing their health behaviors and lifestyles
	Establish effective relationships with patients and their families to effect and sustain behavioral change using evidence-based counseling methods and tools and follow-up
	Collaborate with patients and their families to develop evidence-based, achievable, specific, written action plans such as lifestyle prescriptions
	Help patients manage and sustain healthy lifestyle practices, and refer patients to other health care professionals as needed for lifestyle-related conditions
Use of office and community support	Have the ability to practice as an interdisciplinary team of health care professionals and support a team approach
	Develop and apply office systems and practices to support lifestyle medical care, including decision support technology
	Measure processes and outcomes to improve quality of lifestyle interventions in individuals and groups of patients
	Use appropriate community referral resources that support the implementation of healthy lifestyles

Source: Rippe JM. *Lifestyle Medicine*, 3rd edition. Used with permission.

followed by the lifestyle physical examination to further identify chronic disease risk elements, including adiposity, blood pressure, fitness, and relevant laboratory markers.

The lifestyle medicine physician is also responsible for establishing and supporting an interdisciplinary clinical model that utilizes the expertise of multiple health care professionals such as nutritionists and exercise physiologists. The American College of Lifestyle Medicine has played an important role in this area by establishing a "Lifestyle Assessment Short Form," which is available through the American College of Lifestyle Medicine. This Assessment Form focuses on such issues as nutrition, exercise, sleep, and weight management, as well as mental health, smoking and substance use, and motivational change. Such a Form can play a very important role in helping the clinician streamline obtaining important information related to lifestyle habits and actions and health.

15.8 LIFESTYLE MEDICINE AND OPTIMAL SLEEP

Multiple daily habits and practices significantly impact on both short- and long-term health and quality of life (14). In other chapters of this manual, we will deal specifically with physical activity, nutrition, weight management, and others. However, some energy should also be devoted to the issue of sleep.

Sleep is often underappreciated as an important health consideration and is an area that is central to the practice of lifestyle medicine. It is important to understand that adequate sleep is fundamental to good health. In fact, disturbed sleep is associated with a wide range of chronic disorders, including cardiovascular disease, other metabolic conditions, inflammatory conditions, and even cancer diagnoses. For this reason, it is important for lifestyle medicine practitioners to focus significant attention on sleep.

We know, for example, that inadequate sleep is associated with weight gain, obesity, and various associated metabolic disorders. Inadequate sleep is also associated with increased risk of cardiovascular disease as well as mood disorders, inflammatory disorders, and some cancers. For all of these reasons, it is important that clinicians focus on sleep as a component of an overall lifestyle medicine assessment.

Ways to approach sleep include inquiring about the number of hours of sleep in a 24-hour period. For most individuals, 7–9 hours of sleep is appropriate. Sleep duration of less than 6 hours or more than 9 hours both are associated with adverse health consequences and chronic diseases.

Subjective quality of sleep should also be assessed, including soundness of sleep. If an individual reports poor quality of sleep, including difficulty falling asleep, maintenance of sleep, or early awakening, all of these should be examined in more detail. Poor sleep quality is also associated with increased risk of motor vehicle and other accidents. Estimates of the association between drowsiness and automobile accidents have ranged from 2% to 2.5%, all the way up, in some estimates, to 15–20% of accidents.

There are a variety of lifestyle medicine interventions that can assist in improving duration and quality of sleep such as controlling the temperature in the bedroom.

Some research suggests that gradual decrease in ambient temperature while sleeping improves the quality of sleep. Mindfulness meditation and cognitive medial therapy have also been demonstrated to improve quality and duration of sleep. (See also Chapter 4.) The interaction between other neurological function and sleep has already been discussed in detail in Chapter 11.

15.9 EMOTIONAL HEALTH AND STRESS MANAGEMENT

A key component of lifestyle medicine is emotional health (15). Often this is also a component of managing stress. More details on the aspect of stress management are found in Chapter 4. Assessing and improving emotional well-being can be improved by utilizing a variety of different tools that are available within the field of lifestyle medicine. These include the following:

- Developing a thankfulness journey
- Practicing optimistic thinking
- Learning to live in the present, while not dreading the past or fearing the future
- Learning forgiveness and how to deal with anger
- Practicing positivity and working to enhance happiness. The whole area of positive psychology is explored in more detail in Chapter 4.

Focusing on emotional health is an area that is often ignored in allopathic medicine, but it is a key component of the overall practice of lifestyle medicine.

15.10 HIGH-INTENSITY THERAPEUTIC LIFESTYLE CHANGE

As the field of lifestyle medicine has advanced, the field of high-intensity therapeutic lifestyle change has also emerged (16). In a sense, this field has been available for several decades and is particularly appropriate for individuals who wish to devote their entire practice to the area of lifestyle medicine. Within the field of lifestyle medicine, the most compelling evidence for its effectiveness comes from studies where lifestyle medicine treatment is applied at higher levels of intensity than many clinicians are able to practice. Conceptually, high-intensity therapeutic lifestyle change has become the specialty component of lifestyle medicine.

Intensive Therapeutic Lifestyle Change (ITLC) utilizes intensive total immersion approaches to change rather than the more gradual incremental change commonly recommended by clinicians. ITLC includes comprehensive multifactorial lifestyle change approach. In many instances, this treatment may begin in a residential facility where meals are prepared, exercise is scheduled multiple times a day, and educational activities are conducted, while plenty of sleep is included. Thus, with these various modalities, patients spend 4–8 hours in contact with the intervention staff on most weekdays for a period of a few weeks.

Following return to home, the patient is provided with supportive interventions which may be conducted by phone or online for several weeks or months. Most impressive results from ITLC have demonstrated significant decreases in the risk of heart disease as well as other chronic diseases. Examples of clinicians who have utilized ITLC include the Pritikin Program, the McDougall Program, and the Ornish Program.

15.11 PHYSICIAN HEALTH PRACTICES AND LIFESTYLE MEDICINE

The multiple benefits of lifestyle medicine also extend to physicians who utilize these modalities in their own lives. Certainly, such modalities as regular physical activity, proper nutrition, weight management, tobacco cessation, and healthy sleep, all are relevant to physicians as well as their patients. An additional benefit for physicians practicing lifestyle medicine modalities is that multiple research studies have shown that physicians who follow these habits are much more likely to counsel their patients in these areas than are physicians who do not (17).

One, additional benefit from practicing lifestyle medicine modalities has emerged in the medical literature over the past decade. Within medicine, there is an increasing problem with physician burnout. In fact, in one study, over 50% of physicians surveyed had some evidence of burnout. There are emerging data that individuals who practice self-care behaviors, such as those found in lifestyle medicine, are more likely to be happy in their lives and experience less burnout. More research is emerging at the current time about the connection between lifestyle medicine and reduced risk of burnout.

15.12 CONCLUSIONS

As the field of lifestyle medicine has continued to advance, it is important to have a clear understanding and definitions about this discipline. A number of organizations have provided definitions of lifestyle medicine and have increased the clarity with which the field is framed. An important aspect of lifestyle medicine is that it is based on the same level of high evidence that is found throughout allopathic medicine. Thus, lifestyle medicine may be distinguished from other types of medicine such as alternative medicine, complementary medicine, or integrative medicine because of the high level of evidence that underpins such components of lifestyle medicine as proper nutrition, regular physical activity, weight management, and many others. As the field has matured, competencies have been developed for practitioners of lifestyle medicine and guidelines for how to employ lifestyle medicine in a clinical practice have also been developed. In addition, for individuals who wish to become specialists in lifestyle medicine, the field of high-intensity therapeutic lifestyle change has also emerged and has shown dramatic results in decreasing risk factors for a variety of chronic diseases.

15.13 CLINICAL APPLICATIONS

* Lifestyle medicine is supported by an enormous body of evidence which underpins it and is comparable to the evidence-based foundation of allopathic medicine.

- Clinicians interested in practicing lifestyle medicine should take advantage of the published core competencies in lifestyle medicine as well as the published clinical processes to develop a lifestyle medicine clinic.
- For those who wish to specialize in advanced lifestyle medicine, the field of high-intensity therapeutic lifestyle change has also emerged.

REFERENCES

1. Rippe JM (ed.). *Lifestyle Medicine* (3rd edition). CRC Press (Boca Raton), 2019.
2. Rippe JM. (ed.). *Lifestyle Medicine*. Blackwell Science, Inc. (London), 1999.
3. Wynder E. Cancer Control and Lifestyle Medicine. *Present and Future of Indoor Air Quality. Proceedings of the Brussels Conference.* 1989; 3–13.
4. Egger G, Binns A, Rossner S. Introduction to Lifestyle Medicine. In: Egger G, Binns A, Rossner S, eds., *Lifestyle Medicine* (1st edition). McGraw-Hill Australia Pty Ltd. (Sydney, NSW), 2007.
5. American College of Lifestyle Medicine. https://lifestylemedicineconference.org. Accessed July 8, 2020.
6. Morton D, Rankin P, Kent L, et al. The Complete Health Improvement Program (CHIP): History, Evaluation, and Outcomes. *American Journal of Lifestyle Medicine.* 2016;10:64–73.
7. Ornish D, Brown SE, Scherwitz LW, et al. Can Lifestyle Changes Reverse Coronary Atherosclerosis? The Lifestyle Heart Trial. *Lancet.* 1990;336:129–133.
8. Lianov L, Johnson M. Physician Competencies for Prescribing Lifestyle Medicine. *JAMA.* 2010;304:202–203.
9. American Heart Association. https://www.heart.org/. Accessed July 8, 2020.
10. The Lifestyle Medicine Global Alliance. https://lifestylemedicineglobal.org/. Accessed July 8, 2020.
11. American Journal of Lifestyle Medicine. https://journals.sagepub.com/home/ajl. Accessed July 8, 2020.
12. Guthrie G. Definition of Lifestyle Medicine. In: Rippe JM, ed., *Lifestyle Medicine* (3rd edition). CRC Press (Boca Raton), 2019.
13. Edshteyn I. Lifestyle Medicine Clinical Practice. In: Rippe JM, ed., *Lifestyle Medicine* (3rd edition). CRC Press (Boca Raton), 2019.
14. Gurley V. Sleep as Medicine and Lifestyle Medicine for Optimal Sleep. In: Rippe JM, ed., *Lifestyle Medicine* (3rd edition). CRC Press (Boca Raton), 2019.
15. Nedley N, Ramirez F. Emotional Health and Stress Management. In: Rippe JM, ed., *Lifestyle Medicine* (3rd edition). CRC Press (Boca Raton), 2019.
16. Kelly J. High Intensity Therapeutic Lifestyle Change. In Rippe JM, ed., *Lifestyle Medicine* (3rd edition). CRC Press (Boca Raton), 2019.
17. Frank E, Holmes D. Physician Health Practices and Lifestyle Medicine. In: Rippe JM, ed., *Lifestyle Medicine* (3rd edition). CRC Press (Boca Raton), 2019.

16 Lifestyle Medicine for the Older Adult Population

KEY POINTS

- Multiple studies have shown that cognitive function may decline as part of the aging process. However, lifestyle habits and actions such as regular physical activity and proper nutrition can positively impact on cognition.
- There is a decrease in muscle function and strength associated with aging. These can also be ameliorated to some degree by regular physical activity, including both aerobic physical activity and resistance strength training as well as nutritional strategies based on general guidance for healthy nutrition and adequate levels of protein and vitamin D.
- Dietary quality is directly related to both physical and cognitive function in later years. Clinicians should emphasize these options as healthy lifestyle practices for all patients, particularly those above the age of 65.
- Advancing years are often accompanied by declines in sensory perceptions such as taste, smell, vision, dexterity, and mobility, which may necessitate added attention to dietary behavior in older patients.

16.1 INTRODUCTION

Individuals over the age of 65 comprise approximately 13% of the U.S. population. These numbers are projected to reach 72.1 million (19% of the total population) by the Year 2030 (1). This age group is the most rapidly growing of all population segments in the United States (1).

A large and persuasive body of scientific information supports the concept that a variety of lifestyle measures yield multiple health and quality of life benefits for people over the age of 65 (1,2). Since the aging population in the United States is rapidly growing, finding cost-effective mechanisms for improving the health and forestalling disabilities in this age group assumes great importance. The role of various lifestyle measures is central to the health, well-being, and quality of life for people over the age of 65 (3).

Over the past decade, our views of the population over the age of 65 have changed dramatically. This has also given rise to the concept of "successful aging" (SA), which will be discussed further in this chapter (3).

The purpose of this chapter is to provide a summary of recent scientific information related to a variety of lifestyle measures for the elderly population. These measures have been clearly shown to improve the health and longevity of individuals in this population and reduce the risk of chronic disease as well as assist in the

treatment of already present diseases and lower the risk of any injury or falls resulting in the risk of developing chronic disabilities in the elderly population.

16.2   AGE-ASSOCIATED COGNITIVE DECLINE AND
ITS ALLEVIATION BY LIFESTYLE MEASURES

There are a variety of age-related effects on various organ systems. The brain also
experiences age-related changes (4). The brain experiences a progressive decline in
volume with increasing age after the age of 30. It has been estimated that decline
in brain volume is approximately 0.3% per year, resulting in about a 15% reduction
in brain volume between the ages of 30 and 80 (5). In addition, the brain experiences a gradual reduction in the ability to replace lost neurons in the process of
neurogenesis. Neurosynapses and networks also show age-related decline as well
as neurotransmitter activity at synapses. In addition, a variety of vascular changes
which reduce cerebral blood flow also occur with aging. All of these factors have the
potential to contribute to adverse neurological changes (6).

The changes in the brain may be associated with decline in cognitive processes, including memory, learning ability, problem-solving, and executive control. These decreases in cognitive function in the aging brain may range from
relatively minor changes in age-related memory (ARMI), mild cognitive impairment (MCI), and various forms of dementia, including Alzheimer's disease (AD).
Various lifestyle measures such as controlling risk factors for vascular disease,
including elevated blood pressure, diabetes (T2DM), and dyslipidemia, are all
strongly influenced by regular lifestyle measures. In addition, physical activity,
especially aerobic exercise of sufficient intensity and volume to increase aerobic
fitness, has been repeatedly shown to result in improved cognitive function in the
elderly population.

The Physical Activity Guidelines for Americans 2018 Scientific Report (PAGA
2018) recommends 150–180 minutes per week of moderate intensity physical
activity (7). This is the same recommendation given for all adults. These levels
of physical activity also result in a decrease in other diseases which become more
prevalent in the aging population, such as cardiovascular disease (CVD), T2DM,
and a variety of cancers. The recommended doses of physical activity may need to
be adjusted if the elderly population has previously been sedentary or is very unfit.
Similar recommendations have also been given by the American College of Sports
Medicine (ACSM).

These levels of physical activity have been shown to reduce the risk of MCI
and dementia. The precise mechanisms for the improvement of cognitive function
are not completely understood. Regular physical activity may promote neurogenesis, including the generation of new neurons and synapses, lowering the risk of
cerebral vascular narrowing and decline, and may also significantly contribute
toward improving cognition. Various lifestyle measures may also increase the level
of "cognitive reserve" (8). Cognitive reserve can also be enhanced by continuing to encourage the elderly population to engage in volunteer work and social
engagements.

16.3   REDUCING THE AGE-ASSOCIATED RISK OF SARCOPENIA

Skeletal muscle declines with age (9). Skeletal muscle constitutes the largest soft tissue mass in the human body. It constitutes about 40% of the total lean body mass in the average, healthy young man and about 25% in a comparably aged young woman (10). Skeletal muscle and mass and strength generally peak at the age of mid-20s–30. This is then generally followed between ages 30 and 50 by a progressive decline of about 1% a year, until the age of 70 at which time the rate of loss accelerates to about 3% per year (10).

When there is a significant amount of muscle loss, it can lead to frailty. This condition is commonly accompanied by a term called "sarcopenia," which is defined as loss of two or more standard deviations of muscle mass below the mean (20–30 years old) of the same sex and ethnicity. Sarcopenia can represent a significant decline in metabolism and also frailty, leading to significant functional decline. It is currently estimated that 13–24% of adults over the age of 70 and 50% of those over the age of 80 have sarcopenia (11).

A variety of biological mechanisms seem to underline sarcopenia. These include reduction in muscle fiber number and size, molecular and biochemical changes, some cell death (apoptosis), inflammation, accumulation of damaged muscle protein, reduced anabolic hormone activities, and reduced levels of blood supply.

Numerous studies have consistently demonstrated that a sedentary lifestyle contributes to sarcopenia and frailty. Conversely, exercise training even in older, physically frail individuals has been demonstrated to improve muscle mass and strength as well as muscular and cardiorespiratory endurance. Even though most of the data on these issues is in individuals over the age of 50, regular physical activity throughout the lifespan can forestall sarcopenia.

The recommendations for physical activity in individuals over the age of 70 include resistance strength training two to three days a week utilizing both upper and lower body exercise via machinery, weight lifting, and/or elastic bands. In addition, moderate to vigorous aerobic activity of 150 minutes per week as recommended by the PAGA 2018 is also recommended. Low-impact exercise, which also has a low risk of injury, including walking, stationary cycling, and swimming, is recommended. In addition, flexibility and balance training can be conducted as a component of warming up and cooling down and is useful to reduce the risk of falls and associated injuries.

A variety of biological mechanisms are thought to underlie the benefits of exercise or physical activity in individuals over the age of 70. These include reduced apoptosis, reduced oxidative stress, reduced anti-inflammatory effects, improved insulin/glucose dynamics, and enhanced quality and quantity of muscle protein and mitochondria. Besides, regular physical activity can result in enhanced muscle blood supply (9). In addition to physical activity, nutritional strategies may also help with age-related loss of muscle. A variety of recommendations have been made in this area:

- Follow national guidelines for a healthy, balanced diet.
- Ensure adequate food intake.

- Meet the requirements for good quality protein.
- Maintain an adequate circulating vitamin D level from sun exposure, diet, and other supplements.
- Adequate intake of food sources with exogenous antioxidants.

16.4 AGING SUCCESSFULLY: PREDICTORS AND PATHWAYS

As more data have accumulated on mechanisms for enhancing and helping the quality of life in individuals over the age of 65, the concept of "successful aging" (SA) has achieved increased prominence (3). Currently, it is estimated that in the United States, an alarmingly low percentage of individuals over the age of 65 are aging successfully. The Health and Retirement Study showed that only 11.9% of older adults can be categorized as aging successfully. Other studies have shown similar low percentages of aging successfully.

A number of definitions and models of successful aging have been proposed. Perhaps the most utilized model was put forth by Rowe and Kahn. They defined criteria, including the following three key characteristics as the basis of their SA model: the low risk of disease and disease-related disability, high mental and physical function, and active engagement with life. In order to be considered aging successfully, older adults need to display high levels in all three of these characteristics. As more research and interest has occurred in the area of SA, it has become clear that adoption of many of these factors optimally would begin to take place earlier in life and this has led to a life course approach to the study of SA. This, in turn, has led to research that shows a variety of pathways that can result in successful aging.

Perhaps the most important component of SA is regular exercise or physical activity. Physical activity has the potential to serve as a primary vehicle for enhancing or maintaining each of the three characteristics identified for SA in Rowe and Wade. In addition, a large body of research has identified that physical inactivity is a key factor for reducing the risk of a number of chronic medical conditions, which further underscores the importance of regular physical activity (12,13). The PAGA 2018 Scientific Report recommends 150 minutes of moderate to vigorous intensity physical activity per week. This would clearly enhance the likelihood of individuals aging successfully.

In addition, other lifestyle practices also play important roles in SA. Cognitive training and stimulation have been demonstrated to improve cognitive function in both healthy older adults and those already experiencing mild cognitive impairment. Dietary influences are also important. Both the adequacy and quality of food consumed by older adults influence the ability to age successfully. A number of studies have demonstrated the impact of an inadequate diet on physical health. Recommendations for older adults may be found in a variety of sources, including the Dietary Guidelines for Americans 2015–2020 (14). Also see subsequent sections in this chapter.

Social engagement and volunteerism have also been demonstrated to contribute to SA. It is important to emphasize that health care professionals can play an important role in promoting SA among older adults. Health care providers are viewed by the majority of older adults as a primary source of health information and therefore have the credibility and ability to play an influential role in getting older adults to embrace a healthier lifestyle. Unfortunately, the percentage of adults over the age of 65 who report receiving counseling about health-promoting activities, such as regular physical activity, is very low (approximately 31%). This, despite the fact that a number of studies have shown that physician-based counseling, particularly as it relates to physical activity, smoking cessation, alcohol consumption, and nutrition, is a powerful tool and can be conducted in counseling sessions as short as 3–5 minutes. Failure to provide this type of information for older adults constitutes a wasted opportunity since over 70% of older adults in the United States see their physician at least once a year and it is likely that individuals over the age of 65 see their physicians even more regularly than that.

16.5 THE ROLE OF PHYSICAL ACTIVITY IN THE WELL-BEING OF OLDER ADULTS

As already indicated, physical activity is associated with multiple benefits for individuals over the age of 65 (2). In particular, physical activity has been routinely shown to improve cognitive function and lower cognitive decline. In addition, regular physical activity helps with the age-related risk of sarcopenia and frailty. In addition, regular physical activity improves physical function and reduces age-related loss of function in the aging population.

The PAGA 2018 Scientific Report demonstrated that there was an inverse dose-response relationship between the volume of aerobic physical activity and the risk of physical function limitations in the aging population. According to the National Health Interview Survey conducted during 2001–2007, 22.9% of older adults aged 60–69 reported limitations such as great difficulty or inability to do basic tasks of life (e.g., walk 0.25 mile or lift a 10-pound bag of groceries) (2). At the same time, 42.9% of adults aged 80 or older reported significant limitations in this area. The PAGA 2018 Scientific Report also indicated that physical activity could prevent or delay disability. Based on multiple studies, including randomized controlled trials (RCTs) and cohort studies of aerobic activity, muscle strengthening and balance, and/or multicomponent physical activity programs, there is strong evidence that demonstrates that physical activity improves physical function and reduces age-related declines in function.

Cohort studies of physical activity have suggested that there is approximately a 50% reduction in major functional limitations which may occur in individuals who are regularly physically active. This is particularly important since this population is rapidly growing.

In addition, physical activity has the significant benefit of helping to prevent falls. Falls can present multiple medical challenges to individuals over the age of 65 and often herald the end of independent living. Regular physical activity has been demonstrated to decrease the likelihood of a fall. The PAGA 2018 concluded that there was strong evidence that multicomponent physical activity programs can significantly reduce the risk of injury from severe falls that may result in bone fracture, head trauma, open wounds, and soft tissue injury or other injuries requiring medical attention or admission to the hospital. A number of RCTs have consistently reported that fall-related injuries in bones are reduced by 32–40% and bone fractures by 40–66% among individuals over the age of 65 who are physically active. There is also evidence that adults over the age of 85 obtain similar benefits from regular physical activity programs.

These results have significant public health implications. Up to 25% of individuals over the age of 65 years fall in the United States every year. Falls are the leading cause of fatal injury and the most common cause of non-fatal trauma related to hospital admissions for older individuals. The effectiveness of physical activity programs to lower the risk of falls has significant public health relevance not only because of the high prevalence of falls, but also because this represents a cost-effective approach to fall prevention.

16.6   NUTRITION FOR OLDER ADULTS

The changes in the recommended daily allowance (RDA) by the Food and Nutrition Board of the Institute of Medicine starting in 1999 brought more precise recommendations for individuals above the age of 50 years (15). Recommendations for vitamin D, calcium, and vitamin B6 are higher for individuals over the age of 70. Dietary Reference Intakes (DRI) for vitamin D increased from 600 IU per day for females and males between ages 51 and 70 to 800 IU per day for both females and males above the age of 80. The DRI for calcium increased from 1000 and 1200 mg/day for females and males, respectively, between 51 and 70 years of age, to 1200 mg/day for both females and males above the age of 70. The DRI for vitamin B6 increased from 1.3 and 1.4 mg/day for females and males, respectively, between the ages of 51 and 70 years of age, to 1.5 and 1.7 mg/day for both females and males, respectively, over the age of 70.

Dietary quality is directly related to optimal physical and cognitive function in older adults. Some nutrient requirements have increased, as already indicated, but most of the others stay the same. Energy requirements in older individuals typically decline, increasing the importance of nutrient-dense food choices. Changes in sensory perception and the onset of chronic diseases may necessitate added attention to diet composition in older adults. Alterations in social environments and living situations make it important to monitor the ability and desire to obtain and consume a high-quality diet for older Americans (15).

- *Nutrients of concern:* In the 2015 Dietary Guidelines for Americans Advisory Committee Report, vitamin D, calcium, potassium, and fiber were all considered nutrients of concern for older individuals as well as younger adults. In addition, because of under-consumption of these nutrients, however, there were some nutrients where the dietary guidelines were concerned about over-consumption. These included sodium, saturated fat, and added sugar.
- *Special dietary considerations for older adults:* The way the body handles nutrients can change with advancing age (15). Many individuals experience

a decline in gastric hydrochloric acid secretion, which can result in a decline of vitamin B12. Other factors such as decreased function of the cardiovascular system, including heart, blood vessels, and kidneys, can put additional stress on normal demands for everyday life.

In addition, there are other factors which may impact on adequate nutrition for older individuals. For example, taste and smell typically are diminished in older individuals, which may make food less palatable. In addition, diminished vision, dexterity, and mobility can make food acquisition and preparation difficult and significantly alter the variety and quality of foods consumed.

In addition to declines in physical capacity associated with the aging process, older adults may have declines in social factors such as companionship, mental state, and economic issues, all of which can make adequate nutrition more difficult to achieve. Finally, there are a number of physiological changes which may be of particular concern for older adults. For example, salivary secretions decrease with increasing age and dentition may be adversely affected by aging, such as loss or extraction of teeth or poorly fitting dentures. In addition, a number of chronic illnesses are more prevalent in older adults, including CVD, osteoporosis, type 2 diabetes (T2DM), hypertension, immune function, and cancer, all of these can create additional challenges for adequate nutrition among older adults.

16.7 CONCLUSIONS

A number of physiological and mental changes are associated with aging. Changes in cognition, muscle mass, and a variety of other changes can be particularly challenging for individuals over the age of 65. However, multiple lifestyle practices can significantly improve both the health and quality of life for individuals over the age of 65. The study of successful aging has demonstrated that individuals who participate in regular physical activity and healthy nutrition as well as cognitive training and social engagement such as volunteer work can all contribute in significant ways to both health and emotional well-being in the older population. It is incumbent upon all clinicians to understand the changes that are typically associated with the aging process and how various lifestyle habits and practices such as physical activity, proper nutrition, and social engagement can lead to both improved health and quality of life for individuals over the age of 65.

16.8 CLINICAL APPLICATIONS

- Aging may be associated with decline in both cognitive function and muscle mass and strength. Lifestyle habits and practices can help ameliorate these.
- Aging may also be associated with decreases in dietary quality. Clinicians should check for these issues in all older patients.
- Attention should be given to ensure adequate nutrient intake in older patients since the amount of food consumed typically declines with age.

- Clinicians should inquire about such issues as taste, smell, vision, dexterity, and mobility to make sure that older patients have the capacity to achieve adequate nutrition.
- The study of successful aging has demonstrated that factors such as regular physical activity, social engagement, and high mental and physical function are all important components of health and quality of life in the older population.

REFERENCES

1. Centers for Disease Control and Prevention. Healthy Aging for Older Adults, 2007. http://www.cdc.gov/aging. Accessed July 8, 2020.
2. Physical Activity Guidelines Advisory Committee. *2018 Physical Activity Guidelines Advisory Committee. 2018 Physical Activity Guidelines Advisory Committee Scientific Report. Older Adults.* U.S. Department of Health and Human Services (Washington, DC), 2018.
3. Rose D. Aging Successfully Predictors and Pathways. In: Rippe JM, ed., *Lifestyle Medicine* (3rd edition), CRC Press (Boca Raton), 2019.
4. Leon A. Aging-Associated Cognitive Decline and Its Attenuation by Lifestyle. In: Rippe JM, ed., *Lifestyle Medicine* (3rd edition), CRC Press (Boca Raton), 2019.
5. Raz N, Rodrigue K. Differential Aging of the Brain: Patterns, Cognitive Correlates, and Modifiers. *Neuroscience & Biobehavioral Reviews.* 2006;30:730–748.
6. Whalley L, Deary I, Appleton C, et al. Cognitive Reserve and the Neurobiology of Cognitive Aging. *Ageing Research Reviews.* 2004;3:169–182.
7. Physical Activity Guidelines Advisory Committee. *2018 Physical Activity Guidelines Advisory Committee Scientific Report.* U.S. Department of Health and Human Services (Washington, DC), 2018.
8. Gorelick P, Furie K, Iadecola C, et al. Defining Optimal Brain Health in Adults: A Presidential Advisory from the American Heart Association/American Stroke Association. *Stroke.* 2017;Oct, 48(10) e284–e303. .
9. Leon A. Reducing Aging-Associated Risk of Sarcopenia. In: Rippe JM, ed., *Lifestyle Medicine* (3rd edition). CRC Press (Boca Raton), 2019.
10. Leon A. Attenuation of Adverse Effects of Aging on Skeletal Muscle by Regular Exercise and Nutritional Support. *American Journal of Lifestyle Medicine.* 2015;9:1–13.
11. Fielding R, Velias B, Even S, et al. Sarcopenia: An Underdiagnosed Condition in Older Adults. Current Consensus, Definition, Prevalence, Etiology, and Consequences. International Working Group on Sarcopenia. *Journal of the American Medical Directors Association.* 2011;12:249–256.
12. Rowe JW, Kahn RL. Human Aging: Usual and Successful. *Science.* 1987;237:143–149.
13. Rowe JW, Kahn RL. *Successful Aging.* Dell Publishing (New York), 1998.
14. U.S. Department of Agriculture and U.S. Department of Health and Human Services. *Dietary Guidelines for Americans, 2015–2020.* U.S. Government Printing Office (Washington, DC), 2015.
15. Lichtenstein A. Optimal Nutrition Guidance for Older Adults. In: Rippe JM, ed., *Lifestyle Medicine* (3rd edition). CRC Press (Boca Raton), 2019.

17 Heath Promotion

KEY POINTS

- The field of lifestyle medicine has many areas in common with health promotion; in fact, health promotion is a key area within lifestyle medicine.
- Lifestyle medicine physicians can play a very important role in helping individuals make positive lifestyle decisions to improve their own health.
- Lifestyle medicine physicians can also play a critically important role in recognizing that health decisions involve not only the individual but also the community and built environments and workplace settings.

17.1 INTRODUCTION

The field of health promotion and lifestyle medicine play important roles in helping individuals improve their health and well-being. These fields have been shown to identify early indicators of chronic disease and provide interventions to lower these risks. Health promotion and lifestyle medicine share the goal of helping individuals not only lower their risk of chronic disease, but also improve their quality of life. While many aspects of health promotion have come from the standpoint of companies, lifestyle medicine continues to expand concepts from health promotion by giving physicians tools for early-stage treatment opportunities.

The purpose of this chapter is to provide a summary of key issues related to health promotion and their interaction with lifestyle medicine. More details about each of these areas may be found in the superb section on Health Promotion edited by Dr. Dee Edington who has been an international leader in this area for many years in the major textbook that I edited, *Lifestyle Medicine*, 3rd edition (CRC Press, Boca Raton, 2019).

17.2 MOTIVATION AS MEDICINE

Changing behaviors from unhealthy ones to healthy ones is a complex task that may be difficult for some people to achieve, but it is possible. A key area is how to enhance motivation in individuals to participate in this process. Physicians can play a very important role in helping create conditions and encourage behaviors and settings that will enhance motivation.

There are many tools and theories available which can help people on the path to healthier living. Many of these theories of how to enhance behavior change are research proven. These are handled in much more detail in Chapter 4.

The essence of motivation for change involves helping individuals to adopt reasons for acting or behaving to enhance their health. Lifestyle habits such as poor diet, lack of exercise, obesity, and smoking lead to significant increases in heart disease. If we could change these factors, we could see an 80% reduction in heart disease, a 90% reduction in diabetes, and a 60% reduction in cancer (1–3). The key is helping people actually make those changes in their daily lives. Some of this motivation must emanate from internal qualities that individuals have (4). This has also been called "autonomous" motivation. Motivation is further divided into "intrinsic," which involves doing things purely for their own sake, and "extrinsic," which relates to changing things that individuals do not find inherently interesting or enjoyable.

A key to autonomous motivation is establishing ways to blend both internal and external motivation. It is essential to respect the point of view of the patient. This is also a key component of the field of motivational interviewing (MI), which is described in more detail in Chapter 4. MI involves employing a different approach that has typically been involved in medical care (5). In typical medical care, physicians are seen as experts and their role is to give advice or administer some form of treatment. In MI, the physician forms a partnership with each patient, which recognizes the need, wants, and desires of the patient. This involves the physician approaching patients with passion and listening deeply to understand the individual's personal goals to add purpose and meaning in their lives. These are the essential elements of MI. This technique has been shown to be highly effective in helping individuals control their blood pressure, increase intake of fruits and vegetables, enhance adherence to diet and exercise modification programs, diabetes management, and smoking cessation.

17.3 HEALTH PROMOTION: HISTORY AND EMERGING TRENDS

In the mid-20th century, health promotion was based on general public health issues helping people to develop lifestyles to maintain and enhance their state of well-being (6). As the field has progressed, it has taken on more of an individual health-oriented focus. This is typically an area where lifestyle medicine has made significant contributions.

This evolution has basically catalyzed the change from a focus on "wellness" to health and productivity. This has also engendered new tools and frameworks designed to blend both community health and individual health into the field of population health involving both individual and community health.

Tools that have helped in the area of lifestyle medicine include the understanding of how lifestyle habits interact with epigenetics as well as behavioral techniques underscoring how social connections impact on health as well as on mind-body issues and behavioral economics.

Health care financing and delivery innovations also have occurred, including the Affordable Care Act (ACA) and broader use of value-based incentivized health reimbursement arrangements in health savings accounts. All these trends have been further accelerated by growing understanding among the patient population that both quality and costs are important, particularly in the area of reversing or decreasing the likelihood of disease.

All these efforts have expanded the field of health promotion to also include behavioral medicine, epidemiology, exercise physiology, and nutrition. Finally, the role of physicians, particularly through involvement in lifestyle medicine, has helped accelerate the interaction between health promotion and lifestyle medicine.

17.4   THE EMPLOYERS' ROLE IN LIFESTYLE MEDICINE

As both fields of health promotion and lifestyle medicine have continued to advance, employers have played an increasingly aggressive role in helping to take care of the health and pay attention to lifestyle habits among their employees (7). There are multiple reasons why companies are involved in this area. First, health care costs among employers have increased dramatically. For example, in the decade between 2006 and 2016, annual employee health care costs increased by 58% (8). These are simply unsustainable cost increases. In addition to fiscal concerns, companies are also becoming involved in positive lifestyle measures simply because it is the right thing to do.

It is simply good business for a company to improve quality and lower costs. The power of lifestyle decisions in lowering the risk of costly chronic diseases such as heart disease (CVD) and type 2 diabetes (T2DM) is supported by literally thousands of studies. Companies have increasingly looked for health care partners and physicians who have an understanding and commitment to improving lifestyle behaviors. In some instances, this has taken the place of onsite clinics, while in other situations employers have insisted that their health care insurers adopt a more pro-active stance to help rein in costs of various chronic diseases—often through including lifestyle measures such as diabetes and heart disease prevention programs as a key component of the overall insurance offered to the company. It is estimated that over half of large employers now have an emphasis on controlling costs through this type of measure.

17.5   LEVERAGING THE VALUE OF HEALTH

As lifestyle medicine and health promotion have continued to gain in application and sophistication, a substantial opportunity exists for health care providers to positively improve health and reduce illness in populations and in groups of individuals (9). Published studies continue to demonstrate the economic benefits of lifestyle medicine at a time when costs of traditional medicine and health care have become virtually unsustainable. In recent years, health care reform discussions in the United States have focused on both cost-effective delivery and better patient outcomes. A number of new conceptual models have been advanced to achieve these goals. One of them is the Patient-Centered Medical Home (PCMH) (10) and another is the Accountable Care Organization (ACO) (11). Both of these concepts contain a central emphasis on encouraging physicians, hospitals, and other stakeholders to be more accountable to the care system. This provides an opportunity for the principles of lifestyle medicine to take hold in a variety of situations.

Employers, for example, have become much more active participants in helping to manage the health of their employees. A number of these models also emphasize shared accountability between companies and local health care systems. These models include patients, providers, and purchasers of care.

These partnerships provide yet another opportunity for practitioners of lifestyle medicine. A number of organizations have arisen to help in this effort. For example, the U.S. Preventive Medicine Organization provides multi-site Diabetes Prevention Programs (DPP) as does the YMCA of the USA (12). Other organizations are likely to emerge in the future.

Frameworks are also available to show how a positive return on investment may be generated for people who improve their lifestyle and health. For example, the Edington Risk Model divides risk levels into 15 health risk factors and defines low, medium, and high risk categories (13). In one study, individuals in a high risk category who followed positive lifestyle measures were reduced from 11% to 6% in the population and in the medium risk category were reduced from 29% to 23%, while the low risk category was increased from 60% to 71%. These kinds of changes which have been demonstrated by both the U.S. Preventive Medicine Organization and by Parkinson et al. at the University of Pittsburgh Medical Center have resulted in enormous cost-savings (14).

17.6 INTERNATIONAL HEALTH AND LIFESTYLE

Health, well-being, and risk factor reduction have become global issues for countries and also for multinational employers (15). This is largely due to the risk of non-communicable diseases (NCDs) which have very significant components of physiological, environmental, and behavioral factors. These include CVD, cancer, chronic respiratory disease, and T2DM among others.

NCDs result in deaths of 40 million people around the world each year which amounts to more than 70% above all deaths. The cumulative economic impact of these diseases is estimated to be 30 trillion dollars by the year 2030. CVD, cancers, respiratory disease, and T2DM account for 80% of all premature NCD deaths globally and the vast majority of these deaths occur in low- and middle-income countries.

A variety of health risk factors related to lifestyle have been measured by the Organization for Economic Cooperation and Development (OECD) (16). These include mental health issues, tobacco usage, obesity, and lack of physical activity. The United States, when compared to other developed countries, fares poorly with regard to various diseases, especially those related to lifestyle (17). The Institute of Medicine in 2013 reported that when the United States was compared to 16 other high-income countries, "Americans have shorter lives and experience more injuries and illnesses than people in other high income countries." In this study, Americans were found to have the highest infant mortality rate, the highest incidence of death related to alcohol and other drugs, and the highest rate of obesity and T2DM and the second highest rate of CVD. On the positive side, the United States had the second lowest rate of smoking and better control of cholesterol and high blood pressure. Clearly, these findings show that there is an enormous issue and a substantial opportunity to apply lifestyle medicine principles.

17.7 THE COMMUNITY AS A CATALYST FOR HEALTHIER BEHAVIORS

The environments in which individuals live play a very significant role in their overall health. For this reason, communities across the United States are beginning to include excellent venues for people to live and work as part of their overall economic development strategy (18). This emphasis has been called "place making," which focuses on environments and person-centered approach to community development that can have a positive impact on lifestyle, well-being, and healthy decision-making.

Diverse disciplines also contribute to this effort. Physicians can play a significant role in helping to emphasize the valuable role of environment and place in overall health. This effort emphasizes systems and environmental changes to make the healthiest and the easiest choices and represents another outreach effort in which practitioners of lifestyle medicine can play a critically important role. This emphasis was a key component for the Centers for Disease Control and Prevention (CDC) Health Impact in Five Years Initiative as well as the United Nations sustainable development goals. An organization which has been a recognized leader in this area is the Robert Wood Johnson Foundation (RWJF), which has long played a visionary role in the Healthy Places Movement.

17.8 FUTURE DIRECTIONS OF HEALTH PROMOTION: THE ROLE OF THE PHYSICIAN

As health promotion and lifestyle medicine have become more pervasive and sophisticated, future opportunities for lifestyle medicine physicians have expanded. One area that is particularly promising is the emerging emphasis placed on lifestyle decisions and their impact on non-communicable diseases and the expanded definition of health. In 1986, for example, WHO said that health is a "resource for every day life not the objective of living. Health is a positive concept emphasizing social and personal resources as well as physical capacities." This definition is much broader than the notion of health that has been central to American medicine for the last 60 years which is based on the absence of disease. As we move to the future, helping patients understand the critically important role of lifestyle decisions to prevent disease in the first place will become an increasingly important area.

In order for individuals to make and sustain lifestyle changes, healthy choices must also be easy choices. These may include built environments in the community that are more amenable to physical activity. Such environments will also help individuals with the increasing obesity epidemic. Finding everyday solutions to provide fresh produce in communities, particularly in food "deserts," will also be important. In the future, physicians need to understand and promote how individual health and community health interact with each other. Physicians should not only learn methods to assistant patients in sustainable behavior change (see Chapter 4) but also be aware of how the individual interacts with the community.

17.9   CONCLUSIONS

The field of health promotion has evolved significantly over the past 25 years. The emergence of lifestyle medicine offers an opportunity to further advance health promotion and provides multiple opportunities for physicians who have an interest in, and potential to become experts in, lifestyle medicine to help not only with individual health but also the health of communities. Physicians who are skilled in promoting lifestyle habits and actions as key components of short- and long-term health and quality of life can play a critically important role in helping to ameliorate the overwhelming problem of non-communicable diseases.

17.10   CLINICAL APPLICATIONS

* Physicians can play a very important role in individual patient health and population health.
* Helping individuals understand how their daily habits and actions impact on their health is an important role for physicians interested in lifestyle medicine.
* As health care costs have risen steeply, lifestyle medicine can play a critically important role in helping to mitigate costs while improving patients' lives through positive daily habits and actions.

REFERENCES

1. Lee I, Shiroma E, Evenson K, et al. Accelerometer-Measured Physical Activity and Sedentary Behavior in Relation to All-Cause Mortality: The Women's Health Study. *Circulation.* 2018;137:203–205.
2. Hu F, Willett W. Diet and Coronary Heart Disease: Findings From the Nurses' Health Study and Health Professionals' Follow-Up Study. *Journal of Nutrition, Health and Aging.* 2001;5(3):132–8.
3. Knoops K, de Groot L, Kromhout D, et al. Mediterranean Diet, Lifestyle Factors, and 10-Year Mortality in Elderly European Men and Women: The HALE Project. *JAMA.* 2004;292(12):1433–1439.
4. Pitts J. *Motivation as Medicine. Lifestyle Medicine* (3rd edition). CRC Press (Boca Raton), 2019.
5. Fitfield P, Suzuki J, Minski S. *Motivational Interviewing and Lifestyle Change. Lifestyle Medicine* (3rd edition). CRC Press (Boca Raton), 2019.
6. Parkinson M. *Health Promotion: History and Emerging Trends. Lifestyle Medicine* (3rd edition). CRC Press (Boca Raton), 2019.
7. Shurney D. *The Employer's Role in Lifestyle Medicine Why, How, and What in Leveraging the Value of Health. Lifestyle Medicine* (3rd edition). CRC Press (Boca Raton), 2019.
8. Kaiser Family Foundation. 2016 Employer Health Benefits Survey. 14 September 2016. http://www.kff.org/report-section/ehbs-2016-section-one-cost-of-health-insurance/.
9. Loeppke R. *Why, How, and What in Leveraging the Value of Health. Lifestyle Medicine* (3rd edition). CRC Press (Boca Raton), 2019.
10. Patient-Centered Medical Home Recognition. https://www.pcdc.org/what-we-do/. Accessed July 13, 2020.

11. Accountable Care Organizations. https://innovation.cms.gov/innovation-models/aco. Accessed July 13, 2020.

12. YMCA of the USA. https://www.ymca.net/. Accessed July 13, 2020.

13. Loeppke M, Eddington D, Beg S. Impact of the Prevention Plan on Employee Health Risk Reduction. *Population Health Management*. 2010;(13)5. https://www.ncbi.nlm .nih.gov/pmc/articles/PMC3128505/pdf/pop.2010.0027.pdf.

14. Parkinson M, Peele P, Keyser D, et al. UPMC MyHealth: Managing the Health and Costs of U.S. Healthcare Workers. *American Journal of Preventive Medicine*. 2014;47:403–410.

15. Burton W. *International Health and Lifestyle. Lifestyle Medicine* (3rd edition). CRC Press (Boca Raton), 2019.

16. Organisation for Economic Co-operation and Development. Non-Communicable Diseases (NCD), 2019. http://www.oecd.org/health/non-communicable-diseases.htm. Accessed July 2020.

17. Organisation for Economic Co-operation and Development. Health at a Glance: 2015, 2015. http://www.oecd-ilibrary.org/social-issues-migration-health/health-at-a-glance -2015_healthglance-2015-en;jsessionid=4fuk5w6cil2cu.xoecd-live-03. Accessed July 2020.

18. Ellery J. *The Community as a Catalyst for Healthier Behaviors. Lifestyle Medicine* (3rd edition). CRC Press (Boca Raton), 2019.

18 Injury Prevention

KEY POINTS

- Injuries are very common in the United States.
- Counseling about injury prevention should be a key component of the practice of lifestyle medicine.
- Injuries are the leading cause of death in ages 1–44, with unintentional injuries being the major component.
- Injuries are the leading cause of years of potential life loss before the age of 65—twice that of heart disease and 1.6 times that of cancers.
- It is important to distinguish between injuries and accidents. The science of injury prevention teaches us that injuries are not accidents; they are predictable and preventable.

18.1 INTRODUCTION

Injuries, including both unintentional injuries and violence-related injuries, are a major public health problem and an area where lifestyle medicine physicians can play a significant role (1,2). Injuries are typically underestimated in all of medicine, including lifestyle medicine. This is because we mistakenly often call injuries "accidents." This suggests that they are random events or even acts of God. There is a large science of injury prevention that shows us that injuries are not accidents; they are predictable and preventable. Clinicians in the area of lifestyle medicine should become knowledgeable in this area and help educate the public on the importance of injury prevention.

The National Academy of Sciences in 1985 pronounced that "injury is the most underrecognized public health problem facing the nation today" (3). Despite this declaration and decades of compelling research, injury prevention receives relatively little attention from physicians and other health care providers compared to other public health issues. In addition to focusing on physical activity, nutrition, tobacco cessation, hypertension, and sexually transmitted diseases, physicians in the area of lifestyle medicine should add preventing injury as part of a comprehensive public health approach to lifestyle change.

- *The burden of injuries:* In the United States, unintentional injury is the fourth leading cause of death for people of all ages and the leading cause of death for children and adolescents as well as the leading cause of years of potential life loss (YPLL) before the age of 65 years—twice that of heart disease and 1.6 times that of cancer (4). Injuries, including unintentional and violence-related injuries, account for 59% of all deaths among people 1–44 years of age in the United States. Each year millions more are injured and survive. In fact, 2.5 million people with injuries are hospitalized and 26.9 million people with injuries are treated in emergency departments and released each year. The costs of injuries are staggering. The total lifetime medical and work lost due to injuries and violence in the United States was $671 billion in 2013 (5). To offset these expenses, there are a number of low-cost safety devices and practices which can return large benefits for small investments (6). Here are a few examples:

- For every dollar spent on child safety seats (CSS), society can save $100 in direct medical costs.
- For every dollar spent on a bicycle helmet, society can save $440 in direct medical and other costs.
- For every dollar spent on a smoke alarm, society can save $15 in direct medical costs.
- *Injury or accident?:* It is important to recognize that injury is not the same as accident. The word "injury" connotes the medical consequences of an event which are both predictable and preventable. In contrast, accidents are not usually considered predictable or preventable.
- *Future directions:* The National Academy of Sciences/Institute of Medicine Report, *Reducing the Burden of Injury* emphasized the importance of using a scientific approach to injury prevention and called on all components of the health care system as well as communities and businesses to support alliances to help reduce injuries. One example of this is that in the area of motor vehicle prevention, more than 35% of injury deaths occur. The drastic reduction in motor vehicle injury deaths during the past 20 years shows what can be accomplished when data are used in decision-making and actions.

The bottom line is that reduction in injuries and costs both to individuals and to the health care system at large are possible, but will need support, collaboration, and partnering from multiple sectors of society, including policymakers, clinicians, and other health care practitioners. For all these reasons, we have devoted this entire chapter to the area of injury prevention.

18.2 TRAFFIC INJURY PREVENTION

Traffic injuries are a leading cause of death in the United States and a major public health problem. A number of evidence-based strategies are available to help ameliorate this problem, but they are not completely implemented. The area of lifestyle medicine offers great promise in helping to reduce the number of injuries and fatalities related to traffic injuries.

Traffic-related injury and lifestyle are inextricably linked. Motor vehicle dominates all other modes of travel in the United States. Over 90% of households own at least one vehicle and 20% of households own more than three vehicles (6). While exposure to being on the road has increased significantly, there has been a long-term decline in the rate of traffic-related deaths per mile driven by over 90% since 1925. Despite this positive statistic, in 2016 the Centers for Disease Control and Prevention (CDC) issued a report comparing the United States to 19 other high-income countries which revealed that the United States had the highest number of motor vehicle crash tests per 100,000 people and per 10,000 registered vehicles.

- *Epidemiology:* Traffic crashes result in more than 30,000 deaths and more than 3 million non-fatal injuries treated in hospital emergency departments each year (7). Traffic deaths vary by age, with the lowest rates among children 0–14 years and the highest rate among those aged 15–24 years and 80 years and older. Fatal crash rates increase notably starting with the age group of 70–74 years old and are highest among drivers 85 years of age and older. The American Highway Traffic Safety Commission (AHTSA) recommends that all physicians counsel their patients on the ability to drive safely. There are a number of effective interventions to improve vehicle safety:
    - *Reduction in alcohol impaired driving:* In 2016, 28% of all traffic deaths involved a driver with a blood alcohol concentration (BAC) of 0.08 g/dL, which is a level illegal in every state. Effective interventions to alleviate this include such things as zero tolerance policies, minimum legal drinking age laws, sobriety checkpoints, lower BAC, ignition interlocks, server intervention training, alcohol screening, and brief intervention and alcohol pricing strategies.
    - *Occupant protection:* Occupant restraints, including lap and shoulder belts and CSS as well as booster seats, are among the most effective injury prevention interventions available. Seat belts reduce the risk of death and serious injuries in crashes by about half. CSS are 71% effective in reducing fatalities among infants and are 54% effective among toddlers (8). Effective types of occupant protection include seat belts, CSS, booster seats, and rear seating positions. In addition to protecting occupants within motor vehicles, motorcycle helmets are highly effective in reducing fatal injuries, as are bicycle helmets. Since motor vehicle crashes are the leading cause of death among teenagers in the United States, graduated driver licenses which require apprenticeship of supervised practice (learner's permit stage) provide a fallback provisional license and are highly effective in lowering teenage motor vehicle fatalities.
- *Emerging considerations:* Older adults have become increasingly prevalent in the United States. Beginning in 2011, 10,000 people in the United States reached the age of 65 every day (9). This segment is the most rapidly growing portion of the United States population as older adults continue in the workforce and frequently chose to live in their own homes, which can make

driving important for older individuals. Living alone can make driving even more critical for meeting everyday needs. All of these considerations need to factor into counseling from lifestyle medicine physicians with individuals as they age.

18.3 CDC GUIDELINES FOR PRESCRIBING OPIOIDS FOR CHRONIC PAIN

It is estimated that one out of five patients with non-cancer pain or pain-related diagnoses are prescribed opioids (10). Nearly two million Americans aged 12 or older either abused or were dependent on prescription opioids in 2014, according to the CDC. It is estimated that 11% of adults in the United States experience daily pain and millions of Americans are treated with prescription opioids for chronic pain (11). Since pain is endemic in our society, this represents a significant lifestyle issue. Primary care providers report that they have insufficient training for prescribing opioids. During 1999–2016, more than 200,000 people died in the United States from overdoses related to prescription opioids.

With all these facts as background, the CDC issued guidelines for prescribing opioids for chronic pain. The CDC developed these guidelines using the Grading of Recommendations Assessment Development and Evaluation (GRADE) framework. The recommendations were made on the basis of a systematic review of the scientific evidence considering benefits and harms, values and preferences, and resource allocation. What follows are the 12 recommendations from the CDC Guidelines on the appropriate prescribing and use of opioids in treating chronic pain (pain lasting more than three months or past the time of normal tissue healing).

- **Recommendations from the CDC Guidelines**
  - *Determining when to initiate or continue opioids for chronic pain*
  1. Non-pharmacologic therapy and non-opioid pharmacologic therapy are preferred for chronic pain. Clinicians should consider opioid therapy only if expected benefits for both pain and function are anticipated to outweigh risks to the patient. If opioids are used, they should be combined with non-pharmacologic therapy and non-opioid pharmacologic therapy, as appropriate.
  2. Before starting opioid therapy for chronic pain, clinicians should establish treatment goals with all patients, including realistic goals for pain and function, and should consider how opioid therapy will be discontinued if benefits do not outweigh risks. Clinicians should continue opioid therapy only if there is a clinically meaningful improvement in pain and function that outweighs risks to patient safety.
  3. Before starting and periodically during opioid therapy, clinicians should discuss with patients known risks and realistic benefits of opioid therapy and patient and clinician responsibilities for managing therapy.

4. When starting opioid therapy for chronic pain, clinicians should prescribe immediate-release opioids instead of extended-release/long-acting (ER/LA) opioids.

5. When opioids are started, clinicians should prescribe the lowest effective dosage. Clinicians should use caution when prescribing opioids at any dosage, should carefully reassess evidence of individual benefits and risks when considering increasing dosage to ≥50 morphine milligram equivalents (MME)/day, and should avoid increasing dosage to ≥90 MME/day or carefully justify a decision to titrate dosage to ≥90 MME/day.

6. Long-term opioid use often begins with treatment of acute pain. When opioids are used for acute pain, clinicians should prescribe the lowest effective dose of immediate-release opioids and should prescribe no greater quantity than needed for the expected duration of pain severe enough to require opioids. Three days or less will often be sufficient; more than seven days will rarely be needed.

7. Clinicians should evaluate benefits and harms with patients within 1 to 4 weeks of starting opioid therapy for chronic pain or of dose escalation. Clinicians should evaluate benefits and harms of continued therapy with patients every 3 months or more frequently. If benefits do not outweigh harms of continued opioid therapy, clinicians should optimize other therapies and work with patients to taper opioids to lower dosages or to taper and discontinue opioids.

*   *Assessing risk and addressing harms of opioid use*

8. Before starting and periodically during continuation of opioid therapy, clinicians should evaluate risk factors for opioid-related harms. Clinicians should incorporate into the management plan strategies to mitigate risk, including considering offering naloxone when factors that increase risk for opioid overdose, such as history of overdose, history of substance use disorder, higher opioid dosages (≥50 MME/day), or concurrent benzodiazepine use, are present.

9. Clinicians should review the patient's history of controlled substance prescriptions using state prescription drug monitoring program (PDMP) data to determine whether the patient is receiving opioid dosages or dangerous combinations that put him or her at high risk for overdose. Clinicians should review PDMP data when starting opioid therapy for chronic pain and periodically during opioid therapy for chronic pain, ranging from every prescription to every 3 months.

10. When prescribing opioids for chronic pain, clinicians should use urine drug testing before starting opioid therapy and consider urine drug testing at least annually to assess for prescribed medications as well as other controlled prescription drugs and illicit drugs.

11. Clinicians should avoid prescribing opioid pain medication and benzodiazepines concurrently whenever possible.

12. Clinicians should offer or arrange evidence-based treatment (usually medication-assisted treatment with buprenorphine or methadone in combination with behavioral therapies) for patients with opioid use disorder.

Source: Dowell D, Haegerich TM, Chou R. CDC Guideline for Prescribing Opioids for Chronic Pain: United States, 2016 *MMWR Recomm Rep* 2016:65(No. R R-1), 1--49.

18.4   IMPROVING THE CARE OF YOUNG PATIENTS WITH MILD TRAUMATIC BRAIN INJURY: CDC'S EVIDENCE-BASED PEDIATRIC MILD TBI GUIDELINES

A traumatic brain injury (TBI) is a serious public health problem contributing to one-third of all injury-related deaths in the United States each year. TBI is typically caused by blunt force applied to the head or body or a penetrating head injury. TBI can cause a wide range of functional short- or long-term changes, which effect thinking (i.e., memory and reasoning), sensation (i.e., sight and balance), language (i.e., communication and understanding), and/or emotion (i.e., depression, personality changes, and social inappropriateness).

The severity of TBI may range from "mild" (i.e., a brief change in mental status or consciousness as with a concussion) to "severe" (i.e., an extended period of unconsciousness or amnesia after the injury with significant associated brain hemorrhaging).

According to data from the CDC, among children under the age of 17, there were almost 840,000 TBI-related emergency department visits, hospitalizations, and deaths (1,343 per 100,000) in 2004 (12). As a result of these high numbers, the CDC has issued guidelines recommending a stepwise return to activity for children following mild TBI. These are listed in Table 18.1.

18.5   OLDER ADULT FALLS: EPIDEMIOLOGOY AND EFFECTIVE INJURY PREVENTION STRATEGIES

Falls among older adults are a major public health burden in the United States. Each year more than one in four (28.7%) of older adults aged 65 or older sustain a fall. Falls in older adults result in seven million injuries requiring medical treatment or restricted activity at an average cost of $10,000 per medically treated fall.

Beginning in 2011, 10,000 Americans turned age 65 every day and this is likely to continue. By the year 2030, when the last of the Baby Boomers will reach this milestone, 18% of the population of the United States will be 65 or older. People reaching the age of 65 will, on average, live another 19 years. Risk factors for falls are multiple, but significantly increase with age. However, there are other modifiable risk factors which have been identified. For example, a meta-analysis of 22 previous studies showed that individuals over the age of 65 taking various sedatives, neuroleptics,

TABLE 18.1

Stepwise Return to Activity Plan for Children Following Mild TBI

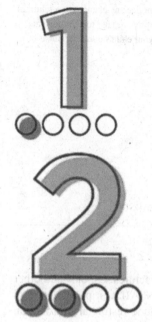

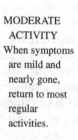

REST Take it easy the first few days after the injury when symptoms are more severe.	Early on, limit physical and cognitive (thinking/remembering) activities to avoid causing symptoms to worsen. Avoid activities that can put them at risk for another injury to the head and brain. Get a good night's sleep and take naps during the day as needed.
LIGHT ACTIVITY As your child starts to feel better, they can gradually return to their regular (non-strenuous) activities.	Find relaxing activities at home. Avoid activities that put your child at risk for another injury to the head and brain. Return to school gradually. If symptoms do not worsen during an activity, then this activity is OK for your child. If symptoms worsen, cut back on that activity until it is tolerated. Get maximum nighttime sleep. (Avoid screen time and loud music before bed, sleep in a dark room, and keep to a fixed bedtime and wake-up schedule.) Reduce daytime naps or return to a regular daytime nap schedule (as appropriate for their age).
MODERATE ACTIVITY When symptoms are mild and nearly gone, return to most regular activities.	Help your child take breaks only if their concussion symptoms worsen. Return to a regular school schedule.

(Continued)

TABLE 18.1 (CONTINUED)
Stepwise Return to Activity Plan for Children Following Mild TBI

	REGULAR ACTIVITY	If you notice any changes or a return of
	Recovery from a concussion is when your child is able to do all of their regular activities without experiencing any concussion symptoms.	symptoms, be sure to communicate with your child's doctor or nurse.

Source: Centers for Disease Control and Prevention, www.cdc.gov/HEADSUP

or antipsychotics had an increased risk of falls and hip fractures. Opioids and other narcotic agents, antidepressants, benzodiazepines, and NSAIDs in people over 75 also increased the risk of falls (14). Other risk factors include vestibular dysfunction which increases the risk of falls by 12-fold.

A variety of strategies have been developed and shown to effectively reduce the risk of falls. In particular, multifactorial interventions which are tailored to individuals have been shown to reduce falls in various clinical trials (13). For example, in one study, exercise plus vision assessment treatment lowered the risk of falls. Environmental assessment, plus calcium supplementation and vitamin D, have also been associated with reduced risk of injurious falls compared to usual care. Various exercise programs, including aerobic exercise, strength, and balance, have also been shown to reduce the risk of falls. Perhaps the most useful, evidence-based guidelines for reducing falls come from the CDC. These guidelines are noted by the acronym STEADI (Stopping Elderly Accidents and Deaths and Injuries). These guidelines can be accessed by going to the CDC STEADI Assessment Tools for Providers and are available at www.CDC.gov/STEADI/index.html.

18.6 PREVENTION OF SUICIDAL BEHAVIOR

Suicidal behavior is part of a larger individual public health category entitled "Self-Directed Violence" (SDV). This includes a variety of violent behaviors, including acts of fatal and non-fatal suicidal behavior and non-suicidal intentional self-harm. In 2016, suicide was the tenth leading cause of death overall in the United States and the second leading cause of death among persons in their 20s and 30s. There are an estimated 500,000 visits to U.S. hospital emergency departments each year for self-directed violence (15,16). Many individuals who engage in suicidal behavior never seek health services. Risk factors for suicidal behavior include substance use disorders, personality disorders, history of prior suicide attempts, physical illness, pain, socioeconomic issues (e.g., poverty and unemployment), family problems, relationship and intimate partner problems, socialized isolation, and easy access to lethal means among those who are at risk.

It is important to note that the national suicide rate has increased steadily during 1999–2015, while the majority of other causes of fatality have declined.

- *Risk and protective factors:* Risk factors for suicidal behavior represent complicated problems and typically are impacted by multiple factors acting at multiple levels, including individual, family, community, and societal over time. Risk factors may vary by age, gender, and culture, while others are universal. Suicide in children, particularly prior to puberty, is a rare event. It is thought that this is due to the fact that the most common risk factors, depression and exposure to drugs and alcohol, typically do not occur until adolescence.

   Adolescence is time of transition and growth. It often includes risk taking and testing, pushing of boundaries, and seeking greater independence. In 2015, suicide was the third leading cause of death among youths aged 10–14 and second among those aged 15–24 (17). Risk factors for suicide during adolescence and young adulthood include mental illness, hopelessness, family history of suicidal behavior, parental divorce and school problems, suicide of a peer or poor problem-solving, as well as easy access to lethal means.

   Middle-aged challenges include problems with jobs or children leaving home, caring for an aging adult, and change in one's own health status such as onset of a chronic illness. Suicide rates in adults aged 25–64 tend to increase during recessions and fall during times of economic expansion.

   Older adulthood may be characterized as a time of more typically stable emotions. Social roles and networks change, as do physical functioning. Among older adults physical illness, loss, and mental illness are common risk factors for suicide. In one review of research for older adult suicides, 71–95% involved mental health conditions, usually depression (18). Another important risk factor for elders is lack of social connectedness with family, friends, and community. Thus, clinicians should focus on discussion and counseling in all of these areas. Protective factors may reduce the likelihood of suicide. Social connectedness is one such powerful protective factor. Another is reduced access to lethal means (e.g., firearms, pesticides and medications).

- *Prevention strategies:* The CDC has released "Preventing Suicide: A Technical Package of Policy Programs and Practices." A summary of the CDC recommendations is found in Table 18.2.

TABLE 18.2

Preventing Suicide: A Technical Package of Policy Programs and Practices

CDC's Technical Package to Prevent Suicide

Strategy	Approach
Strengthen economic supports	• Strengthen household financial security • Housing stabilization policies
Strengthen access and delivery of suicide care	• Coverage of mental health conditions in health insurance policies • Reduce provider shortages in underserved areas • Safer suicide care through systems change
Create protective environments	• Reducing access to lethal means among persons at risk of suicide • Organizational policies and culture • Community-based policies to reduce excessive alcohol use
Promote connectedness	• Peer norm approaches • Community engagement activities
Teach coping and problem-solving skills	• Social-emotional learning programs • Parenting skill and family relationship programs
Identify and support people at risk	• Gatekeeper training • Crisis intervention • Treatment for people at risk of suicide • Treatment to prevent reattempts
Lessen harms and prevent future risk	• Postvention • Safe reporting and messaging about suicide

A summary of the CDC recommendations.
For additional details, clinicians may consult the full document at: https://www.cdc.gov/violenceprevent
ion/pdf/suicideTechnicalPackage.pdf.

18.7 UNINTENTIONAL INJURIES TO DISABLED PERSONS: AN UNRECOGNIZED, YET PREVENTABLE PROBLEM

Individuals with disabilities, including infants, youth, adults, and seniors, are more likely to be injured than other individuals. For example, youth, with and without disabilities, experience similar types of injuries, but the risk of injury is two to three times higher among youth with disabilities (19). Injury prevention program interventions exist for disabled persons, but are not being adapted and implemented as broadly as they should be.

As the population ages with chronic conditions and survival rates increase for birth- and injury-related limitations, the prevalence of disability continues to grow. Individuals with disability constitute 18.7% of the population in the United States or about 56.7 million people.

Disability is an umbrella term for physical, sensory, cognitive, and intellectual impairment, mental illness and chronic diseases characterized by significant activity limitations, participation restrictions, and impairment in body function and/or structure ranging from dyslexia to blindness and paraplegia to cerebral palsy. Clinicians should be aware of the significant and elevated risk of injury in individuals with disabilities.

When an individual has a disability, it is often accompanied by secondary risks where the injury itself can result in a disability. In one survey in Washington State, 87% of respondents who had a disability also reported having a secondary condition resulting from their disability. In addition to coping with daily struggles such as inadequate signage, narrow doorways, inadequate restroom facilities, and absence of ramps or elevators, individuals with disabilities can also experience great financial burden. In one study in New Zealand, the weekly cost of a disability for those with moderate needs range from $204 to $714 and those with high needs range from $719 to $2,568. These expenses can quickly compound if individuals with disabilities acquire secondary health conditions as a result of their disabilities. The role for the clinician is to be aware of the extra burden that individuals with disabilities may suffer and help find mitigation for these problems and conditions.

18.8 CONCLUSIONS

Injuries are a very significant public health problem. In fact, injuries in the United States are the leading cause of death in individuals aged 1–44. Most of these are unintentional injuries. It is important for clinicians to understand that the science of injury prevention teaches us that injuries are not accidents, they are predictable and they are preventable. Physicians practicing in the area of lifestyle medicine should be attuned to the various possible injuries and help with strategies to either lower the risk of injury or assist in the life of those who already have an injury. Traffic injury is one important source of injuries, but other injuries can include addiction and overdose from opioids and mild traumatic brain injury. Lifestyle medicine clinicians should also focus on helping older adults lower the risk of falls, preventing suicidal behavior, and helping to reduce the risk of unintentional injury for disabled persons. All of these are important and often underestimated components of lifestyle medicine.

18.9 CLINICAL APPLICATIONS

- Lifestyle medicine physicians should be tuned into the risks for injuries.
- Counseling to lower the risk of various kinds of injuries has been shown in multiple studies to lower the likelihood that they will occur.
- Clinicians should understand and counsel their patients that injuries are not accidents; they are predictable and preventable.
- Lowering the risk of injury is an important clinical priority.

REFERENCES

1. Sleet D. Injuries and Lifestyle Medicine. In: Rippe JM, ed., *Lifestyle Medicine*. CRC Press (Boca Raton), 2019.
2. Rippe JM. Injury Prevention: A Medical and Public Health Imperative. *American Journal of Lifestyle Medicine*. 2010;4(1):6–7.

3. National Academy of Sciences. *Injury in America: A Continuing Public Health Problem.* National Research Council (Washington, DC), 1985.

4. Ballesteros M, Williams D, Mack K, et al. The Epidemiology of Un-intentional and Violence-Related Injury Morbidity and Mortality among Children and Adolescents in the United States, 1999–2015. *International Journal of Environmental Research and Public Health.* 2018;15(4):616. doi:10.3390/ijerph15040616.

5. Centers for Disease Control. *Web-Based Injury Statistics Query and Reporting System (WISQARS).* National Center for Injury Prevention and Control, (NCIPC) Centers for Disease Control and Prevention (CDC) (producer). Accessed July 10, 2020.

6. Miller T, Levy D. Cost-Outcome Analysis in Injury Prevention and Control. *Medical Care.* 2000;38:562–582.

7. National Highway Traffic Safety Administration. *Traffic Safety Facts 2015: A Compilation of Motor Vehicle Crash Data from the Fatality Analysis Reporting System and the General Estimates System.* US Department of Transportation (Washington, DC), 2017. Report No. DOT HS 812-384. https://crashstats.nhtsa.dot.gov/Api/Public/V iewPublication/812384. Accessed August 19, 2020.

8. National Highway Traffic Safety Administration. *Traffic Safety Facts, Seat Belt Use in 2010.* US Department of Transportation (Washington, DC), 2010. Report No. DOT HS 811 378. https://crashstats.nhtsa.dot.gov/Api/Public/Publication/812378. Accessed August 19, 2020.

9. Administration on Aging, Administration for Community Living. *A Profile of Older Americans.* US Department of Health and Human Services. https://acl.gov/aging-and-dis ability-in-america/data-and-research/profile-older-americans. Accessed: February 1, 2021.

10. Seth P, Rudd R, Noonan R, Haegerich T. Quantifying the Epidemic of Prescription Opioid Overdose Deaths. *American Journal of Public Health.* 2018;108(4):e1–e3.

11. Dowell D, Haegerich T, Chou R. CDC Guideline for Prescribing Opioids for Chronic Pain — United States, 2016. *Morbidity and Mortality Weekly Report.* 2016;65:1–49.

12. Centers for Disease Control. *Traumatic Brain Injury-Related Emergency Department Visits, Hospitalizations, and Deaths—United States.* 2014. https://www.cdc.gov/traum aticbraininjury/pdf/TBI-Surveillance-Report-FINAL_508.pdf?fbclid=IwAR1C8v1yrFlH3 g0vnV9tIIJSgZyKoyf9-ui36oPN0lkvzSmXdeGpTb9oxf0. Accessed August 19, 2020.

13. Bergen G, Stevens MR, Burns ER. Falls and Fall Injuries among Adults Aged >65 Years— United States, 2014. *Morbidity & Mortality Weekly Report.* 2016;65(37):993–998.

14. Thorell K, Ranstad K, Midlov P, et al. Is Use of Fall Risk-Increasing Drugs in an Elderly Population Associated with an Increased Risk of Hip Fracture, after Adjustment for Multimorbidity Level: A Cohort Study. *BMC Geriatrics.* 2014;14(131):1471–2318.

15. Centers for Disease Control and Prevention, National Center for Injury Prevention and Control. Web-Based Injury Statistics Query and Reporting System (WISQARS) Nonfatal Injury Data. 2016. www.cdc.gov/injury/wisqars. Accessed July 10, 2020.

16. US Department of Health and Human Services. Agency for Healthcare Research and Quality. Healthcare Cost and Utilization Project (HCUP). https://www.ahrq.gov/rese arch/data/hcup/index.html. Accessed July 10, 2020.

17. Centers for Disease Control and Prevention, National Center for Injury Prevention and Control. Web-Based Injury Statistics Query and Reporting System (WISQARS) Fatal Injury Data. https://www.cdc.gov/injury/wisqars/index.html. Accessed August 19, 2020.

18. Conwell Y, Duberstein P, Caine E. Risk Factors for Suicide in Later Life. *Biological Psychiatry.* 2002;52(3):193–204.

19. Lee LC, Harrington RA, Chang JJ, et al. Increased Risk of Injury in Children with Developmental Disabilities. *Research in Developmental Disabilities.* 2008;29:247–255.

19 Substance Abuse and Addiction

KEY POINTS

- Substance use disorders are commonly seen in the practice of general medicine and lifestyle medicine.
- Lifestyle medicine practitioners should become knowledgeable about recognition and treatment of substance use disorders such as cigarette smoking, alcohol use disorder (AUD), opioid use disorder, and cannabis use disorder (CUD).
- A variety of treatment options are available, including, in some instances, pharmacologic treatment and, in many others, behavior-based therapies.
- These issues are important for the practice of lifestyle medicine.

19.1 INTRODUCTION

Clinicians who are involved in lifestyle medicine and in primary care will inevitably treat some individuals who are into the habit of smoking, drinking alcohol, and using cannabis or opioids. Knowledge of treatment options and identifying individuals who need assistance are very important medical issues. There are specialists who have been specifically trained in the area of substance abuse and addiction, but lifestyle medicine practitioners should have a general knowledge of available tools and therapies.

There has been some controversy in the past about how to name this field. However, the designation that is currently used in the Diagnostic and Statistical Manual of Mental Health Disorders (DSM), which is produced by the American Psychiatric Association, indicates that the favored term is "substance use disorders" (SUD) (1). The World Health Organization (WHO) has recognized that substance use is one of the most common contributing factors to premature death (2). In 2000, alcohol, tobacco, and illicit drug use combined accounted for over 12% of all deaths worldwide.

Tobacco is the most commonly used substance and the leading cause of premature death around the world. In the United States alone, over 500,000 deaths annually are attributable to tobacco use (3). Alcohol is also frequently consumed in the United States with 86.4% of the population consuming alcohol at least occasionally. Approximately 27% of the U.S. population reports binge drinking and 7% report heavy drinking. Illicit drugs such as cocaine and misuse of prescribed medication such as oxycodone and benzodiazepines as well as cannabis (now legal in most states) are also frequently used in the United States with approximately 10.2% of individuals in 2014 engaged in regular use of such substances. Issues related to recognition and treatment of SUDs form the core of this chapter.

19.2   HISTORY OF ALCOHOL AND OPIOID USE AND TREATMENT IN THE UNITED STATES

Use of intoxicating and potentially addictive substances has been prevalent in human history for millennia. For example, excessive use of alcohol as an illness was described in the 5th century by Herodotus. Opium and other opioids were described as early as 6,000 BC in Mesopotamia. By the 19th century, increasing evidence existed of harm from the use of both alcohol and opioids. By the 20th century, various attempts at addiction treatment had become available. For example, in 1939, Alcoholics Anonymous (AA) was founded. By the early 21st century, excessive opioid use has become an epidemic in the United States. However, by 2016, only 10% of patients with SUDs received the required treatment at a specialty facility (4).

19.3   TOBACCO USE DISORDERS

In the United States, at present about 50% of the adult population (age 18 years and over) and about 4% of youths (aged 12–17 years) are smokers. Smoking rates are higher in males (16.8%) than in females (13.8%) (5). There are also associations with socioeconomic status and education. The higher the level of education and the higher the level of socioeconomic status, the lower the rate of cigarette smoking. In the most recent Diagnostic and Statistical Manual of Mental Health Disorders (DSM5), "tobacco use disorder" was added as a diagnosis in 2013. This aligned tobacco use with other SUDs and helped conceptualize treatment.

The risks of many chronic diseases associated with smoking are directly related to how long the smoker has smoked and the number of cigarettes smoked per day. It is beneficial to quit smoking at any age (6). After quitting, the risk of heart attack drops sharply after just one year and stroke risk drops at about the same time. Risks for cancer of the mouth, throat, esophagus, and bladder are cut in half five years after cigarette smoking cessation and the risk of dying of lung cancer drops by half over ten years.

It is currently estimated that 68% of smokers would like to stop smoking and 55.4% made an attempt to quit in the past year. However, only 7.4% were able to quit for more than six months (7).

Pharmacological aids for smoking cessation include seven medications which are approved by the U.S. Food and Drug Administration (FDA). These include over-the-counter products (nicotine gum, nicotine lozenge, and the nicotine patch) and prescription-only medications (nicotine nasal spray, nicotine inhaler, sustained release bupropion, and varenicline) (8). These nicotine replacement therapies can significantly reduce nicotine withdrawal and have been shown to increase the rate of quitting by 50–70%.

A variety of scientific and community resources have been utilized to attempt to reduce tobacco use and increase smoking cessation. These include individual counseling, group therapy, telephone counseling, and motivational interviewing. Given the medical problems associated with cigarette smoking (9), it is not surprising that the smoking rate is higher among medical patients.

A convenient acronym entitled "F5" for smoking cessation has been developed for use by clinicians (Ask, Advise, Assess, Assist, and Arrange). This acronym can be used as part of brief medical visits.

It is important to recognize that 70% of smokers see some type of primary care physician (PCP) each year. Thus, primary-care-based patient interventions can reach most smokers. Also, hospitalization is considered a teachable moment when the health effects of smoking have caused the patient to require hospitalization.

Community-based approaches may also be utilized, including mass media campaigns, telephone quit lines, and social media such as Twitter and Facebook. In addition, worksite programs may also be helpful. Smoking is more common among unemployed adults. However, nearly 25% of full- and part-time workers smoke. Thus, worksite programs may be very beneficial (10). These include environmental cues, financial and material incentives, and health promotion programs. Various technology-driven approaches are increasingly becoming common. These include internet-based interventions and mobile phone interventions (11).

Smoking cessation is also important in various special populations. For example, 8% of high school students smoke cigarettes. It is important to understand that 90% of smokers begin smoking before the age of 18 (12). Thus, prevention and cessation initiatives in high school students have a high public health priority. Minority and disadvantaged smokers have also been targeted by the tobacco industry, so smoking cessation programs are particularly important in these groups.

Smoking has a negative impact on fetal development, and there are harmful effects of secondhand smoke on children. It is important to help pregnant women stop smoking. It is estimated that currently 55% of smoking women quit when they are pregnant and 40% start smoking again within six months after delivery. Another special population is individuals with chronic mental illness such as depression or schizophrenia since these individuals are two to three times higher than those in the general population to smoke.

A variety of behavioral approaches may be helpful in promoting smoking cessation. For example, the U.S. Department of Health and Human Services promotes exercise as an aid in quitting smoking based on a wealth of clinical trials and acute laboratory-based research.

It is estimated that 3–5% of U.S. adults use e-cigarettes (13). Of these, over 58% also smoke regular cigarettes, while 29% were former cigarette smokers and 11% have never been regular cigarette smokers. There are multiple risks associated with each e-cigarette use. Recently, there has been an alarming increase in vaping-related lung injuries. The exact cause of these lung injuries remains under investigation, but it is clear that vaping does not eliminate risk associated with smoking. Attempts at quitting either through gradual reduction or abrupt quitting both have been tried. However, research has shown that neither method is superior to the other.

19.4   ALCOHOL USE DISORDERS: DIAGNOSIS AND TREATMENT

AUD is very prevalent in the United States. As already indicated, alcohol consumption, at one time or another in people's lives, is highly prevalent in the United States with over 86% of people using alcohol at some point.

In one study, the prevalence of AUD was 13.9% and the lifetime prevalence was 29.1%. Of note, only a small percentage of these individuals actually sought treatment. Among those with a 12-month AUD, only 3.6% sought treatment and of those with a lifetime AUD, only 8.7% sought treatment from health care providers (14).

Most public health authorities characterize stages of addiction to alcohol in a three- or four-stage model. The three-stage model describes AUD as early, middle, and late (15). The early stage is defined by developing tolerance to alcohol. In the next phase, patients have cravings for alcohol and have some symptoms of withdrawal and suffer consequences in their personal or professional life. The final stage, entitled late or end stage, is characterized by loss of control. Individuals in this stage have suffered serious personal and physical consequences of alcohol use.

The diagnosis of AUD as defined by the DSM4 is found in Table 19.1.

Utilizing these criteria, the following subclassifications are made based on how many of these criteria an individual possesses (1):

- Mild: two to three
- Moderate: four to five
- Severe: six or more

A number of populations are particularly important to note in terms of AUD. In patients over the age of 65, there is a high prevalence of AUD. Some studies have reported only 1–3%, but it may be as high as 33%. There is clearly underrecognition of this diagnosis in this population.

Another special population is college students. In one study, 40% of college students were reported for intake of five or more consecutive drinks within the past two weeks. Another special population is physicians. AUD among physicians is quite common. It has been reported that 10–12% of doctors develop a substance use disorder and about 50% of this is AUD (16).

Excessive alcohol consumption carries a wide variety of comorbidities. These include a variety of neurological sequelae, including an increased risk of ischemic stroke. Cardiovascular complications may include cardiomyopathy, atrial fibrillation, ventricular tachycardia, and hypertension. The best well-known physical consequence of alcohol is liver damage which proceeds along the spectrum from ketosis and hepatitis to fibrosis and then cirrhosis. There is also a strong association between alcohol use and cancer risk. Cancers of the following organs have been associated with alcohol use: mouth, esophagus, pharynx, larynx, liver, colon, rectum, and breast. In the urinary system in men, complications may include testicular atrophy and a decrease in erectile capacity. In women amenorrhea, decreased

TABLE 19.1
DSM V Diagnostic Criteria

A problematic pattern of alcohol use leading to clinically significant impairment or distress, as manifested by *at least two of the following, occurring within a 12-month period*:

Impaired Control

1. Alcohol is often *taken in larger amounts* or over a longer period than was intended
2. There is a *persistent desire or unsuccessful efforts to cut down* or control alcohol use
3. A *great deal of time is spent in activities necessary to obtain alcohol,* use alcohol, or recover from its effects
4. *Craving* or a strong desire or urge to use alcohol

Social Impairment

5. Recurrent alcohol use resulting in a *failure to fulfill major role obligations* at work, school, or home
6. Continued alcohol use despite having *persistent or recurrent social or interpersonal problems* caused or exacerbated by the effects of alcohol
7. Important social, occupational, or recreational *activities are given up or reduced* because of alcohol use

Risky Use

8. Recurrent alcohol *use in situations in which it is physically hazardous*
9. Alcohol use is continued despite *knowledge of having a persistent or recurrent physical or psychological problem* that is likely to have been caused or exacerbated by alcohol

Physiological Indicators

10. *Tolerance*, as defined by either of the following:
    a. A need for markedly increased amounts of alcohol to achieve intoxication or desired effect
    b. A markedly diminished effect with continued use of the same amount of alcohol
11. *Withdrawal*, as manifested by either of the following:
    a. The characteristic withdrawal syndrome for alcohol
    b. Alcohol (or a closely related substance such as benzodiazepine) is taken to relieve or avoid withdrawal symptoms

DSM V Diagnostic Criteria for Impairment from Alcohol Use

Source: Chen C, Slatkin S. Alcohol Use Disorders: Diagnosis and Treatment, in: Rippe JM. *Lifestyle Medicine*, 3rd edition. CRC Press, Boca Raton, 2019. Used with permission.

---

ovarian size and infertility have been noted as well as increased risk of spontaneous abortion. It should be noted that alcohol use during pregnancy can result in fetal alcohol syndrome.

A variety of treatments for AUD are available, including detoxification, where withdrawal symptoms may be observed (17). Treatment for this includes benzodiazepines,

which are the mainstream treatment for alcohol withdrawal.

The maintenance of sobriety and relapse prevention are also important. It should be emphasized that if an individual has had AUD, a plan for sustaining abstinence at the onset is important to lower the risk of relapse. The prime risk of relapse is at time points three months to one year from the date of sobriety. Relapse is often considered a part of the process of recovery and should not be considered a treatment failure.

Currently, there are three medications approved by the FDA for treatment of AUD. They are disulfiram, acamprosate, and naltrexone (18). Behavioral treatments are also important and necessary for recovery. These include psychotherapy, behavioral therapy, cognitive behavioral therapy, and family/couples therapy. Finally, mutual help groups are a highly effective form of peer-led support to prevent relapse. Perhaps the most well-known of these is Alcoholic Anonymous. Finally, it may be appropriate to refer someone with AUD to an addiction specialist who can provide clarity about the diagnosis and guide the process of detoxification as well as develop a relapse prevention plan. The website for the American Board of Addiction Medicine (https://www.abam.net/) has a search tool *Find a Doctor* to locate a board-certified addiction specialist in your geographical area.

19.5 DIAGNOSIS AND TREATMENT OF OPIOID USE DISORDER

The diagnosis and treatment of opioid use disorders provides an excellent example of how lifestyle medicine procedures and practices can provide a sound foundation to understand and treat patients who suffer from this chronic medical problem. In 2016 and 2017, life expectancy in the United States dropped for two years in a row. The National Center for Health Statistics attributes this decrease to unintentional injury from drug overdose cases, which makes up the largest share (19). The incidence of opioid overdose deaths has reached epidemic proportions in the United States with nearly 50,000 deaths annually. This makes drug overdose the leading cause of death for those under 50 years of age (20). DSM5 provides the definitive criteria for when an individual should be considered to have opioid use disorder. These criteria are found In Table 19.2.

A wide range of options available for pharmacological treatment of opioid use disorder include methadone maintenance treatment (MMT), buprenorphine office-based treatment, naltrexone, and XR-naltrexone. It is important to note that pharmacotherapy alone is rarely sufficient for treatment of drug addiction. Clinicians have an additional level of responsibility for patients' opioid addiction beyond that of simply prescribing medications. Psychosocial treatment should be utilized as well. Self-help groups such as the 12-Step AA or NA meetings may be helpful. Alternatives include self-management and recovery training (SMART) goals. In addition, motivational enhancement therapy (MET) is designed to help people motivate to change to new behaviors that promote health. This approach has been shown to be helpful for nicotine and AUD. Another innovative approach was derived from MET when it specifically integrated into medical treatment. This is called the Brenda Approach, which is designed to improve treatment retention and medication adherence and can be implemented by a wide range of health care professionals.

The severe opioid epidemic mandates that clinicians be aware of this problem and help people who are suffering from opioid use disorders. Lifestyle modalities such as psychosocial support are important and other modalities which have been useful

TABLE 19.2

Opioid Use Disorder Diagnostic Criteria

A problematic pattern of opioid use leading to clinically significant impairment or distress, as manifested by at least two of the following, occurring within a 12-month period:

1. Opioids are often taken in larger amounts or over a longer period than was intended.
2. There is persistent desire or unsuccessful efforts to cut down or control opioid use.
3. A great deal of time is spent on activities necessary to obtain the opioid, use the opioid, or recover from its effects.
4. Craving, or a strong desire or urge to use opioids.
5. Recurrent opioid use resulting in a failure to fulfill major role obligations at work, school, or home.
6. Continued opioid use despite having persistent or recurrent social or interpersonal problems caused or exacerbated by the effects of opioids.
7. Important social, occupational, or recreational activities are given up or reduced because of opioid use.
8. Recurrent opioid use in situations in which it is physically hazardous.
9. Continued opioid use despite knowledge of having a persistent or recurrent physical or psychological problem that is likely to have been caused or exacerbated by the substance.
10. Tolerance, as defined by either of the following:
    a. A need for markedly increased amounts of opioids to achieve intoxication or desired effect.
    b. A markedly diminished effect with continued use of the same amount of an opioid.
    Note: This criterion is not considered to be met for those taking opioids solely under appropriate medical supervision.
11. Withdrawal, as manifested by either of the following:
    a. The characteristic opioid withdrawal syndrome (refer to Criteria A and B of the criteria set for opioid withdrawal).
    b. Opioids (or a closely related substance) are taken to relieve or avoid withdrawal symptoms.
    Note: This criterion is not considered to be met for those individuals taking opioids solely under appropriate medical supervision.

Specify if:

12. **In early remission:** After full criteria for opioid use disorder were previously met, none of the criteria for opioid use disorder has been met for at least 3 months but for less than 12 months (with the exception that Criterion A4, "Craving, or a strong desire or urge to use opioids," may be met).
13. **In sustained remission:** After full criteria for opioid use disorder were previously met, none of the criteria for opioid use disorder has been met at any time during a period of 12 months or longer (with the exception that Criterion A4, "Craving, or a strong desire or urge to use opioids," may be met).

Specify if:

14. **On maintenance therapy:** This additional specifier is used if the individual is taking a prescribed agonist medication such as methadone or buprenorphine and none of the criteria for opioid use disorder have been met for that class of medication (except tolerance to, or withdrawal from, the agonist). This category also applies to those individuals being maintained on a partial agonist, an agonist/antagonist, or a full antagonist such as oral naltrexone or depot naltrexone.
15. **In a controlled environment:** This additional specifier is used if the individual is in an environment where access to opioids is restricted.

Criteria for Cannabis Use Disorder

Source: Volpicelli J. Diagnosis and Treatment of Opioid Use Disorders, in: Rippe JM. *Lifestyle Medicine*, 3rd edition. CRC Press, Boca Raton, 2019. Used with permission. .

in both alcohol and tobacco cessation such as regular physical activity may also be utilized.

19.6 CANNABIS USE DISORDER AND TREATMENT

Cannabis is the most commonly used psychoactive drug in the United States. Nine percent of the population in the United States aged 12 or older report cannabis use in the past month (21–23). Changes in state laws legalizing cannabis for medical and recreational use have coincided with changes in many perceptions of the use of this substance. Many adults and adolescents increasingly view cannabis as harmless. However, there are significant risks with its use. Evidence suggests that increases in cannabis potency, adult use, and CUD diagnoses are now occurring with 20–30% of users now meeting criteria for CUD. Thus, lifestyle medicine practitioners should be well informed about potential physical, mental, psychological, and psychosocial problems associated with cannabis use.

Cannabis is the most commonly used during pregnancy and evidence indicates that cannabis use is increasing during pregnancy (24). There is limited research available in this area. However, potential risks of prenatal cannabis use exposure include anemia, low birth weight, and need for neonatal intensive care as well as greater frontal cortical thickness and impaired executive functioning during childhood. Recreational cannabis use during childhood is also increasing. One recent survey showed that over 5% of 8th graders use cannabis. Cannabis exposure during childhood may acutely result in lethargy, ataxia dizziness, and respiratory depression.

Concerns also exist about cannabis use during adolescence, including a negative impact on brain development, educational outcomes, cognition and I.Q., life satisfaction and achievement as well as addiction (25,26). With regard to adult use, there are no known cases of fatal overdose from cannabis among adults. However, cannabis users are at increased risk of injury or fatality due to driving while intoxicated. Driving under the influence of cannabis has been shown to substantially increase the risk of fatal or non-fatal motor vehicle accidents.

DSM5 provides specific criteria for making the diagnosis of CUD. These may be found in Table 19.3.

Some symptoms have been reported for cannabis withdrawal. In DSM5, criteria are listed for cannabis withdrawal. These are found in Table 19.4.

With regard to treatment, very few people who met the DSM5 CUD diagnosis received treatment with only 7.2–13.7% doing any type of intervention. The U.S. Preventative Services Task Force recommends screening for health risk behaviors, including substance abuse using a screening, brief intervention, and referral to treatment (SBIRT) model which has been well established for patients who engage in risky alcohol use but its effectiveness for CUD remains unclear.

Chronic pain is very common among U.S. adults. Prescription opioids have been widely prescribed for chronic pain despite inconsistent evidence for benefits. Many medical marijuana patients use cannabis for pain relief and some as a partial or complete substitute for prescription opioids.

TABLE 19.3

DSM-IV and DSM-5 Criteria for Cannabis Use Disorder (CUD)

	DSM-IV Abuse[a]	DSM-IV Dependence[b]	DSM-5 CUD[c]
Hazardous use (e.g., driving under the influence)	X		X
Social/interpersonal problems related to use	X		X
Neglected major roles to use	X		X
Legal problems	X		
Withdrawal			X
Tolerance		X	X
Used large amounts/ longer than intended		X	X
Repeated attempts to quit/control use		X	X
Much time spent using		X	X
Physical/psychological problems related to use		X	X
Activities given up to use		X	X
Craving[d]			X

Source: Aivadyan C, Hasin D. Cannabis Use Disorder and Treatment, in: Rippe JM. *Lifestyle Medicine*, 3rd edition. CRC Press, Boca Raton, 2019. Used with permission

Symptoms of Cannabis Withdrawal.

[a] One or more criteria within a 12-month period.
[b] Three or more criteria within a 12-month period.
[c] Two or more criteria within a 12-month period.
[d] New criterion added in DSM-5.

19.7 SMARTPHONE-BASED TECHNOLOGIES IN ADDICTION TREATMENT

The potential use of smartphones and mobile technologies to improve multiple aspects of health care delivery is increasingly recognized around the world. In November 2016, 77% of Americans at that time owned a smartphone. Smartphones are nearly ubiquitous among younger adults with 92% ownership among adults 18–29 years old. Smartphone devices already offer many uses for substance abuse disorders (27,28). For example, they can provide opportunities for research data collection in populations with various substance use disorders. Smartphones and electronics may offer new insights into the actual experiences of those with substance use disorders. One recent literature review of AUD disorder used smartphones and mobile websites to include motivational interviews and various behavioral theories. This study showed positive outcomes in cognitive changes related to alcohol consumption. Smartphone technologies have also been developed as a component of strategies for smoking cessation. Early generation smoking cessation apps in English

TABLE 19.4

DSM-5 Cannabis Withdrawal

1. Cessation of heavy, prolonged cannabis use (i.e., daily or almost daily use over at least a few months).
2. Three or more of these symptoms within a week after cessation of heavy, prolonged use:
   a. Irritability, anger, or aggression
   b. Nervousness or anxiety
   c. Sleep difficulty (e.g., insomnia, disturbing dreams)
   d. Decreased appetite or weight loss
   e. Restlessness
   f. Depressed mood
   g. At least one of these physical symptoms causing significant discomfort: abdominal pain, shakiness/tremors, sweating, fever, chills, headache.
3. The symptoms cause clinically significant distress or impairment in social, occupational, or other important areas of functioning.
4. The symptoms are not due to another medical condition or another mental disorder, including intoxication or withdrawal from another substance.

Source: Aivadyan C, Hasin D. Cannabis Use Disorder and Treatment, in: Rippe JM. *Lifestyle Medicine*, 3rd edition. CRC Press, Boca Raton, 2019. Used with permission.

did not show positive outcomes for improving smoking abstinence behavior. More research is clearly needed in this area.

Even though recent literature has shown high acceptability for smartphone-based intervention and feasibility in various addiction treatments, the data to date have not found support for evidence-based information to change behavior. Furthermore, there is currently no FDA-approved smartphone app as a medical device for addiction treatments. Clearly, this is an area where more research will be needed in the future.

19.8 PSYCHOSOCIAL INTERVENTIONS FOR TREATMENT OF SUBSTANCE USE DISORDER

Psychosocial interventions can play a very important role in treating a range of drug problems and addictive behaviors (29). A variety of studies have reported efficacy in this area, including behavioral couples therapy, family therapy, cognitive behavioral therapy, community reinforcement approach, contingency management, individual drug counseling, motivational interviewing, 12-Step facilitation, and peer support. All of these interventions can be used across the entire spectrum of substance use disorder treatment.

19.9 CONCLUSIONS

A wide variety of substance use disorders are seen by lifestyle medicine physicians as well as other primary care practitioners. It is clear that cigarette smoking remains a very significant adverse health behavior and is the leading cause of preventable mortality worldwide. Among the substance use disorders, AUD is also prevalent. A variety of lifestyle interventions, including behavioral approaches and, in some instances, exercise, can help in both of these disorders. Recently, opioid use disorder has dramatically increased in the United States and resulted in nearly 50,000 annual deaths, which make this the leading overdose cause of death for individuals under the age of 50. Cannabis use has increased dramatically in the United States, particularly with the legalization of cannabis in many states for recreational and medical use. While many people feel use of cannabis is safe, a number of studies have suggested that there are some significant drawbacks to its regular use. For all of these reasons, it is incumbent on lifestyle medicine practitioners and other primary care physicians to become knowledgeable about the recognition and treatment of substance use disorders.

19.10 PRACTICAL APPLICATIONS

- Lifestyle medicine physicians should inquire about and be able to make the diagnosis of substance use disorders, including use of tobacco, abuse of alcohol, abuse of opioids, and overuse of cannabis.
- Evidence-based tools and recommendations are available from a variety of sources to aid in both the diagnosis and treatment of substance use disorders.
- Given the prevalence of cigarette smoking and alcohol consumption as well as the emerging epidemic of opioid abuse, it is incumbent on lifestyle medicine clinicians to become knowledgeable in these areas.

REFERENCES

1. American Psychiatric Association. *Diagnostic and Statistical Manual of Mental Disorders: DSM-5* (5th edition). American Psychiatric Publishing (Washington, DC), 2013.
2. World Health Organization (WHO). Substance Abuse. 1995. https://www.who.int/topics/substance_abuse/en/. Accessed July 20, 2020.
3. U.S. Department of Health and Human Services. *The Health Consequences of Smoking—50 Years of Progress: A Report of the Surgeon General.* U.S. Department of Health and Human Services, Centers for Disease Control and Prevention, National Center for Chronic Disease Prevention and Health Promotion, Office on Smoking and Health (Atlanta, GA), 2014.
4. Maruti S, Adleman S. History of Alcohol and Opioid Use and Treatment in the United States. In: Rippe JM, ed., *Lifestyle Medicine* (3rd edition). CRC Press (Boca Raton), 2019.
5. Ali R, Hay S. Smoking Prevalence and Attributable Disease Burden in 195 Countries and Territories, 1990–2015: A Systematic Analysis from the Global Burden of Disease Study 2015. *Lancet.* 2017;389(10082):1885–1906.
6. U.S. Department of Health and Human Services. *How Tobacco Smoke Causes Disease: The Biology and Behavioral Basis for Smoking-Attributable Disease: A Report of the Surgeon General.* U.S. Department of Health and Human Services, Centers for Disease Control and Prevention, National Center for Chronic Disease Prevention and Health Promotion, Office on Smoking and Health (Atlanta, GA), 2010.

7. Babb S, Malarcher A, Schauer G, et al. Quitting Smoking among Adults – United States, 2000–2015. *Morbidity and Mortality Weekly Report*. 2017;65(52):1457–1464.

8. Fiore M, Jaen R, Baker T, et al. *Treating Tobacco Use and Dependence: 2008 Update*. U.S. Department of Health & Human Services, Public Health Service (Rockville, MD), 2008.

9. Stead L, Lancaster T. Combined Pharmacotherapy and Behavioural Interventions for Smoking Cessation. *Cochrane Database of Systematic Reviews*. 2012;10:CD008286.

10. Osinubi O, Slade J. Tobacco in the Workplace. *Occupational Medicine*. 2002;17(1):137–158.

11. Shahab L, McEwen A. Online Support for Smoking Cessation: A Systematic Review of the Literature. *Addiction*. 2009;104(11):1792–1804.

12. Singh T, Tobacco Use among Middle and High School Students—United States, 2011–2015. *Morbidity and Mortality Weekly Report*. 2016;65: 361–367.

13. QuickStats: Percentage of Adults Who Ever Used an E-Cigarette and Percentage Who Currently Use E-Cigarettes, by Age Group—National Health Interview Survey, United States, 2016. *Morbidity and Mortality Weekly Report*. 2017;33:892.

14. Grant B, Goldstein R, Saha T, et al. Epidemiology of DSM-5 Alcohol Use Disorder: Results from the National Epidemiologic Survey on Alcohol and Related Conditions III. *JAMA Psychiatry*. 2015;72(8):757–66.

15. Ashwood Recovery at N. The Stages of Alcoholism Explained [Internet]. 2017. https ://www.ashwoodrecovery.com/blog/stages-alcoholism-explained/. Accessed July 16, 2020.

16. Berge K, Seppala M, Schipper A. Chemical Dependency and the Physician. *Mayo Clinic Proceedings*. 2009;84(7):625–31.

17. Kosten T, O'Connor P. Management of Drug and Alcohol Withdrawal. *New England Journal of Medicine*. 2003;348(18):1786–95.

18. Friedmann P. Alcohol Use in Adults. *New England Journal of Medicine*. 2013;364(4):365–373.

19. Dowell D, Arias E, Kochanek K. Contribution of Opioid Involved Poisoning to the Change in Life Expectancy in the United States, 2000–2015. *JAMA*. 2017;318(11):1065–1067.

20. Volpicelli J. Diagnosis and Treatment of Opioid Use Disorders. In: Rippe JM, ed., *Lifestyle Medicine* (3rd edition). CRC Press (Boca Raton), 2019.

21. Substance Abuse and Mental Health Services Administration. *Key Substance Use and Mental Health Indicators in the United States: Results from the 2016 National Survey on Drug Use and Health*. Center for Behavioral Health Statistics and Quality, Substance Abuse and Mental Health Services Administration (Rockville, MD), 2017. https://www.samhsa.gov/data/.

22. Compton W, Han B, Jones C, et al. Marijuana Use and Use Disorders in Adults in the USA, 2002–14: Analysis of Annual Cross-sectional Surveys. *Lancet Psychiatry*. 2016;3(10):954–964.

23. Azofeifa A, Mattson M, Schauer G, et al. National Estimates of Marijuana Use and Related Indicators - National Survey on Drug Use and Health, United States, 2002–2014. *Morbidity and Mortality Weekly Report*. 2016;65(11):1–28.

24. American College of Obstetricians, Gynecologists Committee on Obstetric Practice. Committee Opinion No. 637: Marijuana Use during Pregnancy and Lactation. *Obstetrics & Gynecology*. 2015;126(1):234–238.

25. Volkow N, Baler R. Compton of Marijuana Use. *New England Journal of Medicine*. 2014;370(23):2219–2227.

26. National Institutes of Health. Adolescent Brain Cognitive Development Study. *Alcohol Research*. 2018;Jan 39(1):97. https://addictionresearch.nih.gov/abcd-study. Accessed July 16, 2020.

27. Weissman M. The Institute of Medicine (IOM) Sets a Framework for Evidence Based Standards for Psychotherapy. *Depression and Anxiety.* 2015;32(11):787–789.
28. Carroll K, Onken L. Behavioral Therapies for Drug Abuse. *American Journal of Psychiatry.* 2005;162(8):1452–1460.
29. Haddad S. *Psychosocial Interventions for Treatment of Substance Use Disorders. Lifestyle Medicine* (3rd edition). CRC Press (Boca Raton), 2019.

20 Public Policy and Environmental Support for Lifestyle Habits and Practices

KEY POINTS

- Promoting healthier habits and actions involves not only individual choices, but also support from the community and public policy.
- Environmental supports for increasing physical activity include a variety of strategies such as interacting with schools, promoting the use of parks and other recreational facilities, and other examples where clinicians can play a leading role.
- Clinicians can also play a leading role in promoting factors and facilities that can create a more healthy eating environment not only for their own patients, but also for the community.
- The CDC has recommended a number of public policy initiatives that can help lower the prevalence of obesity and other chronic conditions and diseases. Clinicians can play a central role in promoting these recommendations.

20.1 INTRODUCTION

An enormous literature exists to support the relationship between positive lifestyle habits and multiple health benefits (1). This literature underscores two important concepts. First, positive lifestyle measures can play multiple positive roles in lowering the risk of chronic disease and improving the daily lives of individuals throughout their lifespan. Second, despite the known benefits, the majority of Americans do not participate in many of the positive lifestyle measures where abundant literature supports health benefits. For this reason, this chapter will focus on ways that public policy and environmental support can help support individuals in their efforts to engage in positive lifestyle measures.

A number of frameworks have been utilized to conceptualize factors that impact on lifestyle habits and practices. The Physical Activity Guidelines for Americans 2018 Scientific Report (PAGA 2018) utilized one such framework related to conceptualizing factors that impact on physical activity in the United States. This conceptual framework is shown in Figure 20.1 (2). A similar framework indicating multiple

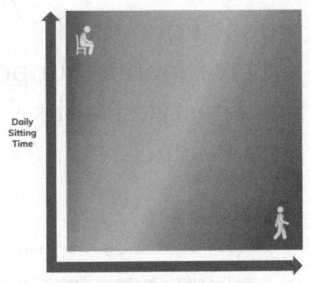

Moderate-to-Vigorous Physical Activity
Risk of all-cause mortality decreases as one moves from light to dark.

FIGURE 20.1 Relationship among moderate-to-vigorous physical activity, sitting time, and risk of all-cause mortality in adults. *Source:* Ekelund U, Steene-Johannessen J, Brown WJ. Does physical activity attenuate, or even eliminate, the detrimental association of sitting time with mortality? A harmonized meta-analysis of data from more than 1 million men and women. *Lancet* 2016;388:1302–1310. 2018 Physical Activity Guidelines Advisory Committee Scientific Report. At the greatest time spent sitting (the top), the risk of all-cause mortality begins.

influences on nutritional behaviors was put forth by the American Heart Association in their Scientific Statement about implementing nutritional guidelines.

As indicated in this figure, multiple influences impact on positive behaviors starting with the individual and then extending to the community, communication environment, as well as the built environment and public policy. This framework will also be explored in more detail later in this chapter under the section on policy and environmental supports for physical activity and active living (see next section).

20.2 LIFESTYLE MEDICINE IN THE ERA OF HEALTH CARE REFORM

The Patient Protection and Affordable Care Act, which is often referred to as the "Affordable Care Act" (ACA), was signed into law on March 23, 2010 (3). The intent of the ACA was to start the process of transforming health care delivery in the United States. There have been a number of modifications since that time.

A number of changes in health care have occurred based on the ACA (3,4). When the ACA started in 2014, over 20 million uninsured individuals obtained coverage. There are some groups of individuals who are not able to participate in the ACA. For example, 4.6 million low-income people are not eligible because their state did not expand Medicaid, 2.2 million are ineligible because their household income is above

400% of the federal poverty line, and 2.1 million are ineligible as a result of having a family member in an employer-sponsored insurance plan deemed affordable by the government. An additional 7.5 million are uninsured due to undocumented status.

One of the major ACA objectives was to develop alternative payment methods. Some of these included accountable care organizations and bundled payment programs (5). However, these types of methodologies appear to have had little measurable impact on health care delivery. The most important programs in the area of lifestyle medicine relate to primary care transformation, episodic care models, and issues focused on the Medicaid population.

The ACA legislation contains elements that could advance lifestyle medicine and primary prevention, but a large segment of the American electorate demonstrated opposition to expanding the government's role in the health care delivery system. For example, almost two-thirds of American citizens under the age of 65 are covered by employer-sponsored health plans. This has remained true even after ACA was inaugurated.

Many of the current metrics in place to define value are very difficult to change. While the United States Medicaid and Medicare Services recognized obesity as a disease in 2014 and the Healthcare Effectiveness Data Information Set (HEDIS) included a measurement of nutrition and physical activity and counseling for patients, children, and adolescents as a recommendation, most U.S. health plans do not use HEDIS for that purpose. Thus, current policies and practices related to the delivery of health care still have not offered adequate incentive (monetary or otherwise) for providers to integrate lifestyle medicine and preventive care into existing practices (5).

As the type of initiative such as ACA moves forward, as it appears inevitable given the rapidly increasing cost of health care in the United States, it is hoped that there will be more opportunity for lifestyle medicine principles and practices to impact on both quality of care and cost.

20.3 POLICY AND ENVIRONMENTAL SUPPORT FOR PHYSICAL ACTIVITY AND ACTIVE LIVING

It is well recognized that the burden of chronic disease in the United States is overwhelming and increasing. To address this burden, researchers and health care practitioners are paying increased attention to environmental and policy issues. One particular area of interest is to increase physical activity, which is a critical component in the prevention of chronic disease (2,6). A number of different approaches have been studied and found to be efficacious in the area of increasing physical activity. The various sources of influence on physical activity are outlined in Figure 20.1 and will be explored in more detail in this section.

- *Individual levels:* The most robust data currently available on effective ways of promoting physical activity comes from initiatives designed to increase physical activity in individuals. This is particularly true of the general adult population, but good data are also available for older adults and post-menopausal women and youths.

  The type of formats used to promote physical activity in individuals typically involves either one-on-one sessions or group-delivered programs involving structured exercises. Educational programs have also been offered. One advantage of these types of programs is that they are very flexible. A downside, however, is that they require a high level of staff involvement and therefore can result in significant cost increases over the long run. Examples of this kind of initiative are personal training and structured exercise classes. The same type of interventions has been employed to target older individuals. These have been shown to have a positive effect on physical activity, when compared to non-exercise controls.

The Physical Activity Guidelines for Americans 2018 Scientific Report (PAGA 2018) rated evidence for individual approaches to promote physical activity as "strong" (2). These types of approaches have also been used for other health-promoting lifestyle activities such as improved diet (e.g., more fruit and vegetables) as well as weight loss behaviors. Similar approaches have been involved and have been shown to be beneficial in post-menopausal individuals, which is a group where adequate physical activity may be difficult to increase or maintain. The most promising of these efforts involve routine strategies, including goal setting and behavioral self-monitoring.

This type of approach has also been found to be beneficial for youth. Benefits are enhanced when incorporating family or delivering physical activity interventions in school settings. In addition, use of school facilities during non-school hours, as well as improving sidewalk and street design for commuting to and from school also appear to be promising strategies.

- *Theory-based interventions to increase physical activity:* Multiple cities have examined various theory-based interventions to increase physical activity. These theoretical frameworks are discussed in more detail in Chapter 4. These include the Health Belief Model (HBM), the Theory of Reasoned Action, Planned Behavior and Integrated Behavior Model, and the Trans-theoretical Model (see Chapter 4 for more details).

- *Community-based interventions to increase physical activity:* A variety of community-wide programs have been undertaken in order to attempt to increase levels of physical activity. Community approaches are based on the understanding that many adults report barriers of participation in regular activity that relate to community issues. For example, a commonly cited barrier is the lack of facilities or safe places to engage in physical activity. Even if health care practitioners encourage physical activity behavior, unless individuals have a place where they can be active, they are often unable to follow such recommendations.

- Various locations have been explored and found to be beneficial. For example, school-based programs have been demonstrated to be highly effective (7,8). Many physical education and health education curricula and programs are now available to provide a framework for promoting youth physical activity. Worksites may also be very valuable places for increased physical activity. This is particularly true since many employed adults spend at least half of their waking hours at work, which makes workplaces a natural place to attempt to increase physical activity.

- Numerous community organizations can also provide facilities and programs with potential to increase physical activity. These include health clubs, dance studios, swimming pools, sports clubs, etc. Non-profit organizations such as YMCAs, YWCAs, and Boys' and Girls' Clubs can also provide places for increased physical activity. In addition, such facilities as parks and trails may be utilized to increase physical activity. A number of research projects have shown that encouraging people to utilize these facilities increases the likelihood of individuals walking or running on trails and parks. Finally, health care delivery models delivered either from primary care clinics or through nurses have also been explored and have shown some benefits for increasing physical activity.

- *Communication environmental level:* The exploding area of new Information and Communication Technologies (ICT) has provided additional modalities for increasing the levels of physical activity. These include wearable activity monitors, telephone-assisted interventions, web-based or internet interventions, computer-tailored print interventions, multiple phone programs and social media, and point of decision prompts and programs to increase access to the indoor and outdoor facilities. A useful summary of all this information can be found in the National Physical Activity Plan (2017 U.S. Report Card on Walking and Walkable Communities).

- *Interventions to reduce sedentary behavior:* Accumulating evidence has emerged that sedentary behavior can have a significant adverse impact on health (9). With this in mind, strategies to promote physical activity should also include ways of reducing sedentary behavior. In youth, reduction in television viewing and other screen time has yielded small, but consistent, positive results in reducing sedentary behavior. With regard to adult interventions, some data suggest that interventions such as education and behavioral approaches to reducing sedentary time may be helpful. With regard to worksite interventions, those which target workers who perform duties primarily while seated may have a significant short-term impact on reducing sedentary behavior (10). Worksite interventions are particularly appealing because they can be implemented during times when physical activity is generally not feasible. Both educational and policy changes designed to reduce prolonged sedentary behavior have been demonstrated to be effective in the workforce. Detailed information concerning many of these initiatives to enhance the likelihood of physical activity may be found in the PAGA 2018 document under the chapter on "Promoting Regular Physical Activity."

20.4   POLICY AND ENVIRONMENTAL SUPPORTS FOR HEALTHY EATING

Consuming food is a matter of survival for all human beings. However, consuming nutritious food is more complicated than we often imagine (11). Eating a diet with adequate fruits and vegetables, along with other nutritious food, has been clearly shown to reduce the risk of many of the leading causes of illness and death such as cardiovascular disease (CVD), type 2 diabetes (T2DM), some cancers, and obesity. Despite these positive health benefits, few adults in the United States meet the nutrition recommendations from the U.S. Department of Agriculture (USDA) 2015–2020 Dietary Guidelines for Americans (12). In fact, less than 10% of adults meet the intake requirements for vegetables and 12% of adults meet the requirements for fruits. Multiple factors impact on people's consumption of fruits and vegetables, including cost, access, and taste preferences. However, these factors get in the way of people's ability to maintain good health and make healthful food choices.

- *Dimensions of access to nutritious food:* There are multiple dimensions related to access to nutritious food. These have been conceptualized by Penchansky and Thomas to include the following five dimensions relevant to nutrition and health (13):

    Availability—This includes the types of restaurants as well as fresh produce available to individuals and families. There is a concept of "food deserts" in the United States, which relates to geographical settings, where it is very difficult for people to obtain nutritious food.

    Affordability—Health professionals should understand that some of the preventive recommendations made may be difficult to follow for cost considerations. A number of reviews have indicated that healthier diets are typically more costly than less healthy diets.

    Acceptability and accommodation—Acceptability refers to food quality, whereas accommodation generally refers to the number of hours that a particular local store is open. A number of studies have shown that these factors into making a choice for nutritious foods.

    Accessibility—A number of studies have offered conflicting viewpoints concerning accessibility. The most reliable concept in this area is car access, travel time, and where participants shop.

- *Disparity/inequities to healthy eating:* The Dietary Guidelines for Americans 2015–2020 has a number of key messages, including reducing calories from added sugars, consuming a variety of foods, replacing solid fats with oils, eliminating refined grains, and moderate coffee consumption. However, these guidelines may be particularly difficult for those in a low socioeconomic status and education levels (14). Another barrier which is found predominantly in African-American populations is access to transportation to grocery stores which sell fresh produce and whole grain options (14–16).

- *Environmental factors:* Multiple environmental factors impact on nutritious eating. Perhaps the most important one is the availability of full-service grocery stores. In fact, in one study, the distance from a grocery store and food pricing were positively associated with obesity. This has led to the conclusion that it may be more important to offer better and more competitive prices for healthy foods compared to less healthy foods and actively market healthier alternatives in order to help people who shop in ways that would improve their overall health.

- *Healthy food policies:* The U.S. Department of Agriculture (USDA) and Health and Human Services (HHS) have developed a variety of programs and policies which are intended to help people to consume healthier foods:

  Food labels—Changes have been made on food labels to make it easier to make informed decisions.

  Restaurant menus—It is important to recognize that one-third of calories from individuals come from foods that individuals do not prepare themselves. In response to this, the Food and Drug Administration established the menu labeling rule which applies to any restaurant establishment that has 20 or more locations (17). These restaurant establishments are required to provide calorie labeling to consumers. Early research has not been promising that this has changed eating behaviors, but at least it is a start.

- *Behavioral economics:* In traditional economic theory, everyday individuals make decisions based on their best interest. Behavioral economics, however, combines the principles of traditional economics with psychology. Individuals tend to overemphasize short-term benefits versus long-term benefits (18–20). This often manifests itself in the area of nutrition with a preference for convenience. For example, American families spent 27% of their food budget in 1962 on restaurant eating versus 46% in 2002. Also, individuals may be attracted to ques such as sight or smell which can temporarily elevate the desire for a specific food item. Another aspect of behavioral economics supports that individuals are highly prone to stick with default options even when better options are available. For example, the automatic side dish is a "default" setting, which adds calories to a meal. For clinicians, understanding behavior economics will help encourage individuals to eat healthier options.

- *Healthy eating recommendations:* The Dietary Guidelines for Americans 2015–2020 (12) and various documents from the American Heart Association and others have been quite consistent with each other, including the following recommendations:
  - Eat a variety of vegetables.
  - Eat more fruits.
  - Eat grains, at least half of which are whole grains.
  - Consume fat-free or low-fat dairy.
  - Consume a variety of healthful protein foods, including seafood, lean meats, poultry and eggs, along with soy products.

- *MyPlate:* Various tools are available to help people conceptualize healthy eating. One from the FDA is the MyPlate Initiative which uses a place setting to illustrate five food groups: fruits, grains, vegetables, proteins, and dairy. This initiative is intended to serve as a reminder about how to eat nutritiously based on individual foods placed on a plate.

20.5 POLICY AND ENVIRONMENTAL SUPPORTS TO CONTROL OBESITY AND WEIGHT GAIN

- *Public health implications:* Obesity was first recognized as a public health issue by the National Institutes of Health in 1985 (19). Data from the CDC indicates that obesity in the United States remains a major public health problem. Obesity now outranks both smoking and drinking alcohol in its adverse effects on morbidity and mortality as well as health costs. For example, obesity is associated with 36% increase in in-patient and out-patient health care costs compared to a 21% increase in spending for smoking and excessive alcohol consumption.

  The goals of the Healthy People 2020 Objectives (21) were to reduce the prevalence of obesity in adults in the United States to 15%. If the American population were able to lose excess body weight, mortality would be reduced by 15%, which corresponds to three years of average life expectancy for every citizen in the United States. The CDC convened an expert panel which identified 24 recommended strategies for obesity prevention. A summary of these strategies are found in Table 20.1.
- *Public policy and environmental strategies:* It is clear that both public policy and environmental strategies will be necessary in order to promote active living, healthy eating, and prevention of obesity. These health strategies may be divided into four areas:
  - Agricultural and food supply policies that support healthy eating
  - Health care delivery policies
  - Educational and school-based policies
  - Urban design, land use, and transportation policies for active living and healthy eating

Factors that impact on obesity are very complicated, as indicated in Figure 20.2.
- *The need for professional health care involvement:* Physicians are identified in many research trials as the leading source of credibility and information in the area of health. When it comes to obesity, the recommendations for clinicians, which were recommended by Utter et al., include the following six recommendations:
  - Eat more fruits and vegetables and fewer foods high in fat and sugar (see http://www.choosemyplate.gov/).
  - Drink more water instead of sugary drinks.
  - Limit TV watching in children to less than two hours a day and do not put a TV in their room.
  - Support breastfeeding.
  - Promote policies and programs at work, at school, and in the community that make the healthy choice the easy choice. This includes policy and environmental support for both healthy eating and active living.
  - Try going for a 10-minute, brisk walk three times a day, five days a week.

TABLE 20.1

CDC Task Force Recommendation for Steps that Communities Could Take to Combat Obesity

- Increase availability of healthier food and beverage choices in public service venues
- Improve availability of affordable healthier food and beverage choices in public service venues
- Improve geographic availability of supermarkets in underserved areas
- Provide incentives to food retailers to locate in and/or offer healthier food and beverage choices in underserved areas
- Improve availability of mechanisms for purchasing foods from farms
- Incentives for the production, distribution, and procurement of foods from local farms
- Restrict availability of less healthy foods and beverages in public service venues
- Institute smaller portion size options in public service venues
- Limit advertisements of less healthy foods and beverages
- Discourage consumption of sugar-sweetened beverages
- Increase support for breastfeeding
- Require physical education in schools
- Increase the amount of physical activity in PE programs in schools
- Increase opportunities for extracurricular physical activity
- Reduce screen time in public service venues
- Improve access to outdoor recreational facilities
- Enhance infrastructure supporting bicycling
- Enhance infrastructure supporting walking
- Support locating schools within easy walking distance of residential areas
- Improve access to public transportation
- Zone for mixed-use development
- Enhance personal safety in areas where persons are or could be physically active
- Enhance traffic safety in areas where persons are or could be physically active
- Communities should participate in community coalitions or partnerships to address obesity

Source: From CDC: Recommended Community Strategies and Measurements to Prevent Obesity in the United States. July 2009. https://www.cdc.gov/obesity/downloads/community_strategies_g uide.pdf

Given the multiple adverse health and economic consequences of obesity, it is vitally important that clinicians help their patients with major individual and public health problems.

20.6 BUILDING STRATEGIC ALLIANCES TO PROMOTE HEALTHY EATING AND ACTIVE LIVING

Health-promoting strategies that include changes in community environments which support increased physical activity and good nutrition are vital to reducing unhealthy behaviors associated with a variety of metabolic diseases and increased obesity prevalence (22–26). Included in the chronic diseases which could be reduced by such changes in environments are CVD, T2DM, arthritis, and some cancers.

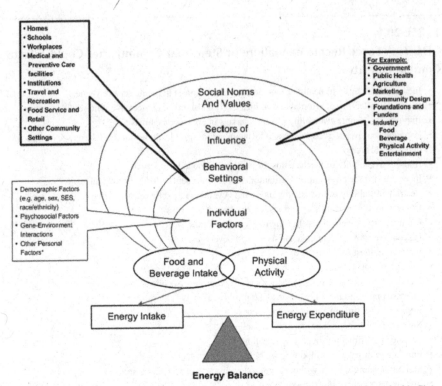

- Homes
- Schools
- Workplaces
- Medical and
  Preventive Care
  facilities
- Institutions
- Travel and
  Recreation
- Food Service and
  Retail
- Other Community
  Settings

For Example:
- Government
- Public Health
- Agriculture
- Marketing
- Community Design
- Foundations and
  Funders
- Industry
  Food
  Beverage
  Physical Activity
  Entertainment

Social Norms
And Values

Sectors of
Influence

Behavioral
Settings

Individual
Factors

- Demographic Factors
  (e.g. age, sex, SES,
  race/ethnicity)
- Psychosocial Factors
- Gene-Environment
  Interactions
- Other Personal
  Factors*

Food and
Beverage Intake

Physical
Activity

Energy Intake

Energy Expenditure

Energy Balance

*Note: Other relevant factors that influence obesity prevention interventions are culture and acculturation; biobehavioral interactions; and social, political, and historical contexts.

FIGURE 20.2   Factors influencing obesity and weight gain. *Source:* Adapted from Centers of Disease Control and Prevention IOM (2007): CDC (2006).

Clinicians have a key role to play in helping to develop strategic alliances to promote these healthy behaviors (27,28). Clinicians remain a source of credibility, expertise, and leadership to help on multiple levels not only with their patients, but also have the ability to lead the creation of environmental and policy changes to improve health throughout the United States. Clinicians can help in bringing organizations and community members together to enhance healthy eating and active living in a community. These have been called "strategic alliances." Coalitions are multidimensional partnerships. There are multiple examples of how this has worked in communities throughout the United States. Physicians should become actively involved in leading such partnerships for the benefit of their patients and the overall health of their community.

20.7   CONCLUSIONS

Many of the changes which will create healthier lives for all patients involve not only the patients' habits and actions themselves, but also the support of the local environment as well as both community resources and national public policy. Such areas as increasing physical activity, promoting healthy eating, and helping to control obesity and weight gain are all examples of where there is an important interaction between the community and the individual. Physicians have a high level of credibility which can allow them to take a leadership role in helping to create the strategic alliances which will be necessary to combat major, non-communicable disease risk factors that are very much prevalent in the United States.

20.8 CLINICAL APPLICATIONS

- Many of the chronic diseases which create adverse health effects are not only individual issues, but also involve the community, environment, and public policy. Clinicians should be involved in all of these areas.
- When counseling individual patients, clinicians should explore what resources are available in the community for both healthy nutrition and physical activity.
- Clinicians should also become involved as credible sources of information and assume a leading position in helping to build strategic alliances which will promote not only individual health, but also environments that make healthy living the easy choice rather than a hard choice.

REFERENCES

1. Rippe JM. *Lifestyle Medicine* (3rd edition). CRC Press (Boca Raton), 2019.
2. Physical Activity Guidelines Advisory Committee. *2018 Physical Activity Guidelines Advisory Committee. 2018 Physical Activity Guidelines Advisory Committee Scientific Report.* U.S. Department of Health and Human Services (Washington, DC), 2018.
3. Hajart A, Weisser S, Wilkerson G, et al. Medicine in an Era of Healthcare Reform—Seven Years of Healthcare Disruption: 2010–2017. In Rippe JM: *Lifestyle Medicine* (3rd edition). CRC Press (Boca Raton), 2019.
4. Blumberg L, Holahan J. Early Experience with the ACA: Coverage Gains, Pooling of Risk, and Medicaid Expansion. *Journal of Law, Medicine & Ethics.* 2016;44:538–545.
5. Doran T, Maurer K, Ryan A. Impact of Provider Incentives on Quality and Value of Health Care. *Annual Review of Public Health.* 2017;38:449–465.
6. Dodson E, Heath G. *Policy and Environmental Supports for Physical Activity and Active Living. Lifestyle Medicine* (3rd edition). CRC Press (Boca Raton), 2019.
7. Stone E, McKenzie T, Welk G, et al. Effects of Physical Activity Interventions in Youth. Review and Synthesis. *American Journal of Preventive Medicine.* 1998;15(4):298–315.
8. Hynynen S, van Stralen M, Sniehott F, et al. A Systematic Review of School-Based Intervention Programs Targeting Physical Activity and Sedentary Behaviour among Older Adolescents. *International Review of Sport and Exercise Psychology.* 2016;9(1):22–44.
9. *2018 Physical Activity Guidelines Advisory Committee. 2018 Physical Activity Guidelines Advisory Committee Scientific Report.* U.S. Department of Health and Human Services (Washington, DC), 2018. Part F. Chapter 2. Sedentary Behavior, F2-1-F2-35.
10. Dodson E, Lovegreen S, Elliott M, et al. Worksite Policies and Environments Supporting Physical Activity in Mid-Western Communities. *American Journal of Health Promotion.* 2008;23(1):51–55.

11. Schmidt C, Maddux E, Hathaway E. *Policy and Environmental Supports for Healthy Eating. Lifestyle Medicine* (3rd ed). CRC Press (Boca Raton), 2019.

12. U.S. Department of Health and Human Services and U.S. Department of Agriculture. *2015–2020 Dietary Guidelines for Americans* (8th edition). http: //health.gov/dietary guidelines/2015/guidelines/. ePub December 2015.

13. Penchansky R, Thomas J. The Concept of Access: Definition, and Relationship to Consumer Satisfaction. *Medical Care.* 1981;19(2):127–140.

14. Thorton L, Crawford R, Ball K. Neighbourhood-Socioeconomic Variation in Women's Diet: The Role of Nutrition Environments. *European Journal of Clinical Nutrition.* 2010;64(12):1423–1432.

15. Timperio A, Ball K, Roberst R, et al. Children's Fruit and Vegetable Intake: Associations with the Neighbourhood Food Environment. *Preventive Medicine.* 2008;46(4):331–335.

16. Rose D, Richards R. Food Store Access and Household Fruit and Vegetable Use among Participants in the US Food Stamp Program. *Public Health Nutrition.* 2004;7:08.

17. U.S. Food and Drug Administration. Calorie Labeling on Restaurant Menus and Vending Machines: What You Need to Know. May 2, 2017. https://http://www.fda.gov /Food/Ingre dientsPackagingLabeling/LabelingNutrition/ucm436722.htm. Accessed July 13, 2020.

18. Jayson L. *The Rise of "Nudge" and the Use of Behavioral Economics in Food and Health Policy.* George Mason University (Arlington, VA), 2015.

19. Liu P, Wisdom J, Roberto C, et al. Using Behavioral Economics to Design More Effective Food Policies to Address Obesity. *Applied Economic Perspectives and Policy.* 2014;36(1):6–24.

20. O'Donoghue T, Rabin M. The Economics of Immediate Gratification. *Journal of Behavioral Decision Making.* 2000;13(2):233–250.

21. Healthy People 2020 Guidelines. https://www.healthypeople.gov/. Office of Disease Prevention and Health Promotion. Washington, DC Accessed July 13, 2020.

22. Wilkerson R, Baker E, Longjohn M, et al. Building Strategic Alliances to Promote Healthy Eating and Active Living. In: Rippe JM, ed., *Lifestyle Medicine* (3rd edition). CRC Press (Boca Raton), 2019.

23. Heath GW. Obesity and Health: Implications of Public Policy. In: Rippe JM, Angelopoulos TJ, eds., *Obesity Prevention and Treatment.* CRC Press (Boca Raton), 2012.

24. Brownson R, Haire-Joshu D, Luke D. Shaping the Context of Health: A Review of Environmental and Policy Approaches in the Prevention of Chronic Diseases. *Annual Review of Public Health.* 2006;27:341–370.

25. Glanz K, Lankenau B, Foerster S. et al. Environmental and Policy Approaches to Cardiovascular Disease Prevention through Nutrition: Opportunities for State and Local Action. *Health Education Quarterly.* 1995;22(4):512–527.

26. King A, Jeffery R, Fridinger F. Environmental and Policy Approaches to Cardiovascular Disease Prevention through Physical Activity: Issues and Opportunities. *Health Education Quarterly.* 1998;22(4):499–511.

27. Compton M. Physicians as Citizens. *Journal of the American Medical Association.* 2004;291(17):2076.

28. Gruen R, Pearson S, Brennan T. Physician Citizens—Public Roles and Professional Obligations. *Journal of the American Medical Association.* 2004;291:94–98.

21 Lifestyle Medicine around the World

KEY POINTS

- Non-communicable diseases (NCDs) exceed communicable diseases around the world.
- Lifestyle practices such as increased physical activity, proper nutrition, including consumption of more fruits and vegetables and whole grains, weight management, avoidance of tobacco products, and avoidance or moderation of alcohol consumption can all play significant roles in combatting the major NCDs around the world.
- Increasingly, physicians and other health care workers are being trained in specific areas of lifestyle medicine to help stem the tide of NCDs around the world.

21.1 INTRODUCTION

The world is in the midst of a pandemic of non-communicable diseases (NCDs). It has been estimated by multiple reliable sources that non-communicable diseases are responsible for over 80% of all morbidity and mortality worldwide (1). The principles and practices of lifestyle medicine are uniquely positioned to help overcome the significant health issues related to NCDs.

While an emphasis on lifestyle medicine as an academic discipline initially was found in the United States, it has now spread throughout the world. The World Health Organization (WHO) has identified NCDs as one of the major emphases in health throughout the world. In fact, the WHO has identified nine major targets to deal with the rapid rise of non-communicable diseases (2). These targets include the harmful use of alcohol, insufficient physical activity, salt/sodium intake, tobacco use and hypertension, stemming the dramatic rise in diabetes and obesity, and seeking ways of lowering the risk of heart attack and stroke. The overarching goal from WHO is to reach a 25% reduction in premature mortality from NCDs by 2025. These include heart disease (CVD), stroke, chronic obstructive pulmonary disease (COPD), and lower respiratory tract infections.

Out of the 38 million deaths due to NCDs in 2012, more than 40% were premature affecting people under the age of 70 years. The majority of premature NCD deaths are preventable, largely through daily habits and actions. Deaths from CVD continue to lead disease categories around the world. It has been clearly demonstrated that such lifestyle modalities as increased physical activity, proper nutrition, and maintaining a healthy body weight (BMI ≤ 25 kg/m^2) all can significantly lower the risk of CVD.

Both obesity and diabetes have a major component of lifestyle in them. It was estimated in 2013 that there were 2.1 billion people worldwide who were obese. This contributes to a wide variety of other metabolic conditions, including cardiovascular disease (CVD), type 2 diabetes (T2DM), and even some cancers as well as other metabolically based diseases (3).

A key to understanding treatment of NCDs is that there are a set of cost-effective interventions to help ameliorate all of these conditions. These all fall within the purview of lifestyle medicine which will be the focus of this chapter.

21.2   THE ROLE OF LIFESTYLE MEDICINE IN LOWERING THE RISK OF NON-COMMUNICABLE DISEASES (NCDS) WORLDWIDE

The mandate of lifestyle medicine is to convey the importance of daily habits and actions on both short- and long-term health and quality of life. I was honored to have named the field "lifestyle medicine" in the academic literature with the publication of my first comprehensive textbook in this field in 1999 (4). In this book, we defined lifestyle medicine as

> involving the integration of lifestyle practice into the modern practice of medicine both to lower the risk factors for chronic disease and, if disease is already present, to serve as an adjunct to its therapy. Lifestyle medicine brings together sound scientific evidence in diverse, health related fields to assist the clinician in the process of not only treating disease, but also promoting good health.

The 3rd edition of this textbook was published in 2019 (5). It represents the collective wisdom of over 200 experts in the area of lifestyle practices and habits and their impact on health. These individuals come from countries all around the world.

While there have subsequently been other definitions of lifestyle medicine, they all are consistent with this initial vision. While lifestyle medicine as a formal academic discipline initially was launched in the United States, it has now grown into a worldwide movement. In fact, Lifestyle Medicine Global Alliance has branches in over 20 countries and virtually every continent of the world. Lifestyle medicine practices and habits are totally consistent with the goals and targets of lowering NCD risk which have been articulated by WHO.

The ongoing development of lifestyle medicine around the world has also been paralleled by the growth of the *American Journal of Lifestyle Medicine* (AJLM). AJLM was founded in 2007 (6). It has grown rapidly since that time. AJLM currently has over 13,000 subscribers and in 2019, over 100,000 full-text articles from AJLM were downloaded. Subscribers to AJLM represent countries around the world. AJLM was founded with the vision of providing a forum for individuals who wish to learn more about lifestyle medicine and to exchange information as well as publish evidence-based articles in areas related to lifestyle medicine. I have had the honor of serving as the editor-in-chief of the *American Journal of Lifestyle Medicine* since its inception.

21.3   NON-COMMUNICATIVE DISEASES (NCDS)

The World Health Organization Status Report on Prevention and Control of NCDs (2014) was framed around nine voluntary target goals. The goal of this important document was to help individual countries develop and implement policies and interventions designed to combat major NCDs within their country. The following nine global targets were identified (2):

- **Global target #1:** *A 25% relative reduction in overall mortality from cardiovascular diseases, cancer, diabetes, or chronic respiratory diseases.*

  CVDs are the leading cause of morbidity and mortality in countries throughout the world. Some countries, such as the United States, have already achieved significant reductions in CVD, but the goal of a 25% reduction is particularly important to achieve in low- and middle-income countries since the majority of premature NCD deaths from CVD occurs in these countries.

- **Global target #2:** *At least 10% relative reduction in the harmful use of alcohol as appropriate within the national context.*

  In 2012, an estimated 5.9% of all deaths (3.3. million) and 5.1% disability adjusted life years (DALYS) were attributed to alcohol consumption. The level of alcohol consumption worldwide is estimated to be 6.2 L of pure alcohol per person per year for individuals aged 15 years and older. The overall level of alcohol consumption is higher in the European region and among Americans. A number of organizations have been active in attempting to lower alcohol consumption. Seventy-six countries have a written national policy on alcohol and 52 have taken steps to lower alcohol consumption.

- **Global target #3:** *Attempt to stem reduction in the prevalence of insufficient physical activity.*

  Insufficient physical activity, according to the WHO, contributes to 3 million annual deaths and 69.3 million DALYS each year. Adults who are insufficiently physically active have a high risk of all-cause mortality compared to those who achieve 150 minutes of moderate intensity activity per week. Regular physical activity reduces the risk of CVD, stroke, diabetes (T2DM), and breast and colon cancer. In 2010, only 22% of adults aged 18 and over were sufficiently physically active. Women were less active than men and older people less active than young people. Globally 81% of adolescents aged 11–17 years were insufficiently physically active. Adolescent girls were less active than adolescent boys. Eighty-four percent of adolescent girls and 78% of adolescent boys did not meet the recommendations from both the WHO and the Physical Activity Guidelines for Americans (PAGA) 2018 Scientific Report of 60 minutes of physical activity per day (7). Much more detail about physical activity and its multiple linkages to good health may be found in Chapter 3.

- **Global target #4:** *A 30% relative reduction in the mean population intake of salt/sodium.*

  Excess consumption of dietary sodium is associated with an increased risk of hypertension and CVD. Globally, 1.7 million annual deaths from CVD have been attributed to excess sodium intake. The AHA and WHO both recommend reduction of salt intake to less than 2300 mg of sodium per day to reduce blood pressure and the risk of CVD and stroke (8). More detail about this aspect of nutrition may be found in Chapter 2.

- **Global target #5** *A 30% relative reduction in prevalence of current tobacco use in people 16+ years.*

  The WHO estimates that 6 million people worldwide die annually from tobacco use and over 600,000 deaths occur due to exposure of secondhand smoke each year. Considerable progress has been made in global tobacco control, but more work is needed in many countries to pass and enforce effective tobacco control measures. In the United States, approximately 15.5% of the adult population continues to smoke cigarettes. While significant progress has been achieved in this area, there still is a considerable way to go.

- **Global target #6:** *A 25% relative reduction in the prevalence of raised blood pressure or contain the prevalence of raised blood pressure according to national circumstances.*

  Elevated blood pressure is estimated to have caused 9.4 million deaths in 2010. High blood pressure is strongly associated with stroke, myocardial infarction (MI), cardiac failure, dementia, renal failure, and blindness. In the United States, aggressive targets of systolic blood pressure less than 120 mmHg and diastolic less than 70 mmHg have recently been recommended by AHA and the American College of Cardiology (9). Multiple lifestyle measures, including reducing the amount of salt in the diet, increasing the intake of fruit and vegetables, controlling weight, regular physical activity, and no more than moderate use of alcohol, have all been shown to help in the reduction of high blood pressure and are key lifestyle measures in this area.

- **Global target #7:** *Halt the rise of diabetes and obesity.*

  Obesity is associated with an increased likelihood of diabetes, hypertension, coronary heart disease (CHD), stroke, and certain types of cancers. Worldwide the prevalence of obesity has nearly doubled since 1980. In 2014, 11% of men and 16% of women aged 18 and older were obese. More than 42 million children under the age of 5 years were overweight in 2013. The global prevalence of diabetes in 2014 was estimated to be 9%. Further research is urgently needed and is undergoing in multiple countries to prevent obesity and diabetes. The key modalities in this fight will be increased physical activity and proper nutrition.

- **Global target #8:** *At least 50% of eligible people receiving drug therapy and counseling (including glycemic control) to prevent heart attacks and stroke.*

CVD was the leading cause of NCD deaths in 2012, resulting in 15.5 million deaths or 26% of NCD deaths. Of these deaths, 7.4 million were due to heart attacks and 6.7 million were due to strokes. Lifestyle medicine interventions to lower the risk of CVD include increased physical activity, proper nutrition, and weight management. These issues are dealt with in more detail in Chapters 2, 3, and 5.

- **Global target #9:** *An 80% availability of affordable basic technologies and essential medicines, including generics, required to treat major, non-communicable diseases in both public and private facilities.*

Essential medicines include aspirin, statins, angiotensin-converting enzyme inhibitors, diuretics, long-acting calcium channel blockers, beta blockers, metformin, insulin, a bronchodilator, and steroid inhalers. Technologies include blood-pressure-monitoring devices, weighing scales, height-measuring equipment, blood sugar and blood cholesterol measurement devices, and urine strips for an albumin assay. These are minimum requirements without which the basic NCD interventions cannot be implemented in primary care.

21.4 LIFESTYLE MEDICINE GLOBAL ALLIANCE

As interest in lifestyle medicine has continued to grow, it has become apparent that the value of various lifestyle medicine modalities can make a major contribution to the fight against NCDs around the world. As a result of this, the Lifestyle Medicine Global Alliance (LMGA) was founded in 2015 (10). The goal of this organization is to build a network of providers, share best practices, educational resources, and research initiatives to advocate for lifestyle medicine on the global stage.

The contribution that lifestyle medicine has to offer is synergistic with public health efforts. This has been recognized by the WHO. The LMGA has been invited to partner with WHO to reduce NCDs by 30% in 2030. The membership in the LMGA has now grown to 17 countries representing virtually every continent. The list of the countries who have joined the LMGA is found in Table 21.1. There are multiple levels of development of lifestyle medicine organizations around the world. The two most prominent ones are the American College of Lifestyle Medicine (ACLM) and the Australasian Society of Lifestyle Medicine. The ACLM has been in existence for 15 years and the Australasian Society for 12 years. Other lifestyle medicine organizations are at various stages of development. It is anticipated that many more organizations will join LMGA in the future.

21.5 CASE STUDIES IN LIFESTYLE MEDICINE

As lifestyle medicine organizations have sprung up around the world, it is useful to examine a few of these organizations at various stages of development. Various country organizations are featured in an ongoing series of columns in the *American Journal of Lifestyle Medicine* entitled "Lifestyle Medicine around the World." Here

TABLE 21.1
Framework for Countries Who Have Joined the Lifestyle Medicine Global Alliance

Level 5 Organizations

(500+ fee-paying members, physician-led, democratically elected leadership, not-for-profit status, published statues/bylaws, organizational bank accounts, paid employees, sophisticated IT infrastructure, including social media, regular conferences, regular IBLM certification exams)

Level 4 Organizations

(200+ fee-paying members, physician-led, democratically elected leadership, not-for-profit status, published statues/bylaws, organizational bank accounts, professional IT infrastructure, at least one LM conference, at least one IBLM certification exam)

Level 3 Organizations

(50+ fee-paying members, physician-led, democratically elected leadership, not-for-profit status, published statues/bylaws, organizational bank accounts, professional IT infrastructure, at least one LM conference)

Level 2 Organizations

(25+ fee-paying members, physician-led, democratically elected leadership, not-for-profit status, published statues/bylaws, organizational bank accounts, website)

Level 1 Organizations

(self-appointed leadership, physician-led, working on Level 2 status)

---

are a few examples of various lifestyle medicine organizations at various stages of development:

- *American College of Lifestyle Medicine (ACLM)* (11): ACLM was the first countrywide lifestyle medicine organization founded. Its vision was first developed by Dr. John Kelley who was impressed by the number of rigorous scientific studies published that showed efficacy of lifestyle interventions in treating and reversing disease. Dr. Kelley was also motivated by the publication of the 1st edition of the comprehensive textbook that I edited, *Lifestyle Medicine*. Dr. Kelley saw the evidence that intensive lifestyle changes could not only prevent disease, but also reverse it. The first general meeting of ACLM was held in March 2004. Since that time, it has grown dramatically. It currently has more than 4000 memberships and has grown 600% between 2013 and 2019.

  ACLM has led the world in promoting the connection between lifestyle habits and practices and reduction in risk of chronic diseases as well as their treatment. This has been done through a variety of educational initiatives as well as annual meetings. The ACLM is governed by a Board of Directors who work in collaboration with a staff of over 20 individuals who operate the main operations of the College and also special projects. The Executive Director of ACLM is Susan Benigas who has been in this role since 2014 and has demonstrated significant leadership and vision in the growth of ACLM as well as fostering growth of other countrywide organizations around the world. More details about the history and advances for ACLM may be found in an article entitled "American College of Lifestyle Medicine: Vision, Tenacity and Transformation," published in the *American Journal of Lifestyle Medicine* (AJLM). AJLM serves as the official journal of ACLM (12).

- *Australasia Lifestyle Medicine Association* (13): The Australasia Lifestyle Medicine Association was the second countrywide organization formed. It now combines both Australia and New Zealand. It was founded in 2006 and formally incorporated in 2008. Its annual meeting in 2018 had grown to 550 individuals. The Australasia Lifestyle Medicine Association has offered a master's degree through a regional university course of study starting in 2008, followed by another in 2010 and, along with ACLM, offers board certification in lifestyle medicine. A key leader in the formation of the Australasia Lifestyle Medicine Association has been Gary Egger who has written an important textbook in this area and has been a leader in articulating the relationship between lifestyle medicine and the relationship to environmental challenges. More details concerning this organization may be found in a column entitled "Lifestyle Medicine in Australia: A Potted History – So Far," published in AJLM (14).
- *British Society of Lifestyle Medicine* (15): The initial vision and impetus for forming this organization came from attendance at the annual conference of the Australasia Lifestyle Medicine Association 2014. In 2016, Rob Lawson announced the formation of the British Society of Lifestyle Medicine (BSLM). In the most recent conference for BSLM, over 400 individuals participated. BSLM plays an active role in education and training and is working with four academic institutions to co-design coaching certificates in lifestyle medicine, a Master of Science in Lifestyle Medicine and Public Health, maintenance courses in lifestyle medicine certification, and courses in well-being and lifestyle medicine at the Bachelor of Science level. BSLM has also facilitated the development of national undergraduate lifestyle medicine courses in medical schools throughout the United Kingdom.
- *Israeli Lifestyle Medicine Society (ILMS)* (16): The Israeli Lifestyle Medicine Society was established in 2012 under the auspices of the Israeli Association for Family Physicians. The initial impetus for ILMS came from the Israeli Association for Family Physicians which asked leaders to coordinate a course in nutrition and lifestyle. This, then, led to more individuals becoming involved in the nationwide promotion of healthy lifestyle. Rapid growth occurred and there were 385 members of ILMS as of June 2019. ILMS is involved in multiple education and training initiatives, including syllabus-based lifestyle medicine courses for family medicine specialists, residents, and medical students. The ILMS has also organized a project in motivational interviewing as well as free online lifestyle medicine courses in Next Generation University and has further initiated a forum on

physicians' health with the Israeli Medical Association. Most recently, the ILMS has been involved in projects encouraging primary care physicians to enhance their clinics by fostering health-promoting lifestyle medicine. A supplement to the ILMS website focuses on this specific initiative.

21.6 CONCLUSIONS

There is no longer any serious doubt that lifestyle practices and habits not only significantly impact the likelihood of developing disease, but also assist in its treatment. This emphasis is buttressed by initiatives not only in the United States, but also around the world. Lifestyle medicine organizations coordinate with a major emphasis of WHO which has listed important targets to help with the enormous burden that lifestyle-related diseases cause all around the world. In addition to working closely with WHO, various lifestyle organizations, including most of which belong to the Lifestyle Medicine Global Alliance, have spawned countrywide lifestyle medicine organizations in numerous countries around the world.

The goal of lifestyle medicine has been to promote the concept that daily habits and actions profoundly influence both short- and long-term health and quality of life. Various lifestyle medicine organizations around the world have also played central roles in the education of physicians and other health care workers to continue the important work of lifestyle medicine.

It is clear that unless we can move the needle to help people adopt positive habits in their daily lives, it will be very difficult to control pandemics such as obesity, diabetes, and CVD. There is overwhelming evidence that lifestyle habits and practices can help ameliorate these chronic conditions as well as numerous other noncommunicable diseases.

21.7 PRACTICAL APPLICATIONS

- The WHO has articulated nine NCDs which can be ameliorated largely through lifestyle habits and practices.
- Lifestyle medicine organizations have sprung up in numerous countries around the world.
- Many physicians and other health care workers are now being trained in the principles of lifestyle medicine.
- Lifestyle medicine modalities such as increased physical activity, proper nutrition, including more fruits and vegetables and whole grains, as well as weight management, avoidance of tobacco products, and avoidance or moderation of alcohol consumption all can play significant roles in helping to combat NCDs.
- As NCDs have become more prevalent than communicable diseases, it is imperative that physicians and other health care workers become knowledgeable and skilled at helping individuals overcome these largely lifestyle-related conditions.

REFERENCES

1. World Health Organization. https://www.who.int/. Accessed July 1, 2020.
2. World Health Organization. Nine Major Targets. https://www.who.int/beat-ncds/take-action/targets/en/. Accessed July 1, 2020.
3. Day S, Jitnarin N, Vidoni M, et al. Epidemiology of Adult Obesity. In Rippe JM, ed., *Lifestyle Medicine* (3rd edition). CRC Press (Boca Raton), 2019.
4. Rippe J. *Lifestyle Medicine*. Blackwell Science, Inc. (London), 1999.
5. Rippe J. *Lifestyle Medicine* (3rd edition). CRC Press (Boca Raton), 2019.
6. American Journal of Lifestyle Medicine. https://journals.sagepub.com/home/ajl. Accessed July 1, 2020.
7. *2018 Physical Activity Guidelines Advisory Committee. 2018 Physical Activity Guidelines Advisory Committee Scientific Report.* U.S. Department of Health and Human Services (Washington, DC), 2018.
8. Gidding S, Lichtenstein A, Faith M, et al. Implementing American Heart Association Pediatric and Adult Nutrition Guidelines: A Scientific Statement from the American Heart Association Nutrition Committee of the Council on Nutrition, Physical Activity and Metabolism, Council on Cardiovascular Disease in the Young, Council on Arteriosclerosis, Thrombosis and Vascular Biology, Council on Cardiovascular Nursing, Council on Epidemiology and Prevention, and Council for High Blood Pressure Research. *Circulation.* 2009;119:1161–1175.
9. Whelton P, Carey R, Aronow W, et al. 2017 ACC/AHA/AAPA/ABC/ACPM/AGS/APHA/ASH/ASPC/NMA/PCNA Guideline for the Prevention, Detection, Evaluation, and Management of High Blood Pressure in Adults: A Report of the American College of Cardiology/American Heart Association Task Force on Clinical Practice Guidelines. *Journal of the American College of Cardiology.* 2018;71:e127–e248.
10. Lifestyle Medicine Global Alliance. https://lifestylemedicineglobal.org/. Accessed July 1, 2020.
11. American College of Lifestyle Medicine. https://www.lifestylemedicine.org. Accessed July 1, 2020.
12. Benigas S. American College of Lifestyle Medicine: Vision, Tenacity, Transformation. *American Journal of Lifestyle Medicine.* 2019;14(1):57–60.
13. Australasian Society of Lifestyle Medicine. https://www.lifestylemedicine.org.au/. Accessed July 1, 2020.
14. Egger G, Egger S. Lifestyle Medicine: The Australian Experience. *American Journal of Lifestyle Medicine.* 2011;6(1):26–30.
15. The British Society of Lifestyle Medicine. https://lifestylemedicineglobal.org/global-aliance/abramev-2/. Accessed July 1, 2020.
16. The Israeli Lifestyle Medicine Society. https://lifestylemedicineglobal.org/global-aliance/israeli-lifestyle-medicine-society-ilms/. Accessed July 1, 2020.

22 The Future of Lifestyle Medicine

KEY POINTS

- The future of lifestyle medicine around the world is extremely bright, filled with multiple opportunities and challenges.
- Non-communicable diseases have significantly increased beyond communicable diseases in almost every region of the world.
- Lifestyle medicine practitioners are ideally suited to play leadership roles as countries around the world attempt to combat non-communicable diseases.

22.1 INTRODUCTION

The future of lifestyle medicine is filled with both enormous opportunities and significant challenges.

There is no longer any serious doubt that non-communicable diseases (NCDs) represent the modern plague, not only in the United States and other industrialized countries, but also in middle-income and low-income countries. There is also enormous evidence that what individuals do in their daily lives such as the amount of physical activity, choice to eat a more nutritious diet, including fruits, vegetables, and whole grains, maintaining a healthy body weight (BMI $\geq$18.5 and $\leq$25 kg/m^2), and avoiding tobacco products all play enormous roles in the likelihood that the individual will develop chronic diseases.

The enormity of the problem of NCDs represents a significant opportunity for physicians skilled in lifestyle medicine to play a central role in helping to reduce this pandemic. The good news is that there is enormous and compelling data on lifestyle practices that individuals can take in their own lives to lower the risk of chronic disease.

The challenge is also great. Despite the overwhelming evidence in this area, it has been extremely difficult to convince individuals to make those changes in their daily lives that have a significant impact on their health. For example, we know that lifestyle habits and actions, such as physical activity 30 minutes per day, healthy weight management (BMI $\geq$18.5 kg/m^2 and $\leq$25 kg/m^2), avoiding tobacco products, and following sound nutrition, including more fruits and vegetables and whole grains, can reduce the risk of heart disease by over 80% and diabetes (T2DM) by over 90% (1,2). Yet, when those practices are grouped together, a number of studies have shown that less than 5% of the population in the United States follows all of the five practices that have been demonstrated to result in these significant declines in two of the most prevalent and costly diseases (3).

Thus, the great challenge for individuals who are practicing lifestyle medicine is to help close the gap between what we know are beneficial habits and actions and what people are actually doing in their lives. While the challenges are great, I remain optimistic that dedicated individuals within the health care professions will rise to these challenges and play a central role in helping individuals combat NCDs.

In a sense, lifestyle medicine practitioners are the "tip of the spear" when it comes to helping people understand how "lifestyle" is truly "medicine." In this final chapter, we will look at some of the ways that lifestyle medicine can play a significant role in the future of health care and overall health for populations around the world.

22.2 THE POTENTIAL OF LIFESTYLE MEDICINE

As lifestyle medicine organizations have sprung up all around the world, it is clear that more and more physicians and other health care workers are recognizing that lifestyle habits and actions are critically important to modern health care.

A central tenet in medicine has always been to practice based on "evidence." The evidence behind lifestyle medicine is literally overwhelming. There are thousands of studies that support the concepts that regular physical activity, proper nutrition, weight management, and avoidance of tobacco all play significant roles in reducing the risk of various chronic diseases such as cardiovascular disease (CVD), T2DM, the metabolic syndrome (MetS), many cancers, and other chronic conditions.

While numerous investigators have played important roles in all of these individual areas, it is clear that the field is coming together under the rubric of lifestyle medicine. Evidence for this comes from many sources. As a cardiologist, I was very pleased to see that one of the councils of the American Heart Association (AHA) that I served on, changed its name from the "Council on Nutrition, Physical Activity and Metabolism" to the "Council on Lifestyle and Cardiometabolic Health" (4). In addition, when the new guidelines from the AHA and American College of Cardiology (ACC) were issued on control of lipids, the first practical tip that was given was to encourage patients to incorporate sound nutritional actions in their daily lifestyle (5).

One key role for lifestyle medicine practitioners will continue to be is to develop educational materials so that the next generation of physicians and other health care workers will become knowledgeable and interested in lifestyle medicine as a key medical discipline.

Numerous organizations such as the American College of Lifestyle Medicine are developing such materials (6). We are also seeing interest groups of medical students and undergraduate students forming to learn more and practice more in the area of lifestyle medicine. All of these initiatives are positive indicators that the medical community is slowly beginning to understand that lifestyle medicine is truly evidence-based and a key component of medicine in the future.

It is also encouraging to see that the WHO has included lifestyle medicine as one of the central organizing concepts as it mobilizes to meet the challenge of NCDs moving forward.

22.3 PHYSICAL ACTIVITY

There are multiple benefits of increased physical activity for virtually every metabolic disease. Not only does regular physical activity reduce risk factors for most metabolic diseases such as CVD, T2DM, and the MetS, but it also decreases the likelihood of many types of cancer and helps in every phase of their treatment. In addition, regular physical activity plays a significant role in improving cognition and reducing the risk of cognitive decline and dementia.

The data supporting the multiple positive roles of physical activity come from many sources. These data have been beautifully summarized in the Physical Activity Guidelines for Americans 2018 Scientific Report (PAGA 2018) (7). It will be incumbent upon all lifestyle medicine clinicians to counsel about increased physical activity in every patient encounter.

Multiple tools to assist clinicians in this area can be found from a variety of sources, including the Exercise Is Medicine (EIM) (8) initiative from the American College of Sports Medicine (ACSM).

Unfortunately, a distinct minority of individuals in the United States and around the world do not achieve enough physical activity to derive health benefits. It has been estimated that only 20–25% of adults in the United States achieve the level recommended by the PAGA 2018. Physical activity among adolescents is even lower with less than 20% of individuals in this age group meeting the guidelines from the PAGA 2018. Adult guidelines from multiple sources are all consistent in recommending 150 minutes of moderate intensity physical activity per week.

An inactive lifestyle is also very hazardous. There has been increased interest in focusing on sedentary behavior and its health risks. Lifestyle medicine clinicians should inquire about both physical activity and sedentary time in every patient encounter.

22.4 HEALTHY NUTRITION

The guidelines for healthy nutrition are consistent across multiple organizations, including the Dietary Guidelines for Americans 2015–2020 (DGA) (9), the American Heart Association (10), and the World Health Organization (11). All of these guidelines focus on increasing the consumption of fruits and vegetables and whole grains and reducing the amount of salt in the diet. Millions of lives could be saved if individuals followed these guidelines. In addition, following these guidelines would help lower the burden of weight gain and obesity. It will be incumbent in the future for all lifestyle medicine clinicians to become knowledgeable in this area and incorporate a discussion of healthy nutrition in every clinical encounter.

22.5 BEHAVIORAL CHANGE

In essence, improving daily habits and actions focuses on helping individuals make positive behavior changes (12). Lifestyle medicine clinicians should be familiar with the literature of what factors influence behavior and also ways that behavior change can be fostered. While many frameworks for health behavior change are available, one technique that would be very helpful for clinicians is to become familiar with is motivational interviewing. Multiple sources exist to help guide clinicians on how to become knowledgeable about motivational interviewing (13). In addition, the profession of coaching has also increased dramatically in the past decade. There are lifestyle coaches available for clinicians to work with their patients in virtually every major geographical area in the United States.

22.6   LIFESTYLE MEDICINE AND CARDIOVASCULAR DISEASE

CVD, coronary heart disease (CHD), and stroke are the third leading causes of death around the world. The pandemic of CVD touches every country in the world. In the United States, the American Heart Association and American College of Cardiology (ACC) have been leaders in identifying how lifestyle measures can help lower the risk of heart disease. Guidance in this area is incorporated in many documents from both the AHA and ACC, including the Practice Guidelines issued in 2013 (14) as well as the Strategic Report for the year 2020 (3).

There is no question that lifestyle practices such as increased physical activity, healthy nutrition, weight management, and avoidance of tobacco products all contribute to lowering the risk of CVD. It is incumbent upon lifestyle medicine physicians to emphasize to every patient that these practices can significantly reduce the risk of heart disease. This will be particularly important moving forward. For example, we know from the Nurses' Health Study and the Physicians' Health Study that over 80% of heart disease can be prevented by adopting a number of lifestyle measures such as increased physical activity, healthy nutrition, weight management, and avoidance of tobacco products (1,2).

We also know that even though progress has been made in some of these areas, we still have a long way to go. In fact, only 25% of adults in the United States engage in enough physical activity to significantly lower their risk of heart disease (7). Moreover, obesity and T2DM, which have enormous lifestyle components, have actually increased in the last 30 years in the United States and could wipe out all of the gains achieved in other lifestyle habits and practices unless we can get a handle on these two epidemics.

The good news is that even small amounts of increased physical activity can substantially lower the risk for heart disease. For example, both the Nurses' Health Study and the Physicians' Health Study showed that adopting even one positive lifestyle factor can reduce the risk of heart disease by 50%. These important facts need to be embodied in every counseling session that clinicians have with patients. These same practices have the potential to be a cost-effective strategy for lowering the risk of heart disease in countries around the world.

22.7   LIFESTYLE MEDICINE AND DIABETES

The prevalence of T2DM has increased significantly in the last 25 years. It is now estimated that 9% of people around the world have T2DM (15). There is a strong correlation between T2DM and obesity. Abundant data show that increased physical activity, healthy nutrition, and weight management all can substantially reduce the risk of T2DM and also assist in its treatment. These factors in the future will need to be emphasized since T2DM is one of the most costly diseases encountered in the United States and around the world.

22.8 LIFESTYLE MEDICINE AND THE METABOLIC SYNDROME

The metabolic syndrome is a cluster of risk factors, including abdominal obesity, elevated triglycerides, depressed HDL, and elevated blood pressure. All of these factors can be ameliorated by lifestyle practices. It has been estimated that 36–38% of adults in the United States already have the metabolic syndrome (16). Framingham Study data show that the majority of CVD occurs in individuals who have multiple risk factors. The National Cholesterol Education Program recommends that individuals who have MetS be treated as though they already have CVD (17). For all of these reasons, it will be important for clinicians in the future to take appropriate measurements to determine if individuals have metabolic syndrome and counsel them about lifestyle measures that can reduce their risk of CVD and T2DM.

22.9 OBSTETRICS AND GYNECOLOGY

Multiple lifestyle factors impact on components of obstetrics and gynecology. For example, it is well known that physical activity increases fertility (18). Regular physical activity can improve multiple aspects of pregnancy and reduce the risks of morbidity to not only the mother, but also the fetus. Moreover, regular physical activity can lower the risk of breast cancer. Many women use their obstetrician as their primary care physician. Therefore, it will be very important for lifestyle medicine practitioners to engage in campaigns to improve lifestyle measures among all women who are seen by obstetricians or gynecologists.

22.10 PULMONARY

Chronic obstructive pulmonary disease (COPD) is one of the four leading NCDs in the world (11). While there are many underlying conditions that cause pulmonary disease, tobacco consumption remains the leading cause of both COPD and lung cancer. The literature supporting the adverse health consequences of tobacco is enormous and should be emphasized in every clinical visit. In the United States, unfortunately, 15.5% of individuals still smoke cigarettes. Worldwide tobacco consumption remains alarmingly high. It will be very important for lifestyle medicine physicians moving forward to engage not only with their patients but also in public policy efforts to lower the prevalence of tobacco consumption and thereby improve overall health, and, in particular, pulmonary health.

22.11 BRAIN HEALTH

As the world population continues to age, brain health has become a much more pressing issue. Lifestyle measures can play a very important role in preserving brain health. In fact, abundant information shows that regular physical activity can help preserve cognition.

In contrast, inactivity is associated with both decreased cognition and decreased mental status and dementia, including Alzheimer's disease. China and the United States have the first and second largest number of people with dementia in the world (19).

Recent collaboration between the AHA and the American Stroke Association (ASA) to launch the "Optimal Brain Health" initiative has brought attention to the close correlation between risk factors for heart disease and diminished brain health (19). It appears that many of the practices that can preserve cognition should be started early in life which makes lifestyle factors even more important. Moreover, lifestyle factors such as increased physical activity, proper nutrition, and lowering the amount of salt in the diet can all lower the risk of stroke, which is one of the major causes of brain disease. For all of these reasons, lifestyle medicine practitioners need to become knowledgeable about how lifestyle factors impact on brain health and include a discussion of this in every counseling session with patients.

22.12   WOMEN'S HEALTH

Multiple lifestyle measures significantly impact on women's health. For example, increased physical activity lowers the risk of CHD as well as a number of different cancers—in particular breast cancer and endometrial cancer (20). In addition, regular physical activity is associated with a decreased risk of weight gain, which increases the risk of CHD. In addition, regular physical activity and proper nutrition both contribute to a decreased risk of T2DM, which is a significant issue particularly in overweight and obese women.

22.13   OVERWEIGHT AND OBESITY

Both overweight (BMI $\geq$25 kg/m^2 through $\leq$30 kg/m^2) and obesity (BMI >30 kg/m^2) are worldwide pandemics. It is estimated that over 2.1 billion people in the world are currently obese (11,21). Obesity is associated with an increased risk of both CVD and T2DM. Weight gain of more than 10 pounds during adulthood is also associated with an increased risk of various chronic diseases. Despite the well-known risk factors associated with obesity, less than 40% of individuals who are obese are counseled by their physicians each year concerning issues of how to control weight. It is very important that lifestyle medicine physicians take the lead in counseling individuals about the risk factors of overweight and obesity. Multiple frameworks and recommendations are available for this both from AHA and The Obesity Society (22). This will be a very significant component of lifestyle medicine moving forward.

22.14   PEDIATRICS

It is now well established that chronic diseases that are typically manifested in adults in their 5th, 6th, and 7th decade and beyond have their roots in childhood. An emerging literature suggests that many chronic diseases actually have their roots *in utero* (23).

An increasing number of children are obese. In fact, pediatric obesity has tripled in the last 25 years in the United States. Conditions such as high blood pressure and T2DM which were very infrequently found in children in the past are now increasingly prevalent in this group (24).

Physical activity has been routinely shown to convey multiple benefits for children, including decreasing the risk of weight gain and obesity as well as improving academic performance and cognition. The PAGA 2018 (7) and the ACSM (25) both recommend that children and adolescents should obtain 60 minutes of moderate to vigorous activity on a daily basis. Lifestyle medicine clinicians should take the lead in emphasizing the importance of physical activity in children. Sadly, less than 20% of adolescents currently achieve these 60 minutes of daily physical activity recommended by the PAGA 2018 and ACSM.

22.15 THE PRACTICE OF LIFESTYLE MEDICINE

As the field of lifestyle medicine has continued to expand around the world, it has become increasingly necessary to provide guidelines and definitions for the practice of lifestyle medicine. A number of organizations have been involved in this area, most prominently the American College of Lifestyle Medicine (ACLM) (6). This organization, which has grown rapidly since its establishment in 2004, has generated a variety of educational materials and supported the development of both certification in lifestyle medicine and student interest groups in this area (26). Details about the Practice of Lifestyle medicine may be found in the section on Lifestyle Medicine edited by former ACLM President, Dr. George Guthrie, in the 3rd edition of my textbook *Lifestyle Medicine* (27).

22.16 LIFESTYLE MEDICINE FOR THE OLDER POPULATION

Individuals over the age of 65 are the most rapidly growing segment of the population in the United States and around the world. By the year 2050, it is estimated that 20% of the population in the United States will be over the age of 65, representing a doubling of the current level (28).

As individuals get into their older years, issues related to lifestyle medicine become increasingly important. A person who has reached the age of 65 can expect to live another 19 years. The PAGA 2018 recommends that the same levels of physical activity for younger adults is highly recommended to individuals over the age of 65. This includes 150 minutes of moderate to vigorous physical activity on a weekly basis and two sessions of strength training per week.

It has become increasingly important for lifestyle medicine physicians to understand the special challenges for people over the age of 65 and address the multiple lifestyle modalities that can assist during these years. These include regular physical activity, weight management, and proper nutrition. Older adults may have a particularly difficult challenge in achieving proper nutrition given various health issues as well as other logistical issues (29).

Recognizing that older adults can have satisfying and fulfilling lives past the age of 65 has given rise to the concept of "successful aging." This is the concept that will help clinicians understand and guide individuals over the age of 65 into various lifestyle measures that will improve their health and quality of life.

22.17 HEALTH PROMOTION

The field of health promotion has grown and deepened particularly in the United States over the last 30 years. An international leader, Dr. Dee Edington, served as section editor in my *Lifestyle Medicine* textbook in this area (30).

Issues of how to keep the workforce healthy are particularly prominent in the area of health promotion. These include regular physical activity and breaking up sedentary occupations so that individuals can get some increased physical activity and also providing healthy nutrition.

A number of studies have emerged showing that economic benefits accrue to companies and health care facilities that pay attention to and promote improvements in lifestyle measures (31). This is particularly important as the cost of health care continues to escalate and now represents over 20% of the U.S. economy.

22.18 INJURY PREVENTION

Lifestyle medicine clinicians frequently underestimate the importance of injury prevention as a key component of lifestyle medicine. Unintentional injuries represent the leading cause of morbidity and mortality for individuals under the age of 44 in the United States (32). This includes motor vehicle accidents and also various other injuries both in the home and in the environment. Included in this are suicide and injuries from gun violence and other terms of violence. Head trauma resulting from bicycle and motor vehicle accidents is also very prevalent in the United States.

One key distinction that the CDC has emphasized is the difference between an unintentional injury and an accident. Too often we think of accidents as being random, whereas a large body of science exists concerning how injuries can be prevented.

It is incumbent upon lifestyle medicine physicians to discuss potential ways that injuries can be avoided for people of all age groups. This is particularly important for people over the age of 70. Falls in this population result in multiple hospitalizations and mortality each year. This will become an increasingly important area as the population continues to age.

22.19 PUBLIC POLICY AND ENVIRONMENTAL SUPPORTS

Multiple factors impact on individuals' ability to improve lifestyle factors such as physical activity and nutrition. These include not only public information campaigns but also the availability and safety of facilities, community, and national and international policies as well as the built environment (33). Lifestyle medicine physicians are uniquely positioned to give credible input and advice in all of these areas and should play an increasing role in these areas in the future.

22.20 LIFESTYLE MEDICINE AROUND THE WORLD

As lifestyle medicine has grown into a movement around the world, it will be important for lifestyle medicine clinicians to join forces and to understand issues related to the various geographical regions and economies around the world. This coordination has already begun with the Lifestyle Medicine Global Alliance and is likely to continue in the years to come (34). I anticipate that many more organizations will form around the world since the problems that are ameliorated with lifestyle medicine modalities are truly pandemics impacting on every country in the world.

22.21 EPIGENETICS

An emerging and intriguing science continues to evolve in the area of epigenetics. The study of epigenetics relates to how the end products of DNA, such as proteins, are impacted on in various ways based on lifestyle practices and habits. There are good data emerging that changes in the epigenetic profile of people contribute to the likelihood that they will develop disease. These are, in turn, significantly impacted by lifestyle habits and practices. It is important for lifestyle medicine clinicians to stay abreast of this emerging literature since it provides important biological roots for why many of the lifestyle medicine components are so powerful.

22.22 EMERGING TECHNOLOGIES

Many emerging technologies will undoubtedly impact on lifestyle medicine in the future. For example, the continuing development of technologies, such as smartphones, Apps, etc., and the increasing power of social media all can contribute to spreading the message of lifestyle medicine modalities and tracking the results of various lifestyle medicine initiatives.

In addition, various wearable technologies increasingly are being utilized in such fields as cardiology to provide real-time data on heart rate and rhythm etc. These emerging technologies can potentially play important roles in encouraging people to pay more attention to positive lifestyle measures. One intriguing example is a blood pressure monitor that can be worn at the wrist which has been shown to provide accurate readings of blood pressure both at rest and during exercise. This technology could encourage people to pay more attention to those lifestyle habits and practices which impact on blood pressure. There are many other examples of this.

22.23 ONGOING AND EMERGING RESEARCH

Lifestyle medicine practitioners should make every effort to stay abreast of research literature in multiple areas that impact on lifestyle modalities. Much of this research is found across many different disciplines, including cardiovascular medicine, diabetes, nutrition, physical activity, exercise physiology, behavior medicine, and many more. While there are many resources for this information, one way to keep abreast of this literature is to subscribe to the *American Journal of Lifestyle Medicine*, which has at its mission bringing this type of literature together in one place for clinicians (35).

22.24   EDUCATIONAL RESOURCES AND EVIDENCE-BASED MEDICINE

As already indicated, a number of initiatives are in progress to provide education in the field of lifestyle medicine. Since the modalities of lifestyle medicine are spread across multiple disciplines, it is important to understand that the evidence behind lifestyle medicine is very robust. This will be increasingly important as lifestyle medicine continues to impact on the rest of mainstream medicine.

22.25   CONCLUSIONS

The future of lifestyle medicine is bright! Many opportunities and challenges exist. The opportunities relate to the power that lifestyle practices such as increased physical activity, healthy nutrition, weight management, and avoidance of tobacco all have on helping to ameliorate the major non-communicable diseases around the world. There is a natural alliance between lifestyle medicine and the WHO. I hope and anticipate that lifestyle medicine practitioners will play an increasingly prominent role in countries around the world by articulating and counseling about the power of daily lifestyle habits and actions on both short- and long-term health and quality of life.

22.26   CLINICAL APPLICATIONS

- It is incumbent upon lifestyle medicine practitioners to understand the power of lifestyle modalities in multiple chronic diseases. These include heart disease, diabetes, cancer, brain health, and many others.
- Multiple education opportunities now exist for individuals to become knowledgeable about specific areas of lifestyle medicine.
- Emerging research in areas such as epigenetics will provide more insight into why lifestyle medicine modalities are so powerful in the area of risk reduction.
- Emerging or current technologies such as smartphones and wearable devices as well as the power of social media will play an increasingly prominent role in generating research data as well as outreach efforts in the area of lifestyle medicine.

REFERENCES

1. Liu S, Stampfer M, Hu F, et al. Whole-Grain Consumption and Risk of Coronary Heart Disease: Results from the Nurses' Health Study. *American Journal of Clinical Nutrition*. 1999;70:412–419.

2. Hu F, Willett W. Diet and Coronary Heart Disease: Findings from the Nurses' Health Study and Health Professionals' Follow-Up Study. *Journal of Nutrition, Health and Aging.* 2001;5(3):132–8.

3. Lloyd-Jones D, Hong Y, Labarthe D, et al. Defining and Setting National Goals for Cardiovascular Health Promotion and Disease Reduction: The American Heart Association's Strategic Impact Goal through 2020 and Beyond. *Circulation.* 2010;121:586–613.

4. American Heart Association. Council on Lifestyle and Cardiometabolic Health. https://professional.heart.org/professional/MembershipCouncils/ScientificCouncils/UCM_3228 56_Council-on-Lifestyle-and-Cardiometabolic-Health.jsp. Accessed July 14, 2020.

5. Grundy S, Stone, N, Baily A., et al. 2018 Guideline on the Management of Blood Cholesterol. A Report of the American College of Cardiology/American Heart Association Task Force on Clinical Practice Guidelines. *Journal of the American College of Cardiology.* 2019;73:24.

6. American College of Lifestyle Medicine (ACLM). http://www.lifestylemedicine.org. Accessed July 14, 2020.

7. Physical Activity Guidelines Advisory Committee. *2018 Physical Activity Guidelines Advisory Committee. 2018 Physical Activity Guidelines Advisory Committee Scientific Report.* Department of Health and Human Services (Washington, DC), 2018.

8. Exercise is Medicine. American College of Sports Medicine. https://www.exerciseismedicine.org/. Accessed July 14, 2020.

9. U.S. Department of Health and Human Services and U.S. Department of Agriculture. *2015–2020 Dietary Guidelines for Americans* (8th edition). December 2015. http://health.Gov/dietaryguidelines/2015/guidelines/.

10. Lichtenstein A, Appel L, Brands M, et al. Diet and Lifestyle Recommendations Revision 2006. A Scientific Statement from the American Heart Association Nutrition Committee. *Circulation.* 2006;114:82–96.

11. World Health Organization. Non-Communicable Diseases. https://www.who.int/news-room/fact-sheets/detail/noncommunicable-diseases. Accessed July 14, 2020.

12. Frates E, Eubanks J. *Behavior Change. Lifestyle Medicine.* 3rd ed. CRC Press (Boca Raton), 2019.

13. Fifield P, Suzuki J, Minski S, et al. *Motivational Interviewing and Lifestyle Change. Lifestyle Medicine* (3rd edition). CRC Press (Boca Raton), 2019.

14. Eckel RH, Jakicic JM, Ard JD, et al. 2013 AHA/ACC Guideline on Lifestyle Management to Reduce Cardiovascular Risk. A Report of the American College of Cardiology/American Heart Association Task Force on Practice Guidelines. *Circulation.* 2013;129:S76–S99.

15. Franz MJ, MacLeod J, Evert A, et al. Academy of Nutrition and Dietetics Nutrition Practice Guideline for Type 1 and Type 2 Diabetes in Adults: Systematic Review of Evidence for Medical Nutrition Therapy Effectiveness and Recommendations for Integration into the Nutrition Care Process. *Journal of the Academy of Nutrition and Dietetics.* 2017;117:1659–1679.

16. Ford E, Giles W, Dietz W. Prevalence of the Metabolic Syndrome among Us Adults: Findings from the Third National Health and Nutrition Examination Survey. *JAMA.* 2002;287:356–359.

17. Third Report of the National Cholesterol Education Program (NCEP) Expert Panel on Detection, Evaluation, and Treatment of High Blood Cholesterol in Adults (Adult Treatment Panel III) Final Report, Washington, DC. *Circulation.* 2002;106:3143.

18. ACOG Committee Opinion Summary, Number 804. Physical Activity and Exercise During Pregnancy and the Postpartum Period. *Obstetrics & Gynecology.* 2020;4:991–993.

19. Gorelick P, Furie K, Iadecola C, et al. Defining Optimal Brain Health in Adults: A Presidential Advisory from the American Heart Association/American Stroke Association. *Stroke.* 2017;48(10):e284–e303.

20. Bassuk S, Manson J. Lifestyle and Risk of Cardiovascular Disease and Type 2 Diabetes in Women: A Review of the Epidemiologic Evidence. *American Journal of Lifestyle Medicine.* 2008;2:191–213.

21. Day R, Jitnarin N, Vidoni M. *Epidemiology of Adult Obesity. Lifestyle Medicine* (3rd edition). CRC Press (Boca Raton), 2019.

22. Jensen M, Ryan D, Apovian, et al. 2013 AHA/ACC/TOS Guideline for the Management of Overweight and Obesity in Adults. A Report of the American College of Cardiology/American Heart Association Task Force on Practice Guidelines and The Obesity Society. *Circulation.* 2014;129 Supplement 2:S102–S138.

23. Sauder K, Dabelea D. *Life Course Approach to Prevention of Chronic Disease. Lifestyle Medicine* (3rd edition). CRC Press (Boca Raton), 2019.

24. Miller J, Boles R, Daniels S. *Pediatric Lifestyle Medicine. Lifestyle Medicine* (3rd edition). CRC Press (Boca Raton), 2019.

25. The American College of Sports Medicine. *ACSM Resource Manual for Exercise Testing and Prescription.* Lippincott Williams & Wilkins (Philadelphia, PA), 2017.

26. Benigas S. American College of Lifestyle Medicine: Vision. Tenacity. Transformation. *American Journal of Lifestyle Medicine.* 2019;14(1):57–60.

27. Guthrie G. *Implementing Nutritional Lifestyle Treatment Programs in Type 2 Diabetes. Lifestyle Medicine* (3rd edition). CRC Press (Boca Raton), 2019.

28. Physical Activity Guidelines Advisory Committee. *2018 Physical Activity Guidelines Advisory Committee. 2018 Physical Activity Guidelines Advisory Committee Scientific Report. Part F. Chapter 9. Older Adults. F-9-F–42.* US. Department of Health and Human Services (Washington, DC), 2018.

29. Lichtenstein A. *Optimal Nutrition Guidance for Older Adults. Lifestyle Medicine* (3rd edition). CRC Press (Boca Raton), 2019.

30. Edington D. *Health Promotion Introduction. Lifestyle Medicine* (3rd edition). CRC Press (Boca Raton), 2019.

31. Shurney D. *The Employer's Role in Lifestyle Medicine. Lifestyle Medicine* (3rd edition). CRC Press (Boca Raton), 2019.

32. Sleet D. *Injuries and Lifestyle Medicine. Lifestyle Medicine* (3rd edition). CRC Press (Boca Raton), 2019.

33. Dodson E, Heath G. *Policy and Environmental Supports for Physical Activity and Active Living. Lifestyle Medicine* (3rd edition). CRC Press (Boca Raton), 2019.

34. Lifestyle Medicine Global Alliance. https://lifestylemedicineglobal.org/. Accessed July 14, 2020.

35. American Journal of Lifestyle Medicine. https://journals.sagepub.com/home/ajl. Accessed July 14, 2020.

Index

Printed in the United States
by Baker & Taylor Publisher Services